OXFORD MEDICAL PUBLICATIONS
Primary Anaesthesia

The Educational Low-Priced Books Scheme is funded by the Overseas Development Administration as part of the British Government overseas aid programme. It makes available low-priced, unabridged editions of British publishers' textbooks to students in developing countries. Below is a list of some other medical books published under the ELBS imprint.

Aitkenhead and Smith
Textbook of Anaesthesia
Churchill Livingstone

Atkinson, Rushman and Davies
Lee's Synopsis of Anaesthesia
Butterworth–Heinemann

Boulton and Blogg
Ostlere & Bryce-Smith's Anaesthetics for Medical Students
Churchill Livingstone

Edwards and Bouchier (editors)
Davidson's Principles and Practice of Medicine
Churchill Livingstone

Kumar and Clark (editors)
Clinical Medicine
Baillière Tindall

Munro and Edwards (editors)
Macleod's Clinical Examination
Churchill Livingstone

Ogilvie and Evans
Chamberlain's Symptoms and Signs in Clinical Medicine
Wright

Souhami and Moxham (editors)
Textbook of Medicine
Churchill Livingstone

Swash
Hutchison's Clinical Methods
Baillière Tindall

Weatherall, Ledingham and Warrell (editors)
Oxford Textbook of Medicine Vols 1 and 2
Oxford University Press

Primary Anaesthesia

EMMANUEL AYIM M.D. Hon. Hamburg, F.F.A.R.C.S. Eng.
Professor of Anaesthetics, in the University of Nairobi, Kenya.

PETER C. BEWES M.B. B.Chir. (Cantab). F.R.C.S. (Eng).
Consultant Surgeon to The Birmingham Accident Hospital: formerly Honorary Surgeon to the Kilimanjaro Christian Medical Centre, Tanzania.

JULIAN F. BION M.R.C.P., F.F.A.R.C.S. Eng.
Senior Anaesthetic Research Fellow, Clinical Shock Study Group, Western Infirmary, Glasgow, Scotland.

CLIVE CORY F.F.A.R.C.S. Eng.
Consultant Anaesthetist, Grantham Hospital. Lately Consultant Anaesthetist at the Kilimanjaro Christian Medical Centre, Tanzania.

JOHN V. FARMAN M.B., Ch.B., F.F.A.R.C.S. Eng
Consultant Anaesthetist, Addenbrooke's Hospital Cambridge. Lately Senior Lecturer in Anaesthesia at the University of Ibadan, Nigeria.

ALAN KISIA M.B., Ch.B., F.F.A.R.C.S. Eng.
Chief Specialist Anaesthetist, Kenyan Ministry of Health

FRANK N. PRIOR M.B.B.S, F.F.A.R.C.S. Eng., D.A.
Consultant Anaesthetist to Guy's and Lewisham Hospitals London. Formerly Professor of Anaesthesia in the Christian Medical College, Ludhiana, Punjab, India.

Edited by
MAURICE H. KING M.D. Cantab., F.R.C.P. Lond, F.F.C.M. Eng.
Senior Lecturer in Community Medicine in the University of Leeds; Lately Staff Member with the German Agency for Technical Cooperation (GTZ) in Nyeri Kenya.

OTHER CONTRIBUTORS DN Biswas, Tom Boulton, James Cairns, Murray Carmichael, Nancy Caroline, Tom Cripps, Gerry Hankins, JD Holdsworth, Georg Kamm, Myint Myint Khin, Tim Jack, Richard Laing, Hatibu Lueno, Robert Macintosh, Tim Mimpriss, Keith Nightingale, Peter Papworth, Andrew Pearson, Nigel Pereira, Hugh Philpott, Divya Patel, Walter Schlabach, Bill Sugg, John Thornton, Andrew Tomlinson, Marten Van Wijhe.

Illustrated by DEREK ATHERTON and IVANSON KAIYAI

OXFORD UNIVERSITY PRESS
OXFORD DELHI KUALA LUMPUR

Oxford University Press, Walton Street, Oxford OX2 6DP
Oxford New York Toronto
Delhi Bombay Calcutta Madras Karachi
Kuala Lumpur Singapore Hong Kong Tokyo
Nairobi Dar es Salaam Cape Town
Melbourne Auckland Madrid
and associated companies in
Berlin Ibadan

Oxford is a trade mark of Oxford University Press

Published in the United States
by Oxford University Press, New York

© GTZ, 1986
Reprinted 1990, 1993, 2000

All rights reserved. No part of this publication may be reproduced,
stored in a retrieval system, or transmitted, in any form or by any means,
electronic, mechanical, photocopying, recording, or otherwise, without
the prior permission of Oxford University Press

This book is sold subject to the condition that it shall not, by way
of trade or otherwise, be lent, re-sold, hired out or otherwise circulated
without the publisher's prior consent in any form of binding or cover
other than that in which it is published and without a similar condition
including this condition being imposed on the subsequent purchaser

British Library Cataloguing in Publication Data

British Library CIP Data
Primary anaesthesia — (Oxford medical publication)
1. Anaesthesia
i. Ayim, Emmanuel   ii. King, Maurice
617'.96   RD81

ISBN 0–19–261592–0 (paperback edn)

Printed by Thomson Press (India) Ltd.

Contents

Foreword   vii

Chapter 1 Introduction   1
1.1 A minimum standard of anaesthesia for everyone.

Chapter 2 Background to anaesthesia   4
2.1 Who gives the anaesthetic? 2.2 Anaesthesia in a health centre. 2.3 How much does anaesthesia cost? 2.4 Standardizing equipment. 2.5 Anaesthetic drugs. 2.6 Premedication. 2.7 Atropine and neostigmine. 2.8 Tranquilisers, diazepam, chloropromazine and promethazine. 2.9 Pethidine and morphine. 2.10 Vasopressors, ephedrine and methoxamine.

Chapter 3 Should disaster occur   10
The ten golden rules of anaesthesia. 3.2 Laryngeal spasm (stridor). 3.3 Wheezing. 3.4 Respiratory arrest. 3.5 Cardiac (cardiopulmonary) arrest. 3.6 Sternal compression.

Chapter 4 Care before, during and after the operation   15
4.1 Fitness for anaesthesia. 4.2 Caring for a patient's airway. 4.3 Monitoring an anaesthetised patient. 4.4 Hypotension during the operation. 4.5 Care after the operation. 4.6 Complications after anaesthesia. 4.7 Recording the course of anaesthesia.

Chapter 5 An introduction to local anaesthesia   23
5.1 Advantages and disadvantages. 5.2 Pre- and paramedication for local anaesthesia. 5.3 Drugs for local and regional anaesthesia. 5.4 Infiltration anaesthesia. 5.5 Infiltrate-and-cut anaesthesia. 5.6 Anaesthetizing a fracture haematoma. 5.7 Infiltration anaesthesia for opening abscesses. 5.8 Surface anaesthesia. 5.9 The complications of local anaesthesia.

Chapter 6 Nerve blocks   29
6.1 Blocking a nerve. 6.2 The block has failed. 6.3 Blocks for the mouth and teeth. 6.4 Pterygopalatine (sphenopalatine) block. 6.5 Blocks for the eye. 6.6 Anaesthetizing the scalp. 6.7 Local anaesthesia for abdominal operations. 6.8 Rectus block. 6.9 Local anaesthesia for Caesarean section (intercostal nerve block). 6.10 Field block for the breast. 6.11 Field block for inguinal operations. 6.12 Hernia block. 6.13 Transvaginal pudendal block. 6.14 Paracervical block. 6.15 Ring block for the penis. 6.16 Anaesthetizing the anus. 6.17 Supraclavicular brachial plexus block. 6.18 Axillary block. 6.19 Intravenous regional anaesthesia (forearm block). 6.20 Blocks for the wrist. 6.21 Blocks for the fingers and toes. 6.22 "Three-in-one block". 6.23 Sciatic nerve block. 6.24 Blocks for the ankle.

Chapter 7 Epidural and subarachnoid anaesthesia   49
7.1 Advantages and disadvantages. 7.2 Lumbar epidural anaesthesia. 7.3 Caudal epidural anaesthesia. 7.4 Subarachnoid (spinal) anaesthesia. 7.5 Subarachnoid anaesthesia with isobaric bupivacaine. 7.6 Hyperbaric subarachnoid anaesthesia. 7.7 Augmented saddle block.

Chapter 8 Dissociative anaesthesia and intravenous analgesia   60
8.1 Dissociative anaesthesia with Ketamine. 8.2 Intramuscular and bolus intravenous ketamine. 8.3 Plain ketamine drip. 8.4 Ketamine drip with relaxants. 8.5 Ketamine in children. 8.6 Intravenous analgesia. 8.7 Intravenous morphine. 8.8 Intravenous pethidine. 8.9 Ketamine and morphine drips.

Chapter 9 Nitrous oxide, air, and oxygen   67
9.1 An introduction to inhalational anaesthesia. 9.2 Using nitrous oxide. 9.3 Using oxygen economically.

Chapter 10 Systems for inhalation anaesthesia   72
10.1 Making the gases go in the right direction. 10.2 Non-rebreathing valves. 10.3 Bellows and Bags. 10.4 Draw-over vapourisers. 10.5 A simple vapouriser. 10.6 The EMO vapouriser. 10.7 The Dräeger AFYA systems. 10.8 The "Ether-Pac" and "Fluo-Pac" vapourisers. 10.9 The Loos "Etherair" vapouriser. 10.10 The Oxford Miniature Vapouriser (OMV). 10.11 An uncalibrated vapouriser (the Bryce-Smith Induction Unit or BSIU). 10.12 The "Cyprane" vapouriser. 10.13 An improvised vapouriser.

Chapter 11 Inhalation agents   85
11.1 The advantages of ether. 11.2 The stages of ether anaesthesia. 11.3 Ether with a vapouriser. 11.4 Ether with an open mask. 11.5 Fires and explosions with ether. 11.6 Halothane. 11.7 Trichloroethylene. 11.8 Chloroform. 11.9 Ethyl chloride.

Chapter 12 Thiopentone   93
12.1 Thiopentone as an induction agent. 12.2 Dangers and disasters with thiopentone.

Chapter 13 Controlled ventilation, and intubation   95
13.1 Controlled ventilation. 13.2 Tracheal intubation. 13.3 How to intubate. 13.4 Intubation through the nose. 13.5 Local anaesthesia for intubation. 13.6 Intubating children. 13.7 Compliance and the blocked tracheal tube.

Chapter 14 Muscle relaxants 108
14.1 Long and short acting relaxants. 14.2 Suxamethonium. 14.3 Long acting (non–depolarising) relaxants. 14.4 A patient fails to breathe after a long acting relaxant.

Chapter 15 Fluid therapy 114
15.1 Intravenous infusions. 15.2 Intravenous lines. 15.3 Replacing fluid before the operation—surgical dehydration. 15.4 Replacing fluid during the operation. 15.5 Fluids after the operation.

Chapter 16 Anaesthesia for special circumstances 123
16.1 The patient with the full stomach. 16.2 Vomiting. 16.3 Regurgitation. 16.4 Preventing vomiting and regurgitation. 16.5 Anaesthesia with a full stomach. 16.6 Obstetric anaesthesia. 16.7 Anaesthesia for hypovolaemic shock. 16.8 Anaesthesia for head injuries. 16.9 Anaesthesia for eye surgery. 16.10 Anaesthesia for oral and facial surgery. 16.11 Anaesthesia for outpatients. 16.12 Anaesthesia with the patient in an unusual position.

Chapter 17 Some medical constraints on anaesthesia 132
17.1 Anaemia. 17.2 Metabolic acidosis. 17.3 Hypertension. 17.4 Congestive cardiac failure. 17.5 Hepatic failure. 17.6 Renal failure. 17.7 Diabetes. 17.8 Respiratory infections.

Chapter 18 Anaesthesia for children 136
18.1 Children are different. 18.2 Which methods are appropriate for children? 18.3 Anaesthetic systems for children.

Chapter 19 Primary Intensive Care 141
19.1 Special care for those in special need. 19.2 Monitoring the central venous pressure (CVP). 19.3 Equipment for mechanical ventilation (IPPV) and respiratory monitoring. 19.4 Caring for a patient on a ventilator in an ICU. 19.5 Measuring the pCO_2 with a modified Campbell–Haldane apparatus.

Chapter 20 Evaluating the quality of anaesthesia 151

Chapter 21 Multiple choice questions 152
21.1 What do you know? One. 1.2 What do you know? Two. 1.3 What do you know? Three. 1.4 What do you know? Four. 1.5 What do you know? Five.

Appendices 159
Appendix A, making your own intravenous fluid. Appendix B, Drugs and equipment. Appendix C, References. Appendix D, Answers to the multiple choice questions.

Index 165

Foreword

The production of this manual of Primary Anaesthesia was sponsored by the German Federal Ministry for Economic Cooperation within the scope of the Technical Cooperation Agreement with the Republic of Kenya, under project number 78.2048.3-01.100. It was compiled by Maurice King in close collaboration with Kenyan and other experts.

The manual contains the collective views of an international group of experts. The methods and techniques described correspond to the state of the art with regard to their feasibility in rural hospitals where sophisticated technical equipment may not be available. The manual cannot, however, replace personal instruction by a qualified expert. Neither the editor nor the publisher may be held responsible for any damage resulting from the application of the described methods. Any liability in this respect is excluded.

Dr. R Korte, GTZ
Department of Health,
Nutrition and population Activities.
German Agency for Technical Cooperation
Postfach 5180D
6236 ESCHBORN
West Germany

Preface

The purpose of anaesthesia is to make surgery possible, painless, and safe. Too often it is none of these things, because there is nobody who can anaesthetize a patient competently. The result is that operations are often not done when they should be done, or they are done dangerously, or painfully, or patients are referred unnecessarily.

This manual was developed to help put this right. It is mainly for those who are not anaesthesiologists, and is no substitute for personal instruction from an expert, or for practical experience. We have done our best to cater for the following readers.

(1) General duty doctors working under the exacting conditions of the district hospitals of the developing world. The methods here are those which are required to do the operations in the surgical manuals that accompany this one—"Primary Surgery", volumes One and Two, from the same publishers..

(2) Medical students who are training to work here. For them this is a book to be owned, and to be familiar with, but not to be learnt by heart.

(3) Anaesthetic assistants will doubtless read this, because they presently have nothing else. But it is not ideally suited to them, because they need a book of their own describing similar methods, but in a different way and including much more anatomy and physiology than we have space for. We have however tried to help them by providing an extensive vocabulary.

(4) Workers in health centres may derive some help from Section 2.2.

(5) Ministries of health in the developing world who want to know how to plan and equip their anaesthetic services.

(6) Anyone who is called upon to anaesthetize in ships, or armies and in disaster areas generally.

(7) Private practitioners anywhere in the world who do minor surgery on their own premises without expert anaesthetic help.

(8) Those anaesthesiologists in the industrial world who have never used ether, or ketamine for the purposes described here.

In short, our main concern is to try to improve the quality of anaesthetic care wherever it is least adequate. In the last two chapters we have however broadened our scope to help those hospitals where care is more than minimal, and who wish to advance.

We have chosen methods which are safe, simple, highly cost effective, and within the reach of the countries of the "South", whose public health expenditures are presently only about $11 per person per year compared with $320 in the "North". This is readily possible, because a good anaesthetic is not necessarily an expensive one.

Finally, our aim is to link educational goals to service needs, and in doing so to improve the average level of anaesthesia throughout a health service. This manual is both a detailed exercise in health service design, and in health service research. It is also a step towards the achievement of one of WHO's more tangible goals—to see that all the technologies for Primary Health Care are described systematically in the languages of all the world's health workers.

Dose schedules are being continually revised and new side effects recognized. Oxford University Press makes no representation, express or implied, that the drug dosages in this book are correct. For these reasons the reader is strongly urged to consult the drug company's printed instructions before administering any of the drugs recommended in this book.

1 An introduction to anaesthesia

1.1 A minimum standard of anaesthesia for everyone

A patient in a district hospital is often in greater danger from the anaesthetic than he is from the operation. Under some circumstances deaths from anaesthesia are unnecessarily frequent, particularly in young children. This is both tragic and unnecessary, because there are now simple, safe, inexpensive, modern anaesthetics for all the operations that are possible in a district hospital, even when the anaesthetist is not a doctor. Among them, they constitute an attainable *minimum* standard of anaesthesia that should be available to everyone. These are the anaesthetics that two thirds of the world's people would consider themselves fortunate to have.

But anaesthesia will not be satisfactory unless medical students are taught both the principles of anaesthesia and at least some of its techniques. Medical students should all be proficient in most of the skills described here. Unfortunately, anaesthesia has lost its place in many undergraduate curricula. Postgraduate surgeons are often not taught anaesthesia either, with the result that an increasing number of their seniors cannot give an anaesthetic, or teach medical students how to give one. Too often, the only people who are taught anaesthesia are future specialist anaesthetists and non–doctor anaesthetists. One of the main purposes of 'Primary Anaesthesia' is to help to reverse this unfortunate trend. Any doctor worthy of the name should be able to give most of the anaesthetics described here.

A variety of alternatives are necessary, because: (1) No single method suits all patients. (2) There are often times when some drug or piece of equipment is missing. For example, bupivacaine is usually considered to be the local anaesthetic of choice, but lignocaine is the agent in most common use, and large stocks of procaine still exist in some countries. We have therefore described a variety of alternatives, even if it makes 'Primary Anaesthesia' seem more complicated than it really is. Just because there are so many ways of anaesthetizing a patient, chance, culture, and policy play a large part in determining which methods are used. Nevertheless, each method has its ideal indications, and one of the features of good anaesthetic care is that a range of methods are employed, each for its proper purpose.

'Primary Anaesthesia' has been criticised from two points of view. Some anaesthetists consider that it is not sophisticated enough, because it does not say enough about nitrous oxide or anaesthetic machines of the Boyle's type. Some non–anaesthetists think it is too sophisticated, partly because tracheal intubation features so prominently, and partly because they may never have heard of some of the methods it describes, which may thus sound more difficult than they really are. Isobaric bupivacaine and non–rebreathing valves, are only two such examples. In fact, the methods which follow are little more than some inexpensive drugs, a few tubes, a vapouriser—and the skills to use them.

Firstly, nitrous oxide. Little is said about this or about anaesthetic machines of the Boyle's type. Instead, our main emphasis is on air as the carrier gas for ether, halothane and trichloroethylene, supplemented by oxygen from a cylinder where necessary, and delivered by a sophisticated modern vapouriser. Here are some reasons why nitrous oxide is not the best choice in the hospitals for which we mainly write.

(1) It is a great disadvantage to have to rely on methods that require simultaneous supplies of both nitrous oxide and oxygen and which you cannot use when cylinders of either of them are empty. But, if air is the carrier gas for ether, and the cylinders of oxygen are empty, you can still use air. Supplies of nitrous oxide are often a major problem, especially when they may have to be paid for with scarce foreign exchange, and when heavy steel cylinders may have to be carried hundreds of kilometers along bumpy roads.

(2) Methods using air as a carrier gas are highly effective, and are adequate for almost all operations that are ever likely to be done in a district hospital. One distinguished anaesthetic specialist in a famous regional hospital said that he had not missed nitrous oxide in over 25 000 anaesthetics.

(3) Although a modern ether vapouriser is a sophisticated device, it provides fewer opportunites for mistakes than a machine of the Boyle's type. When air is used as a carrier gas it is much more difficult for an inexperienced anaesthetist to asphyxiate his patients accidentally.

(4) The more robust and well–tried ether vapourisers are much less likely to go wrong. For example, a team visiting one country after a long period of civil disturbance found all the anaesthetic machines of the Boyle's type out of action, but all the EMO ether vapourisers still working.

(5) Ether, with oxygen added as necessary, is about one tenth the price of nitrous oxide; ether costs about sixty US cents an hour, compared with six dollars an hour for nitrous oxide.

(6) The merits of ether compared with more recently developed anaesthetics, and particularly its safety, are slowly being appreciated in the industrial world, despite the fact that many anaesthetists there have never learnt to use it.

(7) Provided reasonable precautions are taken, ether's potentially explosive properties are not a significant hazard. With air as the carrier gas, ether has been used for years without explosions.

Is tracheal intubation really too sophisticated? There can hardly be any more basic and life saving method in the whole of medicine than inserting a tube into a patient's trachea to keep his airway open, and his last meal out of his lungs. Suitably trained assistants often intubate expertly, so this should surely be an essential skill for any doctor.

It is also been said that Primary Anaesthesia is too detailed. In practice what the reader wants is the details—the relevant ones—and these we have tried to provide, to be looked up when necessary, and not to be learnt by heart.

Ketamine has been a huge advance in district hospital anaesthesia. If necessary, you can use it for most patients. It produces a trance–like state of full unconsciousness and analgesia, while largely preserving the protective reflexes of a patient's airway. Now that the nightmares and hallucinations it causes can be minimised with promethazine or diazepam, and muscular relaxation produced with alcuronium or gallamine, there are few operations you cannot do with it–provided you can pass a tracheal tube.

Some form of local or regional anaesthesia is often very suitable, so several of the more useful blocks have been included here. Regional blocks, in particular are not done nearly as often

THE EMO AND A BOYLE'S MACHINE

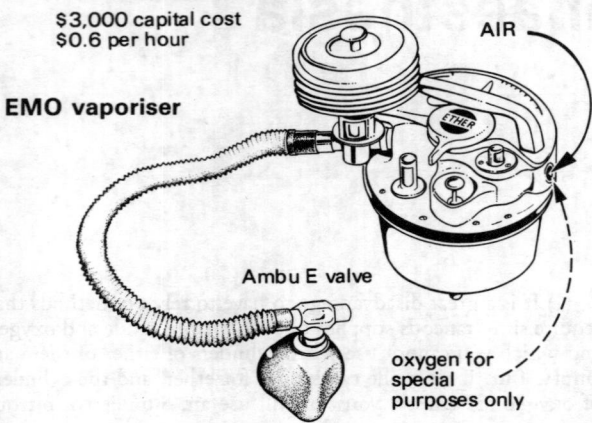

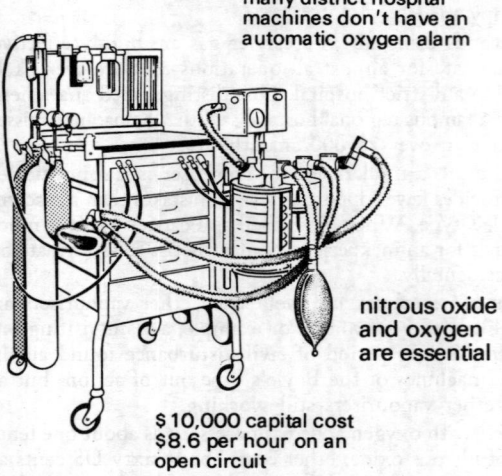

Fig. 1-1 COMPARISONS BETWEEN AN ETHER VAPORISER AND AN ANAESTHETIC MACHINE OF THE BOYLE'S TYPE. A vapouriser is cheaper to buy and to run, and it less easily becomes unserviceable. It does not need oxygen routinely, and can be run without it. *Kindly contributed by Clive Cory.*

as they should be, partly because the instructions for doing them are mostly in specialised texts. We hope that the account we give will fill that gap. In addition to older methods of subarachnoid (spinal) anaesthesia using hyperbaric chinchocaine, we have also described the newer and simpler one, using isobaric bupivacaine.

Great attention has been paid to methods of anaesthetizing children, which are a major shortcoming of many district hospitals, and a field in which the use of paediatric non-rebreathing valves such as the AMBU 'Paedivalve' described in Section 10.2 promises to be useful.

Although some hospitals would do well to achieve even the most minimal of the methods we describe here, many have already achieved these, and wish to progress. With them in mind we have included instructions for the use of a simple ventilator. Although there are some hospitals in which such a ventilator would be lethal, there are others in which it would be lifesaving. If the last chapter on "Primary Intensive Care" seems out of place, it should be remembered that some district hospitals already provide the simpler forms of intensive care most effectively.

What are the limits of the system or methods we describe? Some of them cannot be beaten by any methods anywhere, and are in routine for major procedures in the industrial world. Among them, these methods can anaesthetize almost any patient. Although more complex methods may sometimes give better results in the very old or the very young or the very sick, they will do so only by a small margin. Only such rarities as phaeochromocytoma, porphyria, and malignant hyperthermia lie outside the scope of this system of Primary Anaesthesia.

If the pages which follow provide what appear to be a bewildering variety of alternatives, here are a few hints to help you use them.

BE VERSATILE! USE THE RIGHT METHOD FOR THE RIGHT PATIENT

HOW TO USE THIS BOOK

STYLE You will notice that we use two alternatives styles—the "method style" in which this paragraph is written, and the "narrative style" which is used to start each section. These styles are different typefaces, and serve different purposes.

CROSS REFERENCES These follow the convention of using a full stop for a section (2.3), a dash for a figure (2-3), and a colon for a table (2:3). References to other manuals in the series take the form (S 2.3), for the third section in the second chapter of the accompanying manuals on surgical methods. These are in two volumes, the first starts at Chapter One, and is for all surgical methods other than those for trauma. The second starts at Chapter 50 and is devoted to trauma only.

The names of a few critical suppliers have been given. These take the form of three capital letters, for example, (AMB) is short for AMBU International. They are given in full in Appendix B.

IF YOU ARE A MEDICAL STUDENT, this is a book to be owned and used, not learnt by heart. You should however try to be familiar with all of it, so that you can easily find what you want.

Study the passages which start each section carefully, and read quickly through the "Method" sections. If you think that the practical anaesthetic instruction in your school does not prepare you adequately for the tasks that will face you when you qualify, insist on a few weeks of practical anaesthetic clerkship. Can an arrangement be made whereby you can learn to do regional blocks in the casualty department? If possible, learn to give them with the help of a nerve stimulator.

Make sure you would know immediately what to do in the event of the difficulties and disasters in Chapter 3. A patient's life may depend on taking the necessary action quickly, and there will not be time to look it up!

Take every opportunity you can to learn as many methods as possible under expert supervision. It is very useful to be able to give a local anaesthetic when facilities for general anaesthesia are not available.

IF YOU ARE AN AUXILIARY OR IF ENGLISH IS NOT YOUR FIRST LANGUAGE, look through the vocabulary index with particular care. It will explain the terms you may not know.

IF YOU ARE INEXPERIENCED AND HAVE TO GIVE AN ANAESTHETIC, your choice will probably depend mostly on the drugs and equipment you have, so first see what there is.

If possible, use ketamine, especially if you have to anaesthetize a child.

The safest inhalational anaesthetic to start with is ether from a vapouriser, both for induction and maintenance (11.3). Follow this by learning to induce a patient with thiopentone (12.1).

If your patient has a full stomach, and you cannot intubate him, and he must have a general anaesthetic which produces abdominal relaxation, the safest method will probably be to aspirate his stomach, and then to induce him with ether, while he lies on his side with the table tilted head down (16.5). Have the suction ready—there may still be food in his stomach!

Avoid halothane to begin with.

Resolve to learn how to intubate as soon as you can, and

study carefully what to do if intubation fails. Start by intubating patients when they are deeply anaesthetized with ether. Don't give relaxants until you can give an anaesthetic with a face mask efficiently, and intubate confidently. Become familiar with suxamethonium first, before using a long acting relaxant.

One of the most useful local anaesthetic methods is intravenous forearm block (6.19). Others are finger blocks (6.21), and infiltration anaesthesia for Caesarean section (6.9).

Caudal epidural anaesthesia in non-pregnant adults (7.3), and subarachnoid anaesthesia with isobaric bupivacaine (7.5) should not prove too difficult. Avoid lumbar epidurals to begin with.

IF YOU ARE A DISTRICT HOSPITAL DOCTOR ALREADY RESPONSIBLE FOR ANAESTHESIA, read this manual carefully to see where you might improve the practice in your hospital. Can you improve the postoperative care your patients get? Can you increase the range of anaesthetics your staff give? Which of the basic safety precautions do you or do they regularly neglect?

IF YOU ARE A SPECIALIST ANAESTHETIST your objectives should be: (1) To analyse any data you can find concerning the anaesthetics given in your region. (2) To visit the workers who give them and to see what they actually do. (3) To make an inventory of the resources at your disposal in terms of staff, equipment and finances.

With this information you should be able to: (1) Decide what the priorities are to improve the quality of the anaesthetic care that is given, and remove its major dangers. (2) Decide which methods should be used in your region, and what equipment would be necessary for them. (3) Design an appropriate teaching supervision, and procurement plan to achieve your objectives.

STRIVE TO INCREASE THE QUALITY OF ANAESTHETIC CARE

---

2 Background to anaesthesia

2.1 Who gives the anaesthetic?

All patients *must* be anaesthetized by some competent person. The arrangements for achieving this vary: (1) Some countries recognise only specialist doctor anaesthetists, so that non–doctor anaesthetists do not exist—officially! (2) Other countries recognise that they do not have enough specialist doctor anaesthetists for everyone, and accept that anaesthesia may have to be delegated to non–doctors, who have been *carefully trained.* (3) A further group of countries say they have enough specialist doctor anaesthetists for everyone, but in fact they do not. The result is that patients are often anaesthetized dangerously by untrained staff, and alas, occasionally even by the theatre porter. This is so highly unsatisfactory that all ministries of health are urged to look carefully at just who does anaesthetize the patients in their smaller hospitals. If untrained staff are giving anaesthetics, they must be replaced—by specialist anaesthetists, by well trained general duty doctors, or by trained assistants.

Many assistants anaesthetize excellently. The same anaesthetic routines are repeated many times in the same way, sufficient theory can be learnt, and manual dexterity comes with practice. When something unexpected does happen, the action required can be standardized, and should be automatic. Because good anaesthesia depends so much on practice, trained and experienced non–doctor anaesthetists give excellent service, and are of immense value. Some of them have become so experienced that they give much better anaesthetics than recently qualified doctors, who dare not correct them. Besides, there is a worldwide shortage of specialist anaesthetists, and even in teaching hospitals there are seldom enough of them for everyone who requires surgery. In small hospitals there is usually so much work that a doctor can seldom be spared to act as an anaesthetist. In a developing country the true task of a specialist anaesthetist, including those in teaching hospitals, is to teach, to administer anaesthetic services, to visit and encourage staff in the districts, and to anaesthetize only the most complex and exacting cases himself. Where possible, and this is almost always possible, *he should use only the equipment that he expects other people to use in a district hospital.* It is tragic for operations in a district hospital to be postponed for lack of nitrous oxide or halothane, when an ether vapouriser is available, but an anaesthetic assistant will not use it, because he never used one in his training school!

It is impossible to overestimate the contribution that a well–trained cadre of non–doctor anaesthetists can make to both the quality and quantity of district hospital surgery. About a year's special training is usually considered essential, but some services find that medical assistants can be made into useful anaesthetic assistants in only a 6–week intensive course followed by a 6 weeks' supervision. This must be in a large hospital where much surgery is done and where supervision is easy. If nurses, or, better, basically–trained medical assistants, are given further training in anaesthesia, they have a wider background than staff who have been trained in anaesthesia only. They are also much better able to examine patients preoperatively. When suitably trained, they can become expert at local blocks, they can also give epidural and subarachnoid anaesthetics, they can intubate and they can give relaxants. In some minimally staffed hospitals, theatre staff "trained on the job" routinely give long–acting relaxants.

Most if not all the anaesthetics described here can be given by auxiliaries. But this is not a training manual for them, because they need more theory and explanation that we have space for. This book is primarily for medical students and for doctors. For convenience, we assume that you are giving the anaesthetic yourself, or supervising someone who is only partly trained.

If, for lack of qualified help, you have to be responsible for the anaesthetic and the operation, use local and regional methods where you can. If you have to give a general anaesthetic. secure the patient's airway and make sure that there is a drip running before you start. With a clear airway and a drip, most of your problems will be over. Induce and intubate the patient yourself, and don't operate until anaesthesia is stable. This will save time in the end, and perhaps the patient's life also. Find an intelligent person and make him your assistant. Make sure he monitors the patient's pulse and blood pressure, and tells you about any unexpected changes in its rate, volume and regularity. Teach him to take the blood pressure, and listen with an oesophageal or precordial stethoscope (18.2). He must also replace fluid as it is lost.

All anaesthetists, including anaesthetic assistants, need a helper to change the oxygen cylinder, to work the bag or bellows in an emergency, to measure the blood pressure, to give drugs, to administer cricoid pressure (16.5), and to run for the theatre sister. So try to see that there is always someone around, who can help you by doing these things—competently.

2.2 Anaesthesia in a health centre

Many patients cannot reach a hospital, and have to be treated in a health centre. Such limited surgery as these units can do is often done with the patient in quite unnecessary pain, without any anaesthesia. Which of the methods of Primary Anaesthesia described here are also suitable for use in health centres by auxiliaries, with the minimum of anaesthetic training? There is no sharp distinction between the methods which are suitable for district hospitals and health centres, and much will depend on a health centre's size, the ease with which it can refer patients, and the anaesthetic training its auxiliaries have. You will probably find that the following methods are suitable. For all of them a table which will tip, a sucker, airways, a self–inflating bag and a non–rebreathing valve are essential emergency equipment. If a health centre is going to do surgery it must be properly equipped, and should have an ether vapouriser.

HEALTH CENTRE ANAESTHESIA

Opening abscesses—local infiltration (5.7), ketamine (8.1), open ether (11.4).

Setting fractures—ketamine (8.1), pethidine with thiopentone (8.8).

Toileting and suturing wounds—infiltration anaesthesia (12.1), ketamine.

Evacuating incomplete abortions—pethedine with diazepam cocktail (8.8).

Emergency Caesarean sections—ketamine with local infiltration (6.9).

METHODS WHICH ARE CONTRAINDICATED These include—intravenous forearm block (6.19), and all the methods of general anaesthesia described here.

THE COST OF AN HOUR OF ANAESTHESIA

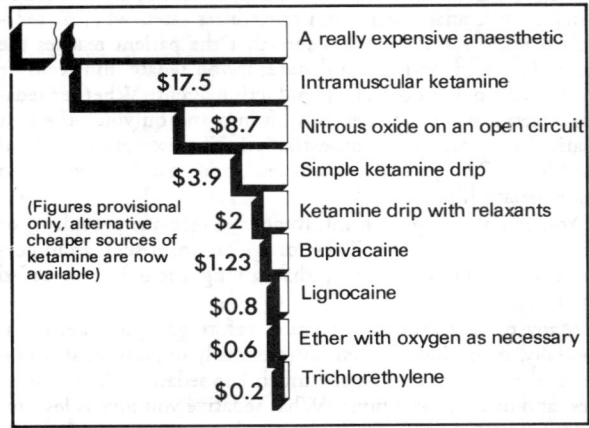

Fig. 2-1 THE COST OF AN HOUR OF ANAESTHESIA. Local and regional blocks are among the cheapest anaesthetics. Ketamine is fortunately becoming cheaper. *Kindly contributed by Clive Cory.*

2.3 How much does anaesthesia cost?

Costs vary from one country to another, depending upon what is manufactured locally, and from year to year. So find out what the cost of different anaesthetics are in your country. Here are some examples from Tanzania in 1978. There, the hourly cost of running a theatre at a district hospital was estimated to be $45. Of this $1 represented the wages of the anaesthetic assistant. Were the anaesthetic to be given by a doctor routinely, the corresponding figure would be much higher. The costs assume that a bottle of intravenous fluid is made locally and costs $0.15, and not $2 as purchased. If fluid has to be bought at the latter figure, the cost of anaesthesia increases greatly.

The cost of a general anaesthetic depends on the carrier gas, the type of circuit and the volatile agent that is used. If nitrous oxide is used, it costs about $9 an hour on an open circuit and $55 on a closed one. When ether is used with air as the carrier gas, an hour of anaesthesia costs $0.25, or about $1 if oxygen is added to produce the same concentration as in an anaesthetic machine of the Boyle's type. The cost falls to $0.6 per hour, if oxygen is only added when necessary.

Large capital savings can be made by using air as a carrier gas. Thus a machine of the Boyle's type costs about $10 000, whereas an ether vapouriser only costs $1,500. In a busy theatre a modern ether vapouriser will pay for itself in about three months.

Halothane is expensive, but only if it is the main anaesthetic agent. If it is used for induction only, it costs $1, or about as much as thiopentone. Trichloroethylene is about a thirtieth of the cost of halothane. Anaesthesia with trichloroethylene only costs $0.20 an hour including the cost of the relaxants, and is not used as often as it should be.

Although ketamine is at present expensive, it can be used economically. Thus 12 mg/kg of intramuscular ketamine gives an adult an hour's anaesthesia for $34. Given intravenously, or by a simple drip, an hour of anaesthesia for an adult requires not less than 280 mg of ketamine at a cost of $7.50. When relaxants are used, only about half as much ketamine is needed and costs $3.70. Fortunately, the patents for ketamine are said to be about to expire, after which it will be cheaper. Cheaper supplies from other manufacturers are already available.

Local and regional anaesthetics are the cheapest, and many anaesthetists would say the best. Subarachnoid (spinal) anaesthesia with cinchocaine, for example, costs $0.20, the maximum adult dose of lignocaine is $1.25, and bupivacaine $0.80.

The most sophisticated anaesthetic described here, although not the most expensive one, is thiopentone followed by suxamethonium, a long-acting relaxant and trichloroethylene. This costs $2.50, and is only a small fraction of what more complicated types of anaesthesia can cost.

2.4 Standardizing equipment

Here is a list on which to base the standardization of anaesthetic equipment for a district hospital. If it has a second theatre for septic cases, much of it should be duplicated, and preferably all of it. We suggest that you look through your Medical Stores Catalogue to see which items might reasonably be included in its next edition. Bupivacaine, for example, might well replace lignocaine, as the standard local anaesthetic. The quantities of each item are those appropriate to the initial equipping of one theatre in a district hospital. The specifications below also indicate the proportions of the different sizes of an item that are needed. For example, many more middle size tracheal tubes are needed than those at either end of the range. To make sure that the pieces fit each other, 15 and 22 mm ISO (International Standards Organisation) cone fittings, and 12 mm corrugated tubing have been specified throughout. Needles have been specified in metric sizes. If you are used to SWG sizes, compare them using Fig. 2-2. Hook-on laryngoscopes are reccommended, in a size which takes the larger American D type battery cells,

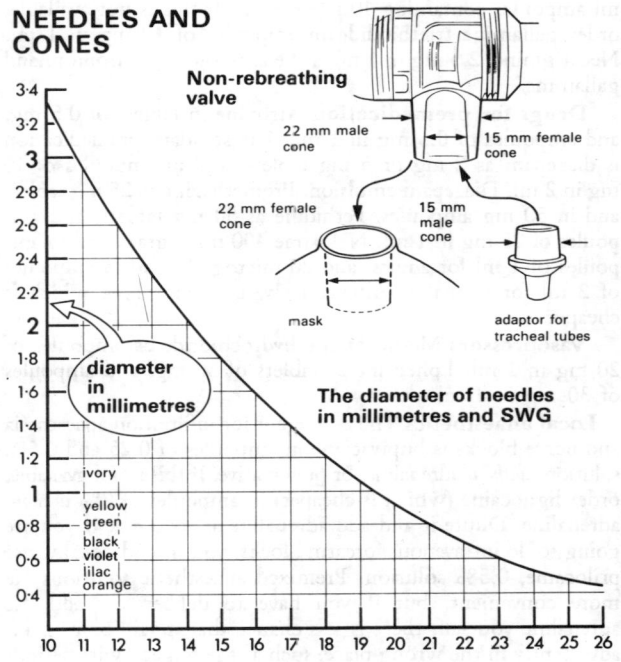

Fig. 2-2 THE SIZES OF NEEDLES AND CONES. In this book all needle sizes are in millimetres. If you are used to SWG sizes (Standard wire gauge), use this conversion graph. You will also see the colours for plastic needle hubs. They apply to the internal diameters, and manufacturers do not always follow them so that they may vary. If all your equipment uses ISO cones, it will fit together.

because these are widely available. In the absence of an international standard for laryngoscope bulbs, 3 volt bulbs with No. 8 ANC threads have been specified. All syringes and needles have Luer fittings. No drugs have been included which need refrigeration. *If you do buy disposable equipment, especially disposable needles, it must be capable of being boiled—you may have to reuse it, perhaps many times.*

All the equipment is summarised in Appendix B. Other sections describe equipment for local anaesthesia (5.1), for subarachnoid and epidural anaesthesia (7.1), for particular vapourisers (10.6 to 10.12), for intubation (13.2), for intravenous drips (15.2), and for children (18.2). Although suction equipment is also needed for surgery, it is listed here.

ALWAYS SPECIFY ISO FITTINGS

2.5 Anaesthetic drugs

Anaesthetic agents. Ether in cans or bottles of 500 ml. Halothane in 250 ml bottles. Trichloroethylene in 500 ml bottles. Ketamine in vials containing 10, 50 and 100 mg/ml. Morphine in 15 mg ampoules. Thiopentone sodium in 0.5 g ampoules to make 20 ml, or in 1 g ampoules to make 40 ml of 2.5% solution. If possible, buy intravenous agents in single—dose ampoules. They are a little more expensive than in multidose containers, but there is less danger of contamination.

Drugs for inducing and reversing muscular relaxation Suxamethonium bromide powder ('Brevedil M') in 50 mg ampoules. This stores better than suxamethonium chloride ('Scoline') solutions, which deteriorate if they are not refrigerated. The most generally useful and cheapest long—acting relaxants for routine use are: (1) alcuronium chloride ('Alloferin') 2 ml ampoules containing 5 mg per ml; or (2) d-tubocurarine in 1.5 ml ampoules containing 10 mg per ml. If this is not available, order gallamine triethiodide in ampoules of 40 mg in 1 ml. Neostigmine, 2.5 mg in 1 ml is the antidote to alcuronium and gallamine.

Drugs for premedication Atropine in tablets of 0.5 mg, and ampoules of 0.6 mg in 1 ml. The standard premedication is diazepam as 2 mg or 5 mg tablets, and in ampoules of 10 mg in 2 ml. Diazepam emulsion. Promethazine as 25 mg tablets and in 50 mg ampoules. Pethidine as 50 mg tablets, and ampoules of 25 mg in 1 ml. Naloxone 400 micrograms/ml in ampoules of 1 ml for adults, and 20 micrograms/ml in ampoules of 2 ml for neonates. Alternatively, use nalorphine which is cheaper.

Vasopressors Methoxamine hydrochloride as ampoules of 20 mg in 1 ml. Ephedrine as tablets of 30 mg, and ampoules of 30 mg in 1 ml.

Local anaesthetics The best agent for infiltration anaesthesia and nerve blocks is bupivacaine in ampoules of 0.25 and 0.5% solution, *without* adrenaline, or preservative. If this is not available, order lignocaine (which is cheaper) in ampoules of 2% *without* adrenaline. Dilute it and add adrenaline as required. If you are going to do intravenous forearm blocks, you should, ideally, use prilocaine, 0.5% solution. Premixed anaesthetic solutions are more convenient, but if you have to deliberately add the adrenaline yourself, there is less chance that it will be used inadvertently in the wrong place, such as the fingers, with serious consequences. A preservative in a multidose ampoule of an anaesthetic solution prevents it becoming contaminated, but makes it unsuitable for intrathecal use where the preservative may damage the cord. For dental anaesthesia you will need lignocaine with adrenaline in cartridges of 1.8 or 2ml. For anaesthetizing the mucous membranes, you will need lignocaine in pressurised aerosol containers delivering 10 mg at each puff, or as a 2% or 4% solution. The 2% solution is safer, especially in children. Adrenaline in ampoules of 1 mg in 1 ml. 0.5% bupivacaine is the drug of choice for isobaric subarachnoid anaesthesia. If you want to give a hyperbaric subarachnoid anaesthetic, order cinchocaine heavy solution with dextrose 6% in ampoules of 3 ml.

2.6 Premedication

All the major anaesthetic agents have their own special methods, and are described in later sections. They also have their limitations and side effects, which you can often minimise by giving other drugs with them as premedication. There are two parts to premedication, *atropinisation,* and *sedation.* Atropine is required to make some anaesthetics and procedures safer, whereas sedation *before the operation* makes sure that the patient reaches the theatre in a calm and tranquil state. If you sedate him well, he will need a smaller dose of the induction agent. Whether sedation is necessary or not depends on him and on you—the best sedation is sympathetic anaesthetist! The exception is local anaesthesia. The patient is conscious, and may be anxious, so *always* sedate him.

You can also give him intravenous diazepam, pethidine, or morphine *at the operation.* These drugs can form such an important part of the anaesthetic, that giving them is best called *paramedication.*

Many patients need no sedation before general anaesthesia, especially, if you induce them intravenously in pleasant surroundings. Very sick patients need much less sedation than healthy ones, and usually need none. What sedative you give is less important than how much you give and how you give it. If possible, sedate a patient orally. Taking a tablet is pleasanter than having an injection, and cheaper, 10 mg of diazepam, for example, costs 50 US cents by injection, but only 3 cents by mouth. Give tablets with 20 ml of water, an hour before operation. Premedicate a patient by injection if he is vomiting, if absorbtion from his stomach is likely to be uncertain, or in a serious emergency.

Don't give opioids, such as pethidine, unless they are necessary to relieve pain, and don't give too much. They depress the respiration and thus slow the uptake of ether. They also alter the pattern of ether anaesthesia, and so obscure some of the signs of anaesthesia. When an opioid is necessary, the standard combination is diazepam 10 mg, and pethidine 50 mg.

If any premedication is going to be useful, it must be timed accurately. Busy or poorly trained ward staff often find this difficult. If ward staff cannot give the right dose of the right drug to the right patient at the right time, you can, if necessary, give the premedication yourself intravenously in the theatre immediately before you operate. Reduce the dose proportionally, and take particular care not to give a strong respiratory depressant.

Giving drugs will be much easier if you always set up a drip, or use a diaphragm needle (15.2). You can use the same bottle of fluid, with separate sterile needles, for more than one patient, so drips need not be expensive.

Give all intravenous injections slowly! The only exception is suxamethonium, which is so short acting that you should to give it quite fast.

GET THE DOSE RIGHT

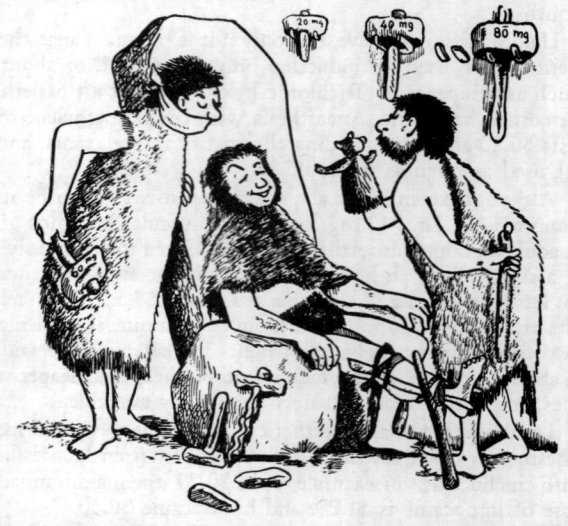

Fig. 2-3 GET THE DOSE RIGHT. *Kindly contributed by Frank Prior from his book "Household hints in Anaesthesia".*

2.7 Atropine and neostigmine

Atropine has several important uses in anaesthesia both before an operation, and during it:

(1) Atropine dries a patient's saliva and makes his bronchial secretions thick and tenacious. Ether and ketamine increase these secretions, sometimes dangerously, so always give atropine before either of these anaesthetics.

(2) Atropine blocks the action of the vagus nerve on the heart, and so prevents the excessive vagal action that may arise during anaesthesia, and especially during intubation. If you don't control this vagal action, it may slow the heart undesirably. Children have a high vagal tone, so always premedicate them with atropine—provided the ambient temperature is not too high (see below). Some anaesthetists prefer not to use atropine routinely, but always have it ready to treat bradycardia.

(3) Atropine minimises the slowing and arrhythmias that halothane, and trichloroethylene sometimes cause. Unfortunately, its protective effect only lasts an hour, so, if the operation takes longer than this, you may have to repeat the dose of atropine. Although the patient's throat may still be dry from the previous dose, atropine will no longer be protecting his heart. The signs that more atropine is indicated, are a pulse that falls to 60 or below, and increasing salivation.

(4) Atropine counteracts the hypotension and bradycardia, and minimises the increased bronchial secretions that are caused by depolarising relaxants, such as suxamethonium.

(5) Atropine also counteracts these same side effects when they are caused by the neostigmine used to reverse non–depolarising relaxants, such as alcuronium (14.3). So always give atropine, either just before you give neostigmine or with it in the same syringe.

In the usual doses for premedication, atropine does not generally dilate the pupil, but in larger doses it may do. This is not important, except that deep ether anaesthesia also dilates the pupil, so that effects of atropine may be confused with those of ether.

Atropine's drying effect on the mucous membranes takes time. It has a stronger effect in reducing secretions if you give it intramuscularly 20 minutes before the operation than if you give it orally or intravenously as the operation begins. If the patient is given atropine much earlier or later the effect of atropine is less, and you may have difficulties. When a patient has been given atropine, he has 20 minutes with an unpleasantly dry mouth—like cardboard. Because of the difficulties of timing, many anaesthetists, compromise and give atropine in the theatre, intravenously with the induction agent. Mix the atropine with the thiopentone or ketamine in the same syringe. If the patient has already been given a dose of atropine earlier in the ward, a second one won't hurt him.

Don't use atropine unless it is indicated. For example, it is not strictly necessary before local, regional, subarachnoid (spinal), or epidural anaesthesia.

Atropine reduces sweating, and in very hot weather it may cause hyperpyrexia in children. If the ambient temperature is above 30°C, don't give it to children under five, and preferably not to those under 15. Even the mildest anoxia may cause cardiac arrest in a hyperpyrexial child.

Neostigmine prevents the normal hydrolysis of acetylcholine by cholinesterase and so allows it to accumulate. Use it to reverse the action of long–acting relaxants such as alcuronium, which prevent the access of acetylcholine to the receptor protein (14.1).

DOSE OF ATROPINE As premedication for ether or ketamine, or to counteract the effects of neostigmine, give 0.02 mg/kg to patients of all ages, the usual adult dose is 0.6 mg intramuscularly, or 1 mg orally 1 to 1½ hours preoperatively. If convenient, mix intravenous atropine with the induction agent.

DOSE OF NEOSTIGMINE Give 0.04 to 0.08 mg/kg. The maximum dose for adults is 5 mg, and the standard dose is 2.5 mg. Mix this with the atropine (0.02 mg/kg) in the same syringe.

DONT GIVE ATROPINE TO FEBRILE CHILDREN IF THE AMBIENT TEMPERATURE IS ABOVE 30°C

2.8 Tranquilisers

Diazepam is a powerful tranquiliser and anticonvulsant. Modest doses make a patient drowsy, and excessive ones make him sleepy or even comatose. Diazepam reduces anxiety, and in ordinary doses does not depress the patient's respiration. But diazepam will depress his response to both carbon dioxide and anoxia, so give it with care if he has respiratory problems. Diazepam also causes 'flat' babies if you use it for Caesarean section. Even so, for most patients diazepam is good premedication for both local anaesthesia and ether.

If possible give diazepam by mouth—it will be absorbed more rapidly than by intramuscular injection. Diazepam *solution* is painful if you inject it into a muscle or intravenously. If by mistake you inject it into an artery, it can cause thrombosis, so use the same precautions as with thiopentone (12.1). If you are fortunate, you have diazepam *emulsion* which is a special preparation that overcomes these disadvantages. You can inject it intravenously, even into the small veins of the hand, without causing pain or thrombosis. But you should if possible give repeated doses (as for tetanus) into a central vein.

If necessary, you can use diazepam as an induction agent, if you give it into a fast running drip. A 'sleep dose' of diazepam depresses a patient's cardiac ouput less than a sleep dose of thiopentone, so diazepam is a good induction agent if he has a severe heart disease; but diazepam takes longer to act than thiopentone, and its effect is longer lasting, so he has more hangover.

A small dose of intravenous diazepam (5 mg), repeated if necessary, is a useful way of controlling the fits that may complicate local, epidural or subarachnoid anaesthesia. These fits are often due to anoxia, so *the first step in treating such fits is to keep him well oxygenated—be sure to ventilate him adequately*. If fits continue after you have done this, give him diazepam.

DOSE OF DIAZEPAM Give 0.15 to 0.25 mg/kg, The usual adult dose is 10 to 20 mg, by mouth one hour before the operation. Crush the tablets and give them with a little water. If you give diazepam two hours before, its effect will have passed its peak, especially if the operation is postponed.
CAUTION ! (1) Undiluted diazepam solution is painful, so minimise the pain by using a big vein. (2) If you dilute diazepam in a small volume, it precipitates and the mixture becomes cloudy. You can safely inject it into a fast running drip, or you can dilute an adult dose in 500 ml. (3) If you give diazepam with pethidine, to produce short periods of anaesthesia (8.8), use separate syringes, because the mixture forms a precipitate. Instead, give the standard dose of pethidine in mg/kg, according to the patient's weight. Then titrate the dose of diazepam until you get the effect you want.

Promethazine has antihistamine, antiemetic and sedative activity, all of which are useful in premedication. It is a weaker sedative than either chlorpromazine or diazepam, and is the best premedication for ketamine. This is its main use in this manual.

DOSE OF PROMETHAZINE Give 1 mg/kg, the usual adult dose is 50 mg, by mouth 2 hours before the operation.

Chlorpromazine is a strong sedative and antiemetic. It reduces anxiety and calms a patient. It also has anticonvulsant and hypotensive effects, so it is contraindicated in shock. Some hospitals use chlorpromazine tablets as their routine premedication. It is cheap and they find that they do not notice its hypotensive effect.

DOSE OF CHLROPMAZINE Intramuscularly, give 0.75 mg/kg, the usual adult dose is 50 mg. Intravenously, give 0.3 mg/kg, the usual adult dose is 25 mg.

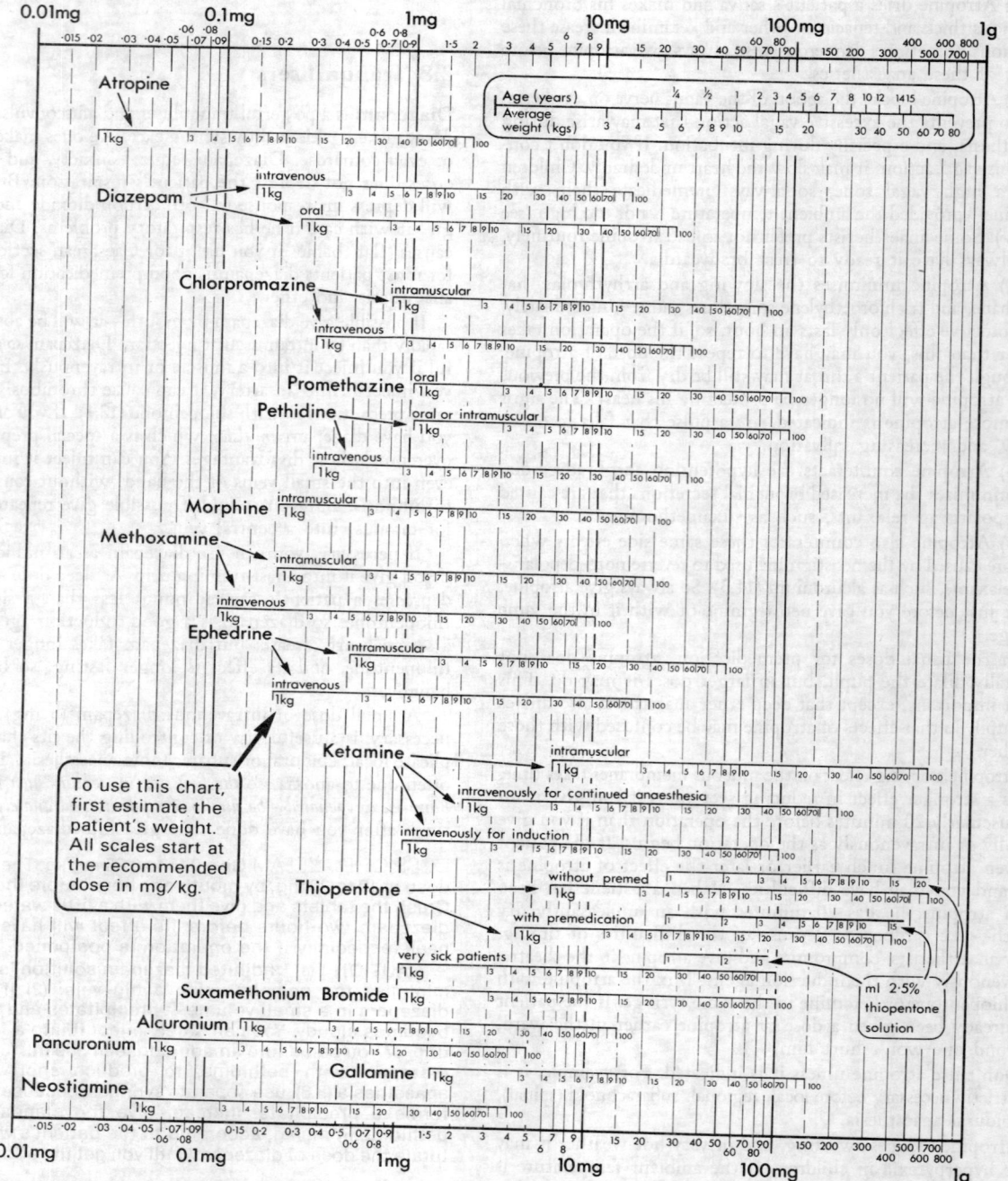

Fig. 2-4 DRUG DOSES FOR ANAESTHESIA. This figure has a scale of vertical lines showing drug doses form 0.01 mg to 1 g. For each drug there is a horizontal weight scale for patients weighing from 1 to 100 kg. Estimate your patient's weight. Find it on the horizontal scale for the drug you want. Most adults weigh about 60 kg, so the usual adult dose is opposite 60 kg on the weight scales. If you are anaesthetizing a child, which of the vertical lines does his weight correspond to? Follow this line to the top or bottom of the figure to read the dose of the drug that he needs.

The 1 kg mark on each horizontal scale shows the dose in mg/kg.

If you don't know the patient's weight, estimate it from his age, using the scale at the top right–hand corner. This is approximate only. Some patients are only a fraction of their expected weight for their age, so be careful.

There is a spare copy of this figure at the end of the book. Tear it out and paste it up on the theatre wall.

Remember that these doses are for patients of average weight, very sick patients need much less, and robust patients much more. Adjust the dose you give to get the response you want.

Do you find this figure confusing? Try these examples. The answers are at the end of Section 2.10.

(1) How many milligrams of oral diazepam would you give to a 40 kg. patient?

(2) About how many ml of 2.5% thiopentone would you give to a 70 kg adult who had not been premedicated?

(3) How many mg of thiopentone would you give a 50 kg patient who had been premedicated?

(4) What is the dose of neostigmine for a 10 kg child?

(5) What is the dose of intravenous ephedrine for a 100 kg adult?

The doses of the long—acting relaxants, particularly alcuronium and pancuronium, are those appropriate for patients who have been given suxamethonium and are to be maintained on ether. Under other circumstances you may need to give slightly larger doses.

2.9 Pethidine and morphine

These are both opioids, or drugs like opium. Until recently, opioids were the standard premedication for most anaesthetics, but, because they depress a patient's respiration, they are not ideal. If you give the patient an opioid and then try to induce him with ether, induction will be much slower. Other drugs, such as diazepam are better.

Pethidine is a powerful central analgesic. It is not a local anaesthetic. If your local block is not quite perfect it will reduce a patient's sensation of pain by acting on his brain. It is also a moderate sedative, so it is useful pre– or paramedication for local anaesthesia. For supplementing regional blocks use it alone, or combine it with intramuscular or intravenous promethazine. If a nerve block is not fully effective, pethidine may dull some of the patient's pain. You can also use pethidine with thiopentone or diazepam to produce intravenous anaesthesia (8.8). You need not titrate the pethidine, but you should titrate the thiopentone or the diazepam to the patient's response.

DOSE OF PETHIDINE Give 1 to 1.5 mg/kg, the usual adult dose is 50 to 75 mg by mouth 2 hours before the operation. Or, better, give it by intramuscular injection 30 minutes before. Or, give an adult 15 to 25 mg intravenously at the operation. If necessary, give additional doses of 10 mg intravenously during it.

Morphine, another powerful analgesic, causes a sense of well being and slight drowsiness. In higher doses than those used for premedication you can use it for paramedication, and for intravenous analgesia. When you use morphine as paramedication for regional blocks, combine it with intravenous or intramuscular promethazine. When you use it for pain, remember that small frequent intravenous doses are better than large infrequent intramuscular ones

DOSE OF MORPHINE For premedication give 0.2 mg/kg, the usual adult dose is 10 to 15 mg.

For paramedication for local anaesthesia, and intravenous analgesia, give up to 0.5 mg/kg.

CAUTION! If you are giving it intravenously, give it slowly, only until you get just the effect you want, as described in Section 8.7.

2.10 Vasopressors

These raise a patient's blood pressure; but because vasopressors act by constricting his blood vessels, they are only useful if his blood pressure has fallen because of vasodilation, for example after subarachnoid or epidural anaesthesia or after an overdose of lignocaine. Vasopressors are useless if the patient's hypotension is caused by haemorrhage. In that case his blood vessels are already fully constricted, so that vasopressors are no substitute for adequate fluid replacement. They are dangerous if hypotension is caused by myocardial failure, because they increase peripheral resistance and so give his heart more work.

Ephedrine is preferred by some anaesthetists to methoxamine, because it stimulates a patient's brain as well as raising his blood pressure. Ephedrine is also more widely available than methoxamine.

DOSE OF EPHEDRINE Give 0.5 mg/kg by intramuscular injection. The usual adult dose is 15 to 45 mg. Give half the dose intravenously for its immediate effect, and half the dose intramuscularly for its delayed effect.

Methoxamine hydrochloride is a pure vasoconstrictor. Intramuscular methoxamine increases a patient's peripheral resistance, and raises his blood pressure for 60 to 90 minutes, without having any effect on his heart or brain. Unlike other vasopressors, such as adrenaline or ephedrine, methoxamine can be safely used with halothane or trichloroethylene or chloroform. It usually remains effective in patients on hypotensive drugs.

DOSE OF METHOXAMINE Give 2 mg intravenously, or 5 to 20 mg intramuscularly. It is good practice to give half the dose intravenously and half intramuscularly. The intravenous dose acts immediatley, but its effect soon wears off. The intramuscular dose takes longer to act, but its effect is more sustained. Don't give more until the first dose has had an opportunity to act. Many anaesthetists always give it intravenously.

If the patient's pulse slows severely after you have given methoxamine, give atropine, and always have atropine ready when you give methoxamine. The increase in peripheral resistance that methoxamine causes may need atropine to reverse it.

Answers to exercises on Figures 2-4 Question one, 10 mg. Question two, between 15 and 20 ml. Question three, 200 mg. Question four, 0.4 mg. Question five, 20 mg. Easy!

3 Should disaster occur

3.1 The ten golden rules of anaesthesia

Before you can give any anaesthetic safely: (1) You must understand the basic care of a patient, before, during and after it. (2) You must know about the disasters that can occur, how to prevent them, and what to do if they do occur. An anaesthetic death is almost always the result of some preventable disaster, and even when it has happened, you can usually treat it, *but only if you recognize it immediately*. (3) You must have the necessary equipment to deal with these disasters.

The disasters that you must do all you can to prevent, and yet be prepared for if they do occur are: (1) The inhalation of stomach contents, following either vomiting or regurgitation (16.2, 16.3). (2) Severe hypotension. (3) Respiratory arrest. (4) Cardiac arrest (3.5). (4) Laryngeal spasm. (5) Bronchial spasm (3.3). (6) Convulsions (5.9). (7) Severe hypothermia in small children (18.1). (8) Machine or oxygen failure is an important cause of disaster if you are using sophisticated equipment dependant on oxygen. (One of the merits of the simple drawover vapourisers described here is that they are less prone to mechanical

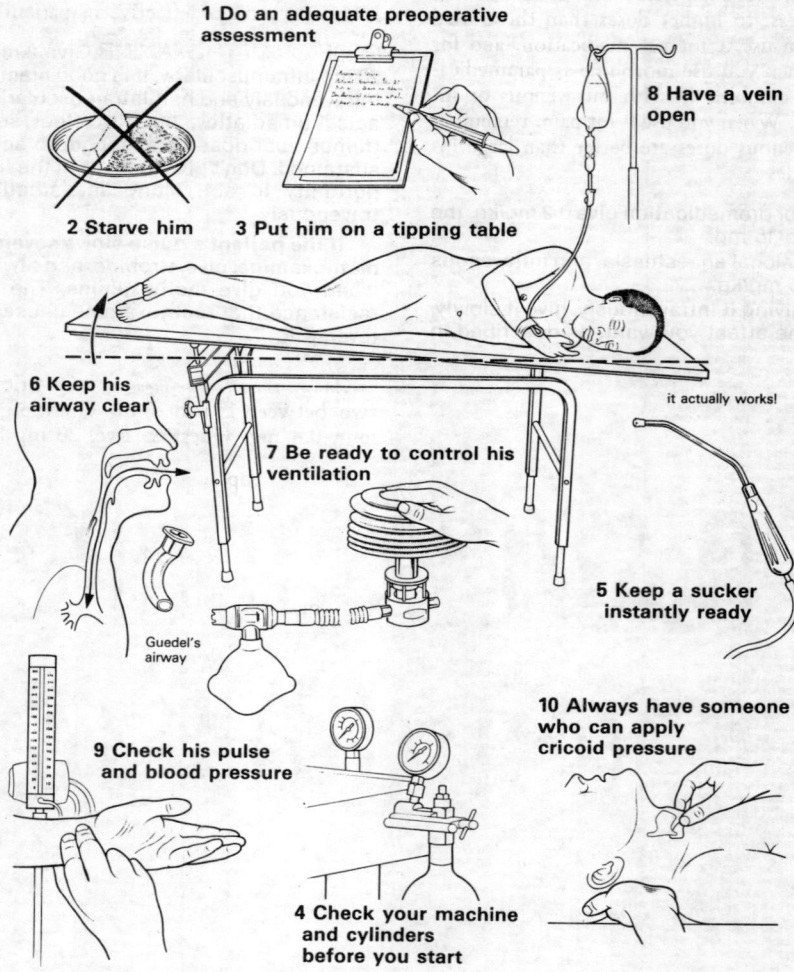

Fig. 3-1 THE TEN GOLDEN RULES. If these rules were always followed there would be far fewer anaesthetic deaths: (1) Assess and prepare a patient adequately. (2) Starve him. (3) Put him on a tipping table. (4) Check the machine and cylinders before you start. (5) Have a sucker ready. (6) Have airways ready. (7) Be ready to control his ventilation. (8) Have a vein open. (9) Monitor his pulse and blood pressure (10) Have someone around who can apply cricoid pressure, and who can be relied on in an emergency. *Kindly contributed by Julian Bion.*

or human error, and do not depend on a supply of oxygen). (9) Fires and explosions with ether and other volatile anaesthetic agents (11.5).

The inhalation of stomach contents is discussed in Chapter 16. Most of the other potential disasters are described here.

You will meet with fewer disasters, and will be better prepared for them if they do occur, if you follow ten golden rules. They apply to all anaesthetics, including ketamine. Even a finger block is no exception, because serious reactions can occasionally follow even a small dose of a local anaesthetic. There may be such a thing as "minor surgery", but there are few "minor anaesthetics". They may be minor one minute, but they can easily become very major the next. So never forget these ten golden rules. Disaster is particularly likely under conditions of stress, such as late at night, or when mass operations are done, as in a tubal ligation 'camp'.

Before you give a patient any general anaesthetic, *including ketamine and "cocktails",* and any but the most minor local ones, follow these rules. They are not a complete system of anaesthesia—that is the whole of "Primary Anaesthesia". They are merely ten of the things that are most often forgotten.

THE TEN GOLDEN RULES

(1) ASSESS AND PREPARE THE PATIENT ADEQUATELY Assess him so that you will not anaesthetize anyone who is asthmatic, acidotic, or grossly anaemic, unknowingly. If he is on any drugs that might interfere with anaesthesia, you must know what they are.

Prepare the patient by correcting dehydration, severe anaemia, cardiac failure or diabetes before you operate.

(2) STARVE HIM, so that if he tries to vomit, his stomach is less likely to be full. Starve him, even if he is having a local anaesthetic, because it may fail so that you have to give him a general one. Remember that you cannot be sure that his stomach is empty, even after 6 hours of starvation.

(3) ANAESTHETIZE HIM ON A TIPPING TABLE, because he may still vomit, even if he is supposed to have been starved, so you must be able to tip him head down. If you do this, his stomach contents are less likely to run into his lungs (16.1). To give *any* anaesthetic on a table which does not tip is negligent. If you are negligent and do anaesthetize him on a table which does not tip and he does vomit, immediately turn him onto his side to protect his airway.

(4) CHECK YOUR DRUGS AND EQUIPMENT before your start, especially if you are using less simple equipment. The equipment to preserve his airway must be ready beside you

(5) KEEP A SUCKER INSTANTLY READY, tested and working, so that if his pharynx fills with vomit, you can suck it out. You will also need suction catheters.

(6) KEEP HIS AIRWAY CLEAR, because it can easily become obstructed. One way to do this is to use Guedel's airway. You will need a range of different sizes.

(7) BE READY TO CONTROL HIS VENTILATION, because almost any anesthetic (including ketamine) may stop him breathing, so that he needs ventilating. To do this you will need a self-inflating bag (10.3), a non-rebreathing valve (10.2) and a face mask. Although you can control his ventilation with these alone, your task will be easier if you can intubate him (13.2). So you should also have a laryngoscope, tracheal tubes, an introducer and suction catheters. Intubation is the only way you can be *sure* to control his airway, and prevent aspiration.

(8) HAVE A VEIN OPEN, because if he has a drip, or an indwelling needle (15.2), you can treat some of the complications that may arise during anaesthesia more easily, and give him both blood and fluids quickly. An "open vein" is an essential precaution in all major operations.

(9) MONITOR HIS PULSE AND BLOOD PRESSURE continually, during the operation and immediately after it, so that you are able to take the necessary corrective action before it is too late. You must recognise cardiac arrest immediately. One of the most effective ways to do this is to strap a precordial stethoscope to his chest and to keep its earpiece always in your ear.

(10) ALWAYS HAVE SOMEONE IN THE ROOM WHO CAN APPLY CRICOID PRESSURE EFFECTIVELY, and will be useful in an emergency.

BITRIS (31 years) has had a postpartum haemorrhage. You are summoned to the delivery room. When you arrive, the anaesthetic assistant has already inserted a plastic intravenous cannula, and saline is running in well. The midwives have the examination set laid out, and the cervical tear set is at hand. She only needs diazepam 10 mg intravenously, and there are no problems. LESSON Have the equipment carefully organised, and the staff trained. If you can do this there will be few problems, and a much smaller chance of disaster.

DISASTERS ARE USUALLY TREATABLE—IF YOU RECOGNISE THEM IN TIME

3.2 Laryngeal spasm

Normal breathing is almost silent—a noise is a sign that something is wrong. Learn to recognise: (1) Stridor, which is caused by partial respiratory obstruction, or by secretions or a foreign body in the patient's throat (complete respiratory obstruction is usually silent). (2) Spasm of his vocal cords (laryngeal spasm). (3) Wheezing from his bronchi as the result of cardiac or bronchial asthma. Don't confuse these last two conditions because they need different treatment.

A patient with *incomplete* laryngeal spasm starts to breathe with a loud noise. His chest heaves, yet almost no air reaches his lungs. He goes blue. Put a hand on his trachea—you will feel it vibrating like the purring of a cat. The more anoxic he becomes, the tighter the spasm, and the louder the noise until his larynx finally relaxes as he is almost dead. Laryngeal spasm sounds alarming, but it usually passes off spontaneously, and is not often fatal.

Laryngeal spasm usually occurs early in anaesthesia while a patient is still only lightly anaesthetized. It can occur: (1) If you suddenly give him too much ether, or any other anaesthetics so give it slowly. (2) If surgery starts when he is too lightly anaesthetized, so take him down to the level of surgical anaesthesia before the operation begins. (3) If an anaesthetic, especially thiopentone, or occasionally ketamine, have enhanced the reaction of his cords to irritants, such as blood or secretions. So never give these drugs unless you have all the emergency equipment. (4) If you traumatise his larynx when you pass or remove a tube, so intubate and extubate him gently. (5) If secretions or blood fall onto his larynx, during induction or recovery, so let him recover on his side, in the recovery position. This will allow secretions to drain from his mouth. Deep anaesthesia and muscle relaxants abolish laryngeal spasm, so there are occasions when you can use them to treat it.

LARYNGEAL SPASM

PRECAUTION (1) When you anaesthetize a patient, always have an 'open vein' so that you can give him an intravenous injection urgently. As you will see below, one of the most useful methods is to give him atropine and suxamethonium intravenously, and to intubate him. You cannot do this if you cannot get into a vein. (2) Preoperative atropine is some help in minimising laryngeal spasm, because it reduces secretions which may fall onto his cords and cause it.

TREATMENT First make sure that airway obstruction (4.2) is not the cause—keep his chin up. Try turning his entire head and body to one side, if there are secretions on his cords, this will let them drain away.

If the operation has started too soon, stop it.

If you are inducing him with ether, give him a breath of

fresh air, and continue inducing him more slowly. At the same time keep his airway clear, and give him oxygen. If he is more deeply anaesthetized, be prepared, as a last resort, to suck any secretions from his pharynx with a catheter.

If spasm does not pass off, have halothane and oxygen ready for his first breath. His spasm will stop as anaesthesia deepens. While he is deeply anaesthetized spray his cords with 4% lignocaine.

If the patient is becoming very blue, give him 100% oxygen. If necessary, as a last resort, quickly give him atropine and suxamethonium. Preoxygenate him, and as soon as fasciculations have stopped, intubate him, connect him to a non-rebreathing valve, and control his respiration.

If laryngeal spasm occurs as he wakes from an anaesthetic, it will be a very disturbing experience, and is usually due to secretions. Turn him onto his side, and suck out his pharynx. Give him oxygen until the spasm passes off. Prevent this happening by sucking out his pharynx under direct vision *before* you remove his tracheal tube.

CAUTION! Don't try to pass a pharyngeal airway, because this will only irritate his pharynx and make the spasm worse.

3.3 Wheezing

Severe wheezing can be caused by: (1) True bronchospasm. It can also be caused by any of the following. So, remember that not every wheeze is caused by spasm of the bronchi. (2) Regurgitation or aspiration of vomit. (3) Left ventricular failure (cardiac asthma). (4) A foreign body in the tracheal tube. (5) A kinked tracheal tube, or a cuff herniating over its end. (6) A patient trying to cough while he is lightly anaesthetized. If he tries to cough when his larynx is forcibly kept open by a tube, all he can do is wheeze. Wheezing from this cause will go as anaesthesia deepens.

Bronchospasm can also present as a "solid chest" which will not expand when you try to inflate it (13.7). When this happens you may not hear any wheezing.

True bronchospasm is a particular danger in asthmatics and chronic bronchitics (17.8), so try not to give them a general anaesthetic, if you possibly can.

TREATING TRUE BRONCHOSPASM

If you assess patients preoperatively, you should be aware of the possibility of cardiac asthma before anaesthesia starts. If they have a history of asthma, beware of bronchospasm.

If a patient starts to wheeze, make sure his tracheal tube is in his trachea. Pass a sterile suction catheter to make sure it is patent.

Give him oxygen. If his tracheal tube is patent, he probably has true bronchospasm. So give him 4 mg/kg of aminophylline intravenously over 5 minutes. If necessary, repeat the dose 10 minutes later, or add it to the drip.

If you have a spray containing salbutamol or any other bronchodilator, use it.

If wheezing persists, give him subcutaneous adrenaline, but only after ether and not after halothane, trichloroethylene, or chloroform.

If he is lightly anaesthetized, lignocaine 3 mg/kg sprayed down his tracheal tube may also help.

If he is already partly anaesthetized with ether or halothane, his bronchospasm may pass off if you continue them—they are both good broncho-dilators.

If you suspect he may have aspirated contents of his stomach, treat him as in Section 16.1.

3.4 Respiratory arrest

If you can control a patient's ventilation, his failure to breathe is hardly a disaster—if you recognise it in time. He can stop breathing because: (1) You have given him too much anaesthetic, perhaps combined with too much opioid premedication. (2) He

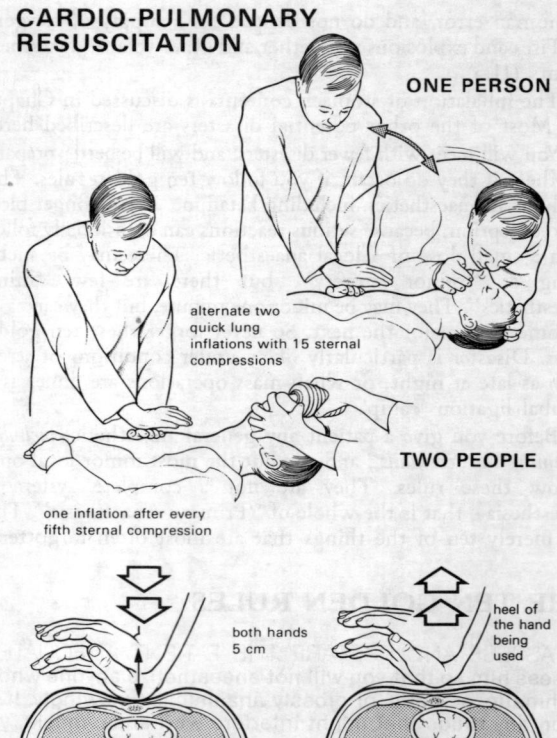

Fig. 3-2 CARDIO–PULMONARY RESUSCITATION. Note that the operator is using the heel of his hand. *Kindly contributed by Peter Safar*

is anoxic, because his airway is obstructed, or the oxygen supply has failed. (3) He is holding his breath. This can happen if you let the surgeon start the operating while anaesthesia is too light. (4) Most seriously of all, his respiration may have stopped because his heart has stopped. He may be dead.

Diagnosing respiratory arrest is usually easy. After too much ether, the patient's respiration fails progressively and he shows the other signs of deep anaesthesia (11.2). When his airway is obstructed, there are the mechanical signs of obstruction (4.2). When the oxygen supply runs out, his skin goes blue (if he is Caucasian), his blood darkens, and his respiration becomes gasping before it finally fails. If his heart stops, he stops breathing suddenly, and he has no pulse or apex beat.

You can restore a patient's ventilation by repeatedly filling his lungs with air, and then letting them empty passively through their own elasticity. This is intermittent positive pressure ventilation (IPPV) or controlled ventilation. In an emergency you can blow up his lungs through his nose or his mouth, but for prolonged ventilation use a tracheal or tracheostomy tube (19.4).

You should always have the equipment for IPPV instantly available, so you should never need to treat respiratory arrest by mouth–to–mouth ventilation. Nevertheless, mouth–to–mouth ventilation is something that everyone should know how to do, because it is lifesaving in many situations outside a theatre. If mouth–to–mouth ventilation fails, because the patient has trismus or fits, you may have to blow through his nose.

BREATHING HAS STOPPED

As soon as you see that a patient is not breathing, check his airway, and his pulse or his apex beat.

If he has stopped breathing because his heart has stopped, goto Section 3.5 quickly.

If necessary, clear his airway.

If he is holding his breath, ventilate his lungs with the bag or bellows, until he starts breathing again. Then deepen the anaesthetic.

If he is deeply anaesthetized, as for example after an overdose of thiopentone, quickly give him a few breaths of oxygen, then pass a tracheal tube, and control his ventilation (13.1). If you cannot intubate him, use a face mask. If you don't have this, ventilate him mouth-to-mouth. Controlled ventilation will be much easier if you have already intubated him. This is one good reason why you should intubate all patients needing prolonged deep anaesthesia, whose respirations might stop.

CAUTION ! If you cannot make his chest expand, or you cannot hear air escaping, ventilation is inadequate, so immediately abandon whatever equipment you are using, and ventilate him mouth to mouth.

MOUTH–TO–MOUTH VENTILATION

Clear the patient's mouth. It may contain vomit or a foreign body. Put two fingers behind his tongue and clear this pharynx. If you have an airway, insert it.

Extend his head fully, with one hand on his forehead, and the other one behind his neck.

If his mouth is closed or his chin is sagging, move your hand from under his neck to support his chin and hold his mouth slightly open.

Take a deep breath, and seal your mouth round his mouth, with a wide open circle and blow forcefully. To prevent air leaking, pinch his nostrils. As you do so, press on his forehead to keep his head extended.

Watch while you blow. If you are successful, you will see his chest expand. Remove your mouth, turn it to the side, and let his chest recoil. Repeat inflation about every 5 seconds in an adult (12 times a minute)—volume is more important than rhythm. Don't blow him up too much. Make his lungs expand as much as they would do if he was breathing normally.

If you meet an obstruction when you blow through his mouth, his neck is probably not extended enough, or his tongue has fallen back. This is the common reason why mouth–to–mouth ventilation fails. If it still fails when you have extended his neck, close his mouth, and blow through his nose. Put one hand under his chin, and close his mouth with your thumb. Take a deep breath (avoid pinching his nose with your lips) and blow. Open his mouth to let him exhale, because his nasopharynx may be obstructed.

VENTILATING WITH YOUR MOUTH

Mouth to mouth

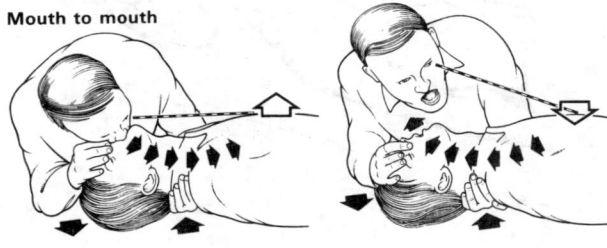

Mouth to nose

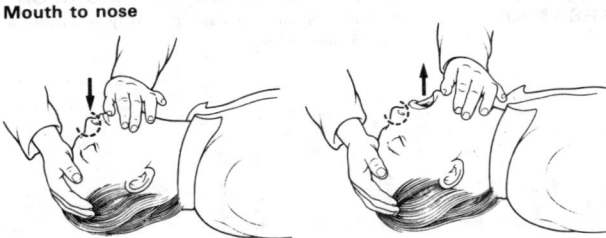

Fig. 3-3 MOUTH–TO–MOUTH AND MOUTH–TO–NOSE VENTILATION. Start mouth–to–mouth, and if this fails try mouth–to–nose. A, and B, extend the patient's head, pinch his nose and watch his chest expand. B, and C, when you ventilate mouth to nose, put one hand on his forehead and hold his chin up with the other one. *Kindly contributed by Peter Safar.*

If blowing through his nose is also unsuccessful, make sure (1) his head is tilted backwards, (2) open his mouth, and (3) grasp the horizontal ramus of his mandible and displace it forwards. Then blow into his mouth again. This is the "triple airway manoevre". It is not easy and is painful, so it is a good test of how unconscious he is.

If the patient is a small child, put your mouth over his nose and mouth, and blow gently with short puffs to avoid rupturing his lungs, about every 3 seconds–20 per minute.

If oxygen is not immediately available, don't delay while you send someone to get it. Your own exhaled air now will be much more useful than oxygen a minute later.

3.5 Cardiac (cardiopulmonary) arrest

This is the most urgent of all disasters. If a patient was previously breathing spontaneously, he stops breathing. His heart and pulse stop, and his pupils dilate enormously. If he has a pale skin, it goes an alarming pale grey.

But if his respiration is being controlled artificially, you can easily overlook cardiac arrest, because the sign that he is not breathing is absent. The blood from his wound may have a dark colour, and his lips and his vocal cords may be dark, but you may not notice any of these things. If he has a dark skin, its colour may change very little. If you are controlling his respiration, the first sign of cardiac arrest is that his pulse stops. *So monitor a patient's heart beat or pulse continuously during controlled respiration.* Use a precordial or oesophageal stethoscope so that you can listen to his heart. Careful monitoring is almost the only way you have of knowing that he is still alive.

A patient's heart may stop because: (1) You have given him too much anaesthetic, especially thiopentone. (2) He has untreated haemorrhage and shock. (3) He has aspirated his vomit, or has regurgitated the contents of his stomach. (4) His tracheal tube is not in his trachea, or is obstructed or kinked. (5) His heart has started fibrillating. This is particularly likely to happen if you are giving him halothane, trichloroethylene, or chloroform, especially if you have not premedicated him with atropine. (6) You are giving him suxamethonium, and he was severely burnt less than three months ago (14.2).

Recognise and start treating cardiac arrest within seconds of it happening. Cardiac massage, and ventilation of his lungs must be established within 3 minutes of the time his heart stops, or his brain will be irreversibly damaged. If he is febrile and toxic, you have even less time.

Remember these steps—"A" is for airway, so quickly check this before you do anything else. "B" is for "breathe" (ventilate) him, so do this with a bag, or if necessary, mouth to mouth. "C" is for "circulate" him, so start sternal compression. "D" is for drugs and fluids. "E" is for an ECG, if you can record one.

"A" IS FOR AIRWAY
"B" IS FOR BREATHE HIM
"C" IS FOR CIRCULATE HIM

A PATIENT'S HEART HAS STOPPED

As soon as a patient stops breathing, or you can no longer feel a peripheral pulse, quickly feel his carotid or femoral arteries. If his abdomen is open, feel his aorta. *The critical sign is that he has no palpable pulse in any major artery.* The other signs of cardiac arrest, unconsciousness, not breathing, and dilated pupils are all altered by the anaesthetic.

If you are giving the anaesthetic for someone else, tell him what has happened. Stop the anaesthetic and give him oxygen only.

Don't waste time trying to take his blood pressure. Shout for help. Note the time, and follow these four steps:

A, CHECK HIS AIRWAY Tilt his head back, lift his neck, or support his chin. Has he regurgitated? Check his tracheal tube. Is it blocked, or kinked?

B, "BREATHE" HIM Ventilate him in the quickest way you can. Use a mask and bag, or ventilate him mouth–to–mouth. Intubating him may take too long, especially if you are not expert. But if other methods fail, and he has no tube in his trachea, insert one. He is unconscious, so no preparation is necessary. Connect the tube to a bellows or self inflating bag. Ventilate him rapidly 3 to 5 times with 100% oxygen, or air if this is not availabe.

Feel his carotid pulse, if it is present, continue inflating him 12 times a minute. If you cannot feel a pulse, "circulate him".

C, "CIRCULATE" HIM Start sternal compression, as in Section 3.6.

CAUTION ! Don't interrupt sternal compression or ventilation. Both should go on continuously, preferably at the same time, because IPPV will maximise his intrathoracic pressure and so enable sternal compression to give a better cardiac output. If you have no help you will have to interrupt them as in Section 3.6.

D, DRUGS AND FLUIDS Give him adrenaline 0.5 to 1.0 mg intravenously, preferably diluted to 10 ml, and repeat it as necessary. This is a method of last resort and some anaesthetists would not use it.

If cardiac arrest has lasted longer than 2 minutes, give him 1 mmol/kg of sodium bicarbonate intravenously. Repeat the dose every 10 minutes until his pulse returns. Severe anoxia causes metabolic acidosis, and bicarbonate corrects it. If you don't have bicarbonate, give him any available intravenous fluid.

E, THE ECG If you have an electrocardiograph and a defibrillator, they are useful, but the four steps above are much more useful.

LATER TREATMENT AFTER SUCCESSFUL RESUSCITATION
Continue ventilating the patient artificially, so as to reduce his arterial carbon dioxide tension. Give him 10% mannitol, 1 g/kg intravenously over two hours to avoid any sudden increase in vascular volume. This will reduce cerebral oedema and promote diuresis. Catheterise his bladder. If his urinary output is less than 50 ml in the first hour, give him frusemide 20 mg, and repeat it later if necessary. Give him 0.18% saline in dextrose in a volume equal to his urinary loss. Continue treatment until the fullest possible recovery of cerebral function has occured. The complications he may have include convulsions, hyperpyrexia, and broken ribs.

3.6 Sternal compression

If a patient's heart has stopped, it may start again, if you compress it sharply between his sternum and his spine. If it does not start immediately, pressing his sternum repeatedly may squeeze just enough blood from it at each compression to keep him alive. The alternative which is to open his chest and massage his heart is messy and is no more effective than sternal compression—provided you are ventilating him.

Although repeatedly compressing his sternum will send some air through his lungs, it will not send enough, so you must ventilate him also. Ventilating him and massaging his heart at the same time needs two people, one for his heart, and other for his lungs. In the theatre, there should always be someone to help you, but if a patient's heart stops elsewhere, you may have to do both these tasks yourself, and interrupt sternal compression to ventilate his lungs. Sternal compression and controlled ventilation may be required immediately at any time anywhere. They are such life–saving procedures that all health staff should know when and and how to do them.

STERNAL COMPRESSION
First, make sure the patient is on a hard surface. You cannot resuscitate someone on a soft bed.

Place the heel of one hand, with your other hand over it, over the lower end of his sternum. Depress it sharply 4 to 5 cm.

Allow his chest to recoil completely. Repeat this once each second.

If you have help, alternate one lung inflation with 15 sternal compressions. Try to compress him once each second, or 60 times a minute. Allow equal time for compression and relaxation.

In children up to the age of 10, use one hand only. In an infant, use two fingers only, and apply them to the middle of his sternum, so as to avoid injuring his liver.

If you are alone, alternate two quick lung inflations with 15 sternal compressions at 80 per minute. Allow equal time for compression and relaxation.

RESUSCITATION ON THE FLOOR

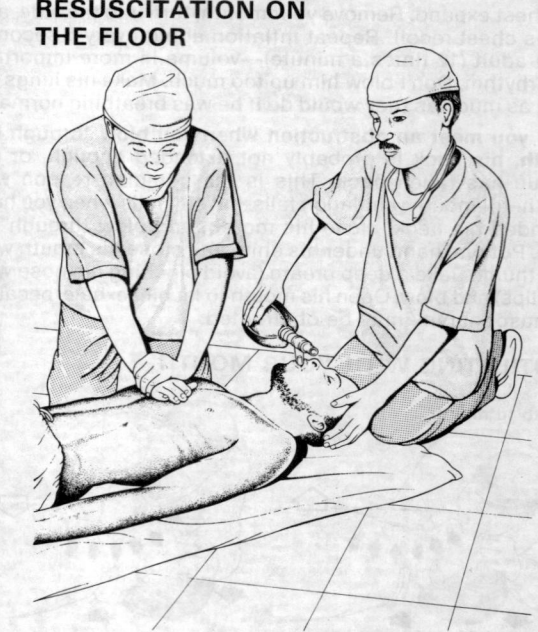

Fig. 3-4 YOU MAY HAVE TO RESUSCITATE SOMEONE ON THE FLOOR. *Notice that he is lying on a hard surface. Kindy contributed by Arthur Adeney.*

4 Care before, during and after the operation

4.1 Fitness for anaesthesia

The purpose of anaesthesia is to keep a patient alive and free from pain, and, having done this, to produce the best possible conditions for surgery. Keeping him alive depends on: (1) preparing him carefully before the operation, (2) maintaining his blood volume and his circulation, (3) securing his airway, and (4) on making sure he is adequately ventilated. A patient is much more likely to withstand the anatomical assaults of surgery if he is physiologically normal before the operation starts. If he is abnormal you must: (1) Know what his abnormalities are and how severe they are, (2) correct them as far as you can, and (3) choose a method of anaesthesia which will minimise their adverse effects. Some patients are at particular risk—the patient with a full stomach (16.1), the patient in shock (16.7), or metabolic acidosis (17.2), or in labour (16.6), the patient with intestinal obstruction (16.1), or cardiac or respiratory failure (17.4), or the child (18.1). They are described elsewhere. Beware also of the following—

Undiagnosed diseases are a great danger. The patient who arrives in the theatre with undiagnosed cardiac failure, or diabetic acidosis is at much greater risk than the patient in whom you have diagnosed and treated these things.

Drugs can also cause problems. The risks of drug medication are often forgotten. For example: (1) Streptomycin, neomycin, kanamycin, and other aminoglycoside antibiotics can prevent or delay a patient recovering from relaxants. (2) Anaesthesia can cause hypotension and collapse if a patient is on long-term steroid medication. Either gradually stop them well before the operation, or give him additional steroids during it. (3) Any general anaesthetic, but especially thiopentone, may cause severe hypotension if he is on hypotensive drugs. (4) Pethidine, morphine, or an anaesthetic, may cause fits or coma if he is on monoamine oxidase inhibitors. Many other drugs can also cause problems.

For these reasons, all patients for anaesthesia should be examined, and have their histories taken, even if the operation is an emergency. It is in these patients that disaster so often occurs. If a patient's history and examination cannot be done by an anaesthetic assistant, you must do it. One practical way of taking the history, especially if this has to be done by an assistant, or through an interpreter, is to use the check list below. Stencil this, and include columns for the answers "Yes" or "No", to each question. The questions are so designed that a fit patient always answers 'No", and any answer "Yes" is abnormal. Include boxes for the patient's weight, his haemoglobin, his blood pressure, the results of urine testing, and the date of a woman's last period. "Yes—no", boxes can also be included for the signing of an operation consent form, for the provision of an identification bracelet, and for the removal of false teeth. The routine use of this check list, or a modification of it, would be an easy way of improving anaesthesia in many hospitals.

If a patient answers "Yes" to any question, find out the details, for example, what treatment is he having? What trouble has he had with a previous anaesthetic? Then consider what pre-operative treatment might improve him. Perhaps he is not fit enough for an anaesthetic, or the operation is not needed? For example, a patient in cardiac failure should probably not have a hernia repair, or he should be refered to an expert anaesthetist. Often, all you need do is to avoid some particularly unsuitable method.

FITNESS FOR ANAESTHESIA
A HISTORY CHECK LIST

Have you had anything to eat or drink in the last six hours?

Will you be going home by yourself? (This is relevant for day cases only. Ketamine, for example, would usually be contraindicated in day cases).

Have you had any serious illness?

Have you had any previous operations?

Have you had any problems with any anaesthetics? (He may, for example, reveal that after a previous anaesthetic, he did not wake up for 18 hours.)

Have any of your family had problems with anaesthetics? (Some anaesthetic problems, such as malignant hyperpyrexia and some forms of cholinesterase deficiency are familial.)

Cardiovascular system Have you had heart disease, rheumatic fever, or high blood pressure?

Do you get breathless on exercise, or at night? Do you get swollen ankles? (Cardiac insufficiency).

Do you faint easily? (Heart block, anaemia)

Do you have anaemia or blood problems? Do you bleed excessively? (Any operation may be contraindicated).

Respiratory system. Do you have bronchitis, asthma, chest pain, or other chest problems? Do you cough? Do you smoke? Do you produce sputum? (If he does, suspect asthma or tuberculosis).

Have you a cold, or other nose trouble at present? (A general anaesthetic may convert an upper into a lower respiratory infection).

Central nervous system. Do you have convulsions or fits? (Fits may occur under ether. Patients taking phenobarbitone or phenytoin may need higher doses of diazepam, or thiopentone).

Drugs. Are you on any medicines (Drugs, tablets, capsules, injections, or inhalations) at present?

Do you have any allergies or reactions to medicines? (A patient reacting to one drug, may cross react to others).

Liver, kidneys. Have you ever been jaundiced? (Poor liver function is a possibility).

Have you ever had urinary or kidney troubles? (Post operative retention of urine, and unsuspected renal failure are possible).

Alcoholism. Try to find out if he is an alcoholic. This will influence the dose of the induction agent he needs, including the dose of ketamine (8.1).

EXAMINATION

Does he have any signs of bronchospasm, acute infection,

or excessive secretions? All these need treating before anaesthesia.

Is he shocked? Shock needs to be corrected before operating.

Is he hypertensive? Anaesthesia can be dangerous if his diastolic pressure is over 120 mm.

Is he dehydrated? As far as possible, correct any electrolyte imbalance before operating. Anaesthetizing a severely dehydrated patient may cause hypotension, coma, and death.

Is he anaemic? Measure his haemoglobin. For the purposes of anaesthesia, "anaemia" starts at a haemoglobin of 10 g/dl, or a haematocrit of 30%. If sickle cell anaemia is common, test for it.

Test his urine. If possible, use a multitest strip. Anaesthesia can be lethal in an uncontrolled diabetic.

PREOPERATIVE CARE

MOUTH If mouth sepsis is gross, remove food debris, and brush his gums with an antiseptic, such as 0.5% chlorhexidine. Look for loose teeth that might be knocked out by a laryngscope during intubation.

STOMACH Give fit patients for elective surgery their last food 6 hours before the operation, provided it contains no meat or fats. They can have a little water only, say 30 ml, not milk, tea, or orange juice, up to 2 hours before the operation.

CAUTION ! Starve a patient who is having any kind of anaesthetic, including local blocks, ketamine, and epidural or spinal anaesthesia.

It is traditional to give a patient no water or fluids of any kind. But if the weather is hot, or the list delayed, this will cause unnecessary suffering if he is late on the list. Let the ward staff give him water, provided it is only water, if he is not going to be operated on until later. Besides making him more comfortable, it will also reduce his need for intravenous fluids during the operation. Babies are a special case (18.1), so are shocked hypovolaemic patients and patients who are dehydrated from diarrhoea and vomiting (15.3).

BLADDER Ask him to pass his urine before the anaesthetic. This will prevent him passing it during induction, and make him less restless and uncomfortable under premedication or local anaesthesia. For some operations, Caesarean section, for example (16.6), catheterisation is essential, and is usually requested by the surgeon.

If the ward staff have difficulty in remembering which patients to starve, have some cards or boards marked "Nothing by mouth" to hang beside their beds. Also, explain to the patient that he should not take anything by mouth before his operation.

EXPLANATION An anaesthetic and an operation may be very ordinary for the ward staff, but they are certain to be a special events in the life of the patient. So reassure him, and explain what is going to happen, this is especially important with subarachnoid or extradural anaesthesia, in which he must cooperate.

4.2 Caring for a patient's airway

One of the hazards of anaesthesia is that it can impair the control of a patient's airway: (1) It relaxes his muscles, including those of his jaw, so that his tongue, or his palate, can fall back and block his pharynx. (2) It abolishes the reflexes that protect his larynx, so that he is at risk from regurgitating his stomach contents, or inhaling his vomit (16.1). Preserving his airway is thus one of the most important anaesthetic skills, and failure to do so one of the commonest causes of death on the operating table.

A patient with a clear airway breathes with very little effort, and usually almost no noise. If his airway is partly obstructed, he breathes noisily, *but if it is completely obstructed, he makes no noise.* You may not notice that he is obstructed, unless you watch the movements of his chest and listen for air going in and out of his mouth. If his airway is obstructed, so that air cannot enter his lungs, his diaphragm can still contract.

This makes his abdomen balloon out when he tries to inhale. This is paradoxical diaphragmatic breathing and is one of the earliest signs of airway obstruction in anaesthesia. Also, the patient's chest is sucked in, and he may regurgitate. He shows "tracheal tug" (11.2) and becomes cyanosed. So diagnose repiratory obstruction early, and treat it promptly.

The most common cause of respiratory obstruction in a patient who has not been intubated is the base of his tongue falling backwards in his throat and blocking it. Use any of the following methods to prevent this happening. With the exception of Fergusson's gag, these are all important nursing skills, so make sure your nurses can do them. Even intubating a patient does not completely prevent respiratory obstruction, as in Fig. 13-16 shows.

EQUIPMENT FOR MAINTAINING THE AIRWAY

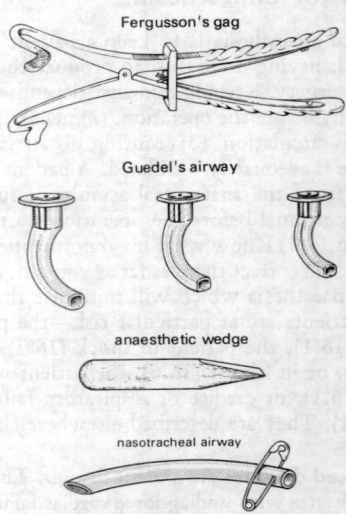

Fig. 4-1 EQUIPMENT FOR MAINTAINING THE AIRWAY.
Guedel's airways are the most useful of these pieces of equipment.
A nasal airway is useful in injuries of the jaw. A wedge and a gag are hardly ever necessary.

• *AIRWAYS, Oral, Guedel, transparent plastic, (a) size 000, two only, (b) size 00, 2 only, (c) size 0, 2 only, (d) size 1, four only, (e) size 2, eight only, (f) size 3, eight only, (g) size 4, four only.* These are life—saving pieces of anaesthetic equipment. Transparent plastic ones are particularly useful because you can see if they are blocked.

• *AIRWAYS, nasal, soft, two only.* If you don't have one, use a short piece of soft tracheal tube, held with a safety pin, as in Fig S 62-2, to prevent it disappearing down the patient's larynx. He cannot easily bite a nasal airway or spit it out, and a suction catheter can easily pass down it. If a patient's jaw has been fractured, it will be easier to pass than a Guedel's airway.

• *GAG, mouth, Fergusson, with Ackland jaws, adult size one only.*

• *GAG, mouth, Fergusson, with Ackland jaws, child size, one only.* These gags are for opening a patient's mouth when his jaw muscles are tightly in spasm. The narrow Ackland jaws make them easy to push between his teeth. The more skillful you become, the less often will you have to use a gag.

• *WEDGE, anaesthetic, boxwood or plastic, with coarse thread one only.* When a patient has clenched his mouth tightly shut, you can force this wedge between his teeth, and use it to lever them open, so that you can insert Fergusson's gag. If a wedge is threaded, you can slowly screw it in. Some anaesthetists never use a gag and rely on pressing their fingers between his molar teeth.

• *TUBES, stomach, plastic, 76 cm. Sizes 10 Ch, 14 Ch, 16 Ch, 20 Ch, 24 Ch, and 30 Ch, two only of each size.* These enable you to empty a patient's stomach before anaesthetizing him and when treating poisoning. Use the largest practical size.

A FOOT OPERATED SUCKER

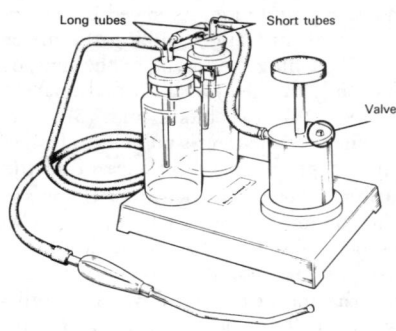

Fig. 4-2 A FOOT OPERATED SUCKER. This is essential, your electric sucker may break down, or there may be no power.

- **SUCTION PUMP, operating theatre, electric with two 1000 ml unbreakable plastic bottles and tubing, state voltage, two only.** These are always breaking down, so the model chosen must be easy to service and spares should be available. If you are going to depend on an electric sucker, *make sure it can actually suck before the operation starts*. A sucker which makes a noise may not necessarily be able to suck.

- **SUCTION PUMP, foot operated, with two wide mouthed 1000 ml unbreakable plastic bottles, rubber bungs, and metal tubes, two only.** This is illustrated in Fig.16-2, and is an automobile pump with the valves in it arranged to suck instead of pumping. Both the surgeon and the anaestetist need a sucker, so two are necessary. A hospital workshop may be able to make one of these suckers by altering the valves of a lorry tyre pump. A foot sucker is much more reliable and more easily repaired than an electric one. *If you use an electric sucker, make sure you have a foot sucker also.*

- **SUCTION TUBES, metal, Yankauer, wide bore, fixed nozzle, three only.** This is the standard suction tube, used at almost every operation. Connect it through a piece of rubber tube to one of the suction pumps above. If you don't have a suction tube, suck with the end of the rubber tube directly.

KEEPING THE AIRWAY CLEAR

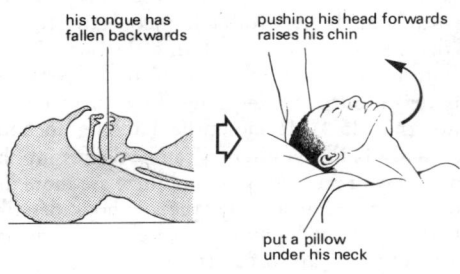

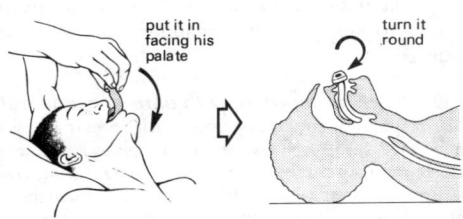

Fig. 4-3 TWO WAYS OF KEEPING A PATIENT'S AIRWAY CLEAR. Tilting a patient's head backwards will usually clear his airway. If this does not, insert Guedel's airway. *Kindly contributed by John Farman.*

KEEPING THE AIRWAY CLEAR

Try these methods in the following order. If one method fails, quickly move on to the next.

FLEX THE PATIENT'S NECK AND TILT HIS HEAD While he is lying flat, grasp his head with one hand and tilt it so that his nostrils point upwards. At the same time, flex his neck forward. Extending his head without flexing his neck is less effective. This combination of movements raises his mandible away from his cervical spine, and lifts his tongue off the posterior wall of his pharynx. A pillow under his head and neck helps to maintain this position.

LIFT HIS CHIN Pull it upwards. This will usually clear the airway of a young adult with a good set of teeth.

LIFT THE ANGLES OF HIS JAW Sit at the head of the table, rest your elbows on it, and lift both the angles of his jaw with your middle fingers. Your thumb and first fingers will then be free, if necessary, to hold the mask, as in Fig. 11-3.

Lifting his chin, if it succeeds, is better than lifting the angles of his jaw, because lifting them can make his jaw stiff, and at worst dislocate it. Lifting the angles of the jaw is for more difficult patients only.

GUEDEL'S AIRWAY If the above methods fail to clear the patient's airway, insert Guedel's airway.

Wet the airway. Open his mouth for a moment, and insert it with its tip pointing towards his hard palate.

Then turn the airway through 180° so that its curve follows his soft palate and the back of his tongue and lifts his tongue forward.

CAUTION ! (1) Be careful not to push his tongue downwards as you insert the airway. (2) Don't insert it during very light anaesthesia, or the patient will cough, retch, or vomit. (3) Even Guedel's airway does not guarantee a clear airway, so you may also need to lift his chin or the angles of his jaw.

NASAL AIRWAY Put a soft wide rubber tube down one of his nostrils, and hold it with a large safety pin as in Fig. S 62-2. This is useful in severe maxillofacial injuries, when opening the patient's mouth may be impossible or painful.

FERGUSSON'S GAG is useful if the patient clenches his teeth shut, and prevents you inserting an airway. Push the gag between his back teeth, and use it to open his jaw. Keep pieces of rubber tube on the ends of the gag to prevent them injuring his teeth. If his teeth are complete, so that you cannot insert a gag, force a wedge between his teeth. Rock it to and fro between them, until they are are far enough apart for you to insert the ends of the gag. The danger of this is that you will break his teeth, but you may have to risk this.

If you don't have a gag or a wedge, press your fingers between his gums behind his molar teeth. This will open his jaws enough for you to pass a laryngoscope. This is less traumatic than using a gag. Many anaesthetists prefer this method and seldom, if ever, use a gag.

GUEDEL'S AIRWAY IN PLACE

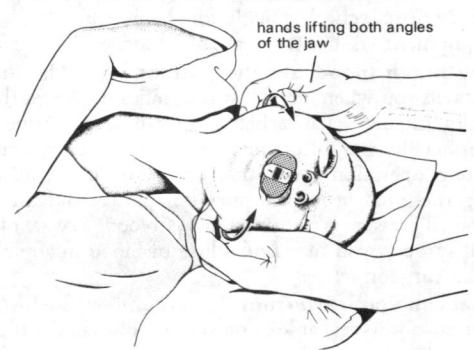

Fig. 4-4 GUEDEL'S AIRWAY IN PLACE. If lifting a patient's chin fails to clear his airway, you may need to lift the angles of his jaw.

INTUBATION If these methods fail to clear the patient's airway, give him a relaxant and quickly intube him, as in Chapter 13.

SUCTION Suck out any secretions from the patient's mouth with Yankauer's sucker, or with a catheter. If convenient, pass the catheter through Guedel's airway.

Suck out his nose by putting Yankauer's sucker into one nostril and pinching his other one closed while you suck. Don't pass a catheter down his nose, or you will make it bleed.

4.3 Monitoring an anaesthetized patient

To monitor an anaesthetized patient is to observe him carefully for the earliest signs of danger. *All patients having anything but the smallest local anaesthetic need monitoring.* This includes general anaesthesia, ketamine (8.1), intravenous analgesia (8.8), and especially epidural (7.2) and subarachnoid anaesthesia (7.4). Here are some of the things to monitor, and where necessary, to record.

The apparatus "Is the patient getting what you think he is getting?" Check the setting and connections of your apparatus. For example, check that you have not left the halothane control on, when he should only be having ether, or that the oxygen has not been turned off by mistake.

Breathing "If a patient is breathing spontaneously, is he breathing normally?" Watch the bellows or bag. The movements of his chest are not a completely satisfactory sign, because his chest can be moving even if his airway is obstructed. So try to observe the movement of air directly, either by listening or with your hand over his mouth. If he is breathing noisily, his airway may be partly blocked. Perhaps his tongue is falling back? If so, pull his jaw forwards. When you have passed a tracheal tube, listen to both sides of his chest, to make sure that you are ventilating both his lungs, and that the tube has not gone into a bronchus. Disconnect the end of the tube from time to time, and listen to him breathing through it. Is there spasm or wheezing? Can you hear any secretions bubbling? Don't forget that even an intubated patient can become obstructed.

Is anaesthesia too light, or too deep? Don't feel you must use a particular percentage of ether for so many minutes. Patients react differently, so adjust the concentration according to the clinical signs. Look at the patient's pupils. If they are big, and react briskly to light, anaesthesia may be too light. If you have given him a relaxant, he may be wide awake. Perhaps you turned the vapouriser off when you refilled it with ether, and forgot to turn it on again? If his pupils do not react to light, either anaesthesia is much too deep, or he is anoxic, or his heart has stopped!

Is the patient adequately oxygenated? The skin colour of a dark patient is no help in monitoring the oxygenation of his blood, so look at his lips, his tongue and his nail beds. Look at his blood as the first cut is made. If it is bright red, this is a good sign. If it is dark purple, this in not necessarily a bad one, because it may be venous. Dark blood in the wound should however alert you. His airway may be blocked, he may be too deeply anaesthetized, or his heart may have stopped. If his colour is not normal, check quickly for the possible causes. Check your equipment. Is his tracheal tube blocked?

How much blood has the patient lost? Make sure the operator tells you when blood loss is significant. Weigh the swabs on a 1 kg kitchen balance before they have had time to dry, and subtract the weight of the same number of dry ones. During a long operation, go round the table to see how much bleeding there has been. You may be able to confirm that his falling blood pressure is caused by loss of blood. Beware of vaginal or rectal surgery, you may find a litre of blood in a bucket between the surgeon's legs!

What can you learn from the patient's pulse? Make sure that you can always feel at least one of his pulses under the drapes. Better, arrange for a limb to project from underneath them, so that you can see and feel it.

Because a normal pulse can vary from 50 to 90, *changes in its rate are more important that its absolute value.* A patient's pulse rate is increased by: (1) anxiety, (2) light anaesthesia, (3) blood loss, (4) some drugs, such as gallamine, (5) dehydration, and (6) arrhythmias. His pulse rate is slowed by: (1) vagal stimulation as the result of intubation, pulling the mesentery or the spermatic cord, stretching the cervix, or the anus, or by pressure on the carotid body or the eye-ball, (2) adequate fluid replacement, (3) hypoxia, (4) heart block, and, (5) some drugs such as halothane. The way a patient's pulse rate changes at any particular moment depends on the balance of all these things.

Is the patient's heart still beating? If you are controlling his ventilation, you must always listen to his heart with a precordial or an oesophageal stethoscope, or monitor his pulse, because they will give you the first warnings of cardiac arrest (3.5).

What can the patient's blood pressure tell you? Don't expect it to tell you all you need to know about his circulation. Interpret it with other signs. For example, a systolic blood pressure of 80 mm is unlikely to be serious, if he has signs of a good cardiac output—a good pulse volume, a warm pink skin and well filled veins. But it may be very serious indeed if he also has signs of a low cardiac output—a weak pulse, cold pale skin and collapsed veins. The volume of his pulse is more useful than its rate, which is often influenced by the drugs you have given him.

Unless you have some reason for wanting to know a patient's diastolic pressure, take his systolic pressure only, and measure it with your fingers on his brachial artery or radial artery. Use the correct size of bag and make sure the cuff completely covers the artery. If you use a dial manometer, check it occasionally, because it can easily be wrong by 20 mm. His blood pressure can be increased by: (1) anxiety, (2) straining at induction, (3) underventilation (carbon dioxide retention), and (4) hypoxia (usually). It can be lowered by any of the causes listed below. These include: (1) blood loss, (2) a very fast or very slow pulse rate, (3) hypoxia (occasionally), (4) pain during light anaesthesia, (5) deep anaesthesia, (6) pulling on the mesentery, (7) subarachnoid and epidural anaesthesia, and (8) being handled too roughly.

Is the patient hypovolaemic? Monitor his capillary and venous filling. Do his capillaries refill easily? Blanch the mucous membrane of his mouth by pressing it with your finger, and see how long it takes to refill. If he has a pale skin you can easily do the same with the capillaries of his nail beds.

Are his nose and forehead cold? These are useful signs of hypovolaemia. Are his fingers warm? Grip one of them. With practice its pulsations will give you a good indication of his peripheral blood flow, but only if the theatre is warm. If it is cold, he will vasoconstrict and you will be unable to feel them.

If he was severely hypovolaemic preoperatively, or you are worried that he may become so during the operation, and you can measure his CVP (19.2), you will find it very useful.

Is his urine output adequate? In a major operation try to monitor this (15.4). It should be 1 ml/kg an hour.

How aware is he? Awareness can be distressing, but there is no simple way of measuring it, and there are more important things to monitor. Fortunately, the methods described here minimise the risk that he will be aware of what is happening to him without you knowing. If you wish, you can use the isolated arm test. Occlude the arterial supply to his arm with a sphygmomanometer for 10 minutes after you have given a systemic muscle relaxant. His arm will not be paralysed and he will be able to respond by signalling, for example with a hand—squeeze.

* *STETHOSCOPE, precordial, with earpiece, one only.* This is an ordinary diaphragm stethoscope but with an extra long tube, and is shown in Fig. 14-3. Always strap it in place before any general anaesthetic. If you have paralysed a patient with a relaxant, and his heart stops, the first sign that this has happened is an absent heart beat. A precordial stethscope is particularly important in babies (18.2).

* *STETHOSCOPE, oesophageal, one only.* If a patient's chest is being operated on, use an oesophageal stethscope instead of a precordial one.

MAKE SURE YOU CAN FEEL AT LEAST ONE PULSE

4.4 Hypotension during the operation

Try to make sure that a patient's blood pressure is normal before the operation starts. It can fall during it for many reasons. Hypovolaemia, unnecessarily deep anaesthesia and too vigorous ventilation are some of the more important ones. The importance of monitoring his circulation has been discussed in Section 4.3.

HYPOTENSION DURING AN OPERATION

If a patient's blood pressure falls during an operation, think of the following causes.

Hypovolaemia, is the most common cause. Replace the blood he loses during the operation (15.4). A fall in blood pressure is a late stage in his adjustment to blood loss. If it falls by 30% during the operation, he needs urgent treatment. *Raise his legs,* but keep his heart on the same level as his head. Speed the rate of the drip. Give him 8 to 10 ml/kg of Ringer's lactate or 0.9% saline, or blood; if this gives some improvement only, but not enough, repeat it. Meanwhile, lighten the anaesthetic.

Hypoxia may make his blood pressure fall, so check his airway, and make sure he is adequately ventilated.

Too much of an inhalation anaesthetic, such as ether, (10% or more) or halothane (2%) will reduce the tone of his blood vessels, and depress his heart, so lighten anaesthesia and give him oxygen.

Ventilation which is too fast or too forceful, will raise his intrathoracic pressure, reduce his venous return, and lower his blood pressure. So ventilate him gently, and allow plenty of time for expiration. The natural panic reaction to hypotension is to ventilate faster and harder. This is harmful.

If a patient has an abnormally fast pulse, (up to 150) he is probably hypovolaemic and needs fluids. If he is an adult, and it is more than 150, he probably has a primary cardiac dysrythmia.

Check the anaesthetic tubing, the connections and the oxygen. If you have corrected fluid losses and the depth of anaesthesia is correct, try carotid massage. Gently press on one of his carotid arteries for 20 seconds.

If his pulse is irregular, give him digoxin 0.5 mg intravenously over 5 minutes. If it is regular, try to avoid treating him until after the operation is over. Many anaesthetists don't like giving cardiac drugs without an ECG, and prefer not to use them.

If a patient has an abnormally slow pulse, (down to 45), he is probably very deeply anaesthetized, so try lightening the anaesthesia. If he is an an adult, and it is less than 45, he probably has a primary cardiac dysrythmia and he may have complete heart block. His slow pulse may be due to excessive vagal action. Try giving him atropine 0.6 mg intravenously to a maximum of 1.8 mg.

Cardiac failure, may be the cause, if his blood pressure remains low after you have excluded or treated the first three causes. Check his central venous pressure by observing his jugular veins. Lift his head and see if the fullness in these veins is above his manubrio–sternal junction. If it is, give him digoxin 0.5 mg. This is the minimum dose. Ideally, he needs 0.75 to 1.25 mg immediately, followed by 0.25 mg 4 hourly under ECG control. If his jugular venous pressure is not raised, he is hypovolaemic and needs more fluids.

The supine hypotensive syndrome, is described in Section 16.6. No mother having a Caesarean section should ever be anaesthetized without being tilted to one side or the other, usually the left.

Suddenly reducing the pressure inside a patient's abdomen, may lower his blood pressure, for example, by draining a large volume of ascitic fluid, or by removing a very large cyst, or by decompressing his gut. A high pressure in his abodmen compresses its capillary vessels and when this is suddenly removed, they dilate and fill with blood. His blood pressure falls severely, and he may need litres of intravenous fluid quickly.

Citrate may accumulate after he has had 4 to 6 units of blood or more, and can cause hypotension. If this might be the cause, give him 1 g of calcium gluconate intravenously (10 ml of a 10% solution). His liver will be able to metabolise the citrate from up to 4 bottles quite easily.

If he is in septic shock, his blood pressure will be low, especially if he also has an associated metabolic acidosis. If so, as well as speeding up his drip, give him 1 mmol/kg of sodium bicarbonate. If this fails to correct hypotension, give him an isoprenaline drip. Titrate the isoprenaline drip against his blood pressure, and stop as soon as possible. He will probably need 4 to 10 drops a minute. Give it in a separate bottle from his other fluids and label it clearly. Isoprenaline is safer than adrenaline, but it is dangerous, even so.

Extradural or subarachnoid anaesthesia, may be responsible, especially if they rise too high.

Too large a dose of lignocaine can also cause hypotension (5.9) so don't exceed the dose in Fig. 5-1.

A surgeon who handles him too roughly, or who pulls on his oesophagus or stomach, will also cause hypotension.

The patient might have had a transfusion reaction from incompatible blood, or be having anaphylactic shock.

If he is on steroids he may be having an Addisonian crisis, and need hydrocortisone succinate 100 mg intravenously.

4.5 Care after the operation

There are many hospitals where care in the theatre is fairly good, but where patients die soon afterwards, quite unnecessarily, from the complications of anaesthesia and surgery. Like the anaesthetic disasters that can occur during surgery, many of those which occur afterwards are treatable—if you treat them early enough, so *observation* is what matters, combined with instant effective treatment. A common disaster starts with a patient's tongue falling back against his throat, causing airway obstruction, followed by cyanosis and cardiac arrest. This is particularly tragic because: (1) it is easily avoidable, and (2) it often occurs in otherwise fit patients. The postoperative aspiration of stomach contents is another common catastrophe.

The safest place for an anaesthetized patient to recover is in the theatre suite itself, so try to ensure that he is awake when he leaves it. You can minimise some of the risks of recovery by leaving his tracheal tube in place until he is out of danger. Where he recovers is much less important than that some competent person should care for him, until he can care for himself. Too often, the care of a postoperative patient is entrusted, either to nobody, or to someone who has never been taught what to do. When complications do occur, they may be so urgent that one nurse cannot care for two patients at the same time, so try to have someone looking after each patient until he is fully conscious. If this is impracticable, try to have one competent person with instantly available help.

Patients can recover equally safely: (1) in a corridor, lobby, or verandah close outside theatre, (2) back in ward, or (3) in a special recovery room or ICU (intensive care unit), but only provided that these places are properly staffed and equipped. The ideal arrangement is a combined intensive care unit and recovery room, continuously and competently staffed, and as close to the theatre as possible. When conditions are difficult and staff are few, care immediately outside the theatre is likely to be best, and care in the ward the most dangerous. If you have to send unconscious patients back to a minimally–staffed ward, make sure they are put in their beds in the recovery position. To lay an unconscious patient on his back is to invite disaster. *He must also lie in the recovery position on the trolley while he is on his way back to the ward.* He can die only too easily on his way there. It has been well said that, if you send him back to the ward looking up to heaven, he will soon be there!

THE RECOVERY POSITION

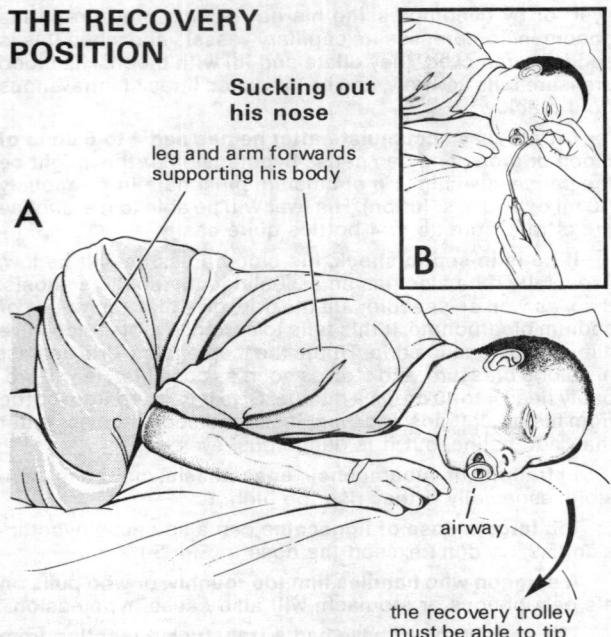

Fig. 4-5 A, THE RECOVERY POSITION is the only safe one for a patient on the trolley on his way to the ward, and in his bed when he gets there. Show your nurses how to place an unconscious patient on his side, with his uppermost arm and leg supporting his body. This position helps to keep his airway clear, it allows his tongue to fall forwards, and it lets blood and secretions drain from his mouth. B, sucking out his nose. Pinch one of his nostrils shut while you suck through the other.
Kindly contributed by John Farman.

SAFE RECOVERY FROM ANAESTHESIA

Here are some instructions to give to the recovery nurse who will be in charge of a patient while he recovers. Teach her: (1) the monitoring procedures described below, (2) the complications to look for, (3) the treatment she should give, and (4) when she should call for help. She must know exactly what to do if his airway is obstructed, or if his heart or breathing stop. She must also be able to get help immediately, and not be afraid to call for it.

EQUIPMENT (1) The bed or trolley on which the patient is lying must be able to tip head down, and should ideally have cot sides, as in Fig. 4-6, so that he can be nursed on his side. If he is brought to and from the theatre in his bed, its foot must be raised on blocks while he recovers. (2) Oxygen with a flowmeter and mask, or a nasal catheter. (3) A sucker, preferably electric, with a Yankauer wide bore pharyngeal suction end. (4) Catheters for tracheal suction. 8, 12 and 14 Ch. (5) A self-inflating bag and facemask. (6) A sphygmomanometer and a stethoscope. (7) A good light. (8) Some means of fetching help.

THE RECOVERY POSITION Put the patient in the recovery position as in Fig. 4-5. If you cannot put him into this position, because he is in traction for example, aspirate his pharynx and stomach while he is still anaesthetized. As always, do this *before* you remove his tracheal tube.

TRANSPORT If an unconscious patient has to be wheeled to another part of the hospital, take him feet first with a nurse following behind to support his chin and maintain his airway. A self-inflating bag, an airway, a wedge, a gag, and a mask should go with him on a shelf underneath the trolley.

RESPIRATION Ask the nurse to look for signs of air passing in and out of his lungs. Show her how to support his jaw from the head of his bed, to feel his warm breath on her hand. Ask her to watch the movements of his chest, and the colour of his skin, mucosa, or nail beds. She can remove the airway as soon as he starts to reject it.

Ask her to count and record his respiratory rate every 15 minutes until recovery is complete.

PULSE AND BLOOD PRESSURE Ask the nurse to take and record his pulse and blood pressure every 15 minutes for half an hour and then every 30 minutes until he is fully recovered.

PERIPHERAL VEINS The state of his peripheral veins is a good guide to his venous pressure, and thus to his blood volume. If these are closed down, and his blood pressure is normal or low, he must be hypovolaemic. Record the state of these veins as "full" or "closed down" on leaving the theatre, and on discharge from the recovery room.

FLUID BALANCE Calculate his input and output during the operation as described in Section 15.5 and enter these on his fluid balance chart in Fig. 15-5.

Record further losses from all routes at regular intervals. Either collect the fluid in a graduated container and record its volume every hour, the loss being the difference between two successive readings. Or, record the contents of the container each hour, and empty it. Make sure the staff know the difference between these two methods, and which they are to use. Twelve hours after a major operation measure his haemoglobin and haematocrit.

Prescribe the fluid he needs for the next 12 hours.

WOUNDS Ask the recovery nurse to inspect the wound at least every 15 minutes. If blood soaks through the dressings, she must tell you immediately.

NERVOUS SYSTEM Ask her to observe: (1) signs of spontaneous movement, and (2) his ability to open his eyes when she asks him to.

RECORDS Continue to record all observations on the anaesthetic record sheet, and note clearly when the operation ended.

CAUTION ! The patient is not out of danger until he is breathing normally, is conscious and has a normal blood pressure.

ALL PATIENTS MUST RECOVER IN THE RECOVERY POSITION

4.6 Complications after anaesthesia

Many patients have postanaesthetic complications of some kind, even if they only vomit. Watch for them and treat them.

"The patient's respiration is obstructed" This is so common and so potentially fatal that every recovery nurse must know what to do. The causes include: (1) His tongue falling backwards. (2) Solid objects, such as loose teeth or food, obstructing his airway. A laryngoscope, a sucker and Magill's forceps must be instantly available to remove foreign objects, and the nurse must know how to use these instruments. (3) Pressure on his trachea, as from bleeding after a thyroidectomy. This may require reintubation, or even an emergency tracheostomy.

"His heart stops" This is the common sequel to respiratory obstruction in a fit patient, and is the main reason why you must prevent respiratory obstruction by the methods given above. It can also follow severe bleeding. Treat it as in Section 3.5.

"His blood pressure falls" Diagnose the reason for this so that you can treat it rationally. It can be caused by: (1) Bradycardia—give him atropine. (2) Hypovolaemia due to bleeding during the operation—raise his legs (not foot of his bed), and give him an infusion. (3) The residual effect of the anaesthetic, particularly halothane. (4) Moving, lifting or turning him too vigorously while he is recovering from anaesthesia. (5) Subarachnoid or epidural anaesthesia extending above L2 and causing a sympathetic block which rises above the level of the sensory block. This will lower his blood pressure and make him very sensitive to changes in position. He might have had a

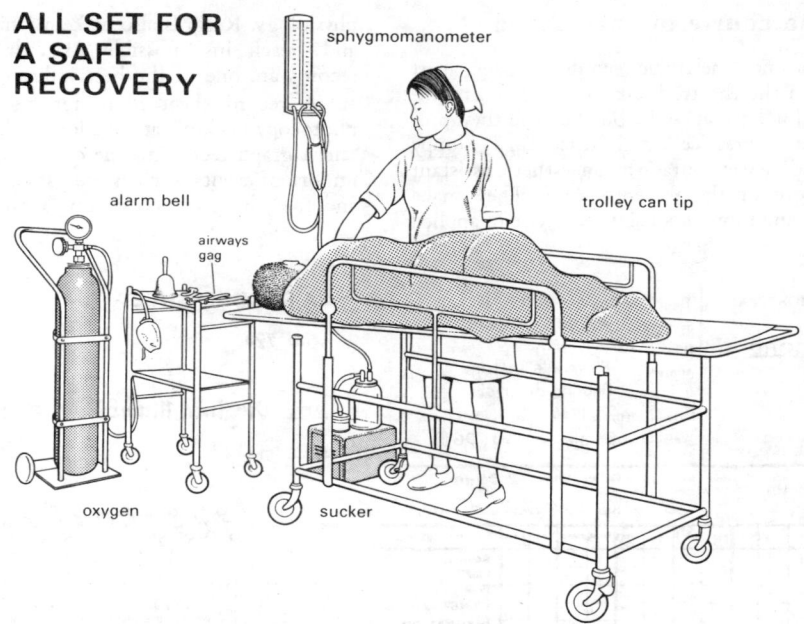

Fig. 4-6 ALL SET FOR A SAFE RECOVERY on a trolley which has sides and can tip. There is an oxygen cylinder and a mask, a bell to summon help, a sphygmomanometer, and a sucker. *Kindly contributed by John Farman.*

transfusion reaction because he has been given incompatible blood. (7) Steroids. If he has been on these and now has hypotension, he needs hydrocortisone 100 mg intravenously.

"His blood pressure rises" This is common and is often accompanied by signs of sympathetic activity, such as tachycardia, sweating and pallor. It may be caused by pain, respiratory depression, a full bladder, overtransfusion or restlessness.

"He fails to breathe adequately" Apnoea caused by respiratory depression is rare but dangerous. Minor degrees of depression often remain unnoticed, so that a patient may seem to be awake and alert, but yet be too weak to overcome even a minor degree of respiratory obstruction. The causes include: (1) Giving him an unsuitable dose of an opioid before, during, or after the operation. You can reverse the effect of most opioids with naloxone (2.5,14.4). (2) Too much thiopentone, especially in repeated doses. (3) Too much anaesthetic agent, especially halothane. (4) Metabolic alkalosis after vomiting or alkali treatment. (5) The most serious causes are due to the complications of relaxants—see Section 14.4.

TREATING RESPIRATORY DEPRESSION

Treatment depends on the cause, so apply any of the specific remedies listed above.

The effects can be serious, so start treating the patient immediately, before completing the diagnosis. In mild cases merely sitting him up in bed will help him greatly, provided he is not hypotensive. Give him oxygen with a mask. Ventilate him with an oxygen–rich mixture, using a mask and self–inflating bag. If necessary, pass a tracheal tube and continue ventilation, manually or with a ventilator.

Are there any surgical reasons which might prevent him breathing adequately? These include, pneumothoraces, broken ribs, spinal injuries, and even tight abdominal bandages.

"Laryngeal stridor occurs as he recovers" This happens as his cough and laryngeal reflexes return, and is usually due to mucus or blood on his larynx. Suck them out and give him oxygen.

"He coughs and wheezes persistently" A gentle cough is more a sign of recovery than a complication. Only persistant coughing matters. The most serious cause is blood, mucus or stomach contents in a patient's lungs. Lay him on his side, head down, suck out his pharynx and give him oxygen. If necessary, ventilate him.

"He becomes cyanosed" This is usually due to respiratory depression, but it can happen from a variety of other causes, even when his ventilation is normal. Give him oxygen.

"He complains of pain" As a patient recovers consciousness, pain is usually his dominant sensation. If necessary give him morphine 0.1 mg/kg, or pethidine 1 mg/kg, every four hours. Ideally, give it intravenously, titrating the dose until you get just the effect you want, as in Section 8.9, or give it intramuscularly. Or, give him bupivacaine as a local block. This will last 6 hours. A caudal epidural block is suitable for perineal operations, and an intercostal block for abdominal ones.

"He has the shakes as he recovers from a general anaesthetic" This is a combination of shivering and skeletal rigidity, and may occur after halothane, or a long operation in a cold theatre. The shakes usually only last a few minutes. Give him oxygen.

"He becomes restless and agitated" A woman or child may cry, and a man may thrash about. The common causes are: (1) pain, (2) hypoxia, (3) a full bladder, (4) a nasogastric tube, (5) backache, and (6) headache. Try to remove the cause; if necessary sedate him.

"He vomits as he recovers" Large doses of opioids, ether or trichloroethylene may be responsible. Vomiting is more common after abdominal operations. After middle ear operations nausea may persist for days. If necessary, give an anti–emetic such as perphenazine 0.1 mg/kg.

"Something quite unexpected occurs during recovery period" Something may happen as the result of quite another disease. For example if a patient is an epileptic, he may have a fit. If something unusual does happen, or he deteriorates suddenly, the recovery nurse must fetch help immediately.

4.7 Recording the course of anaesthesia

In many district hospitals no anaesthetic records are made, apart from a possible entry in the theatre book. Yet records are important, not so much for later analysis, but because they promote good anaesthetic practice, and discourage sloppy undisciplined methods. They encourage an anaesthetic assistant to involve himself more in the patient's care. They make anaesthesia less passive, and more of an active exercise in applied physiology. Records also make meaningful discussions, critisms, and "teach—ins" possible. As with the rest of medicine, good records are one of the best indicators of good care.

A record sheet need not be elaborate—you can easily photocopy or duplicate one locally, like Fig. 4-8. It should contain a graph recording the course of the operation, on which important events, such as the patient's pulse, his blood pressure and the adminstration of drugs can be entered.

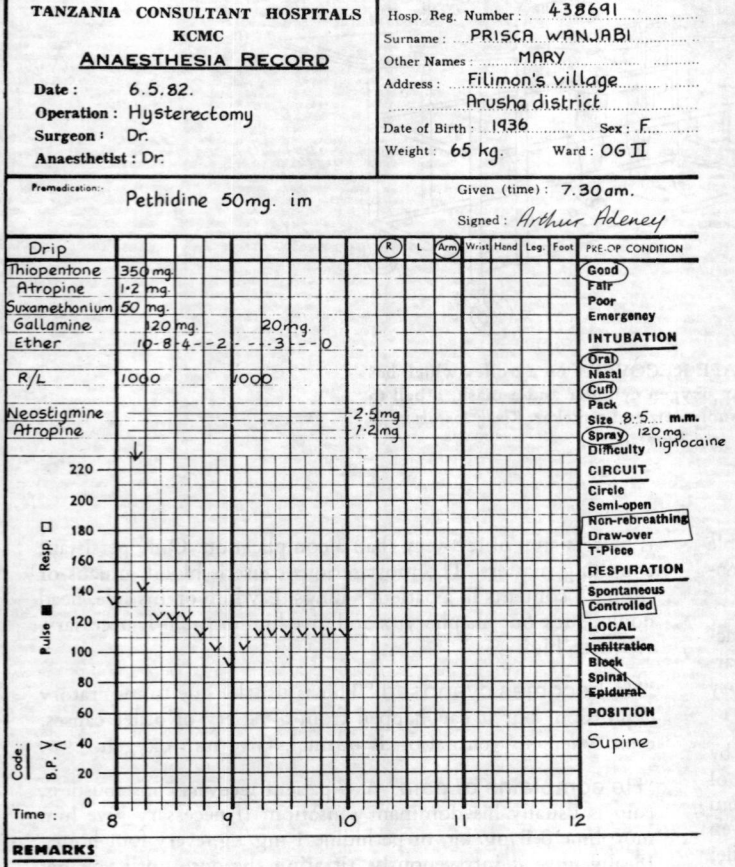

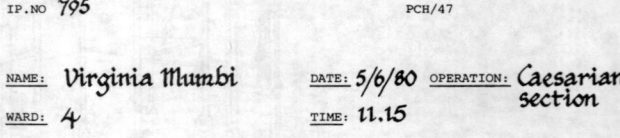

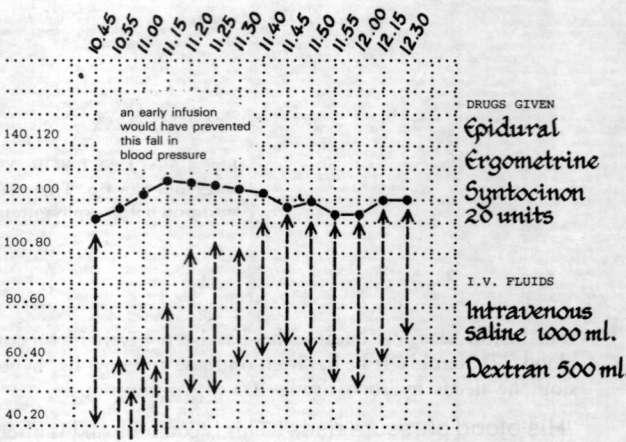

Fig. 4-8 A STENCILED ANAESTHETIC RECORD SHEET has been re-drawn from one of the routine records kept by an anaesthetic assistant trained on the job. It demonstrates a common error, she watched hypotension developing in her patient and then treated it with saline and dextran. Section 7.1 describes how she could have probably have prevented this by preloading the patient with saline. In this hospital saline was so scarce that it could only be used if absolutely necessary. *Kindly contributed by Walter Spellmayer from Tumutumu hospital.*

Fig. 4-7 A PRINTED ANAESTHETIC RECORD SHEET. This record would be improved if it included spaces to include the patient's blood group, his haemoglobin, and any special risk factors. *Kindly contributed by Arthur Adeney.*

5 An introduction to local anaesthesia

5.1 Advantages and disadvantages

Local anaesthesia is: (1) practical, (2) cheap, and (3) safe, especially when trained staff are scarce. (4) If a patient's stomach is full, as it often is after an injury, local anaesthesia is safer that anything but the most expert general anaesthetic. (5) The patient breathes normally. (6) His pharyngeal and laryngeal reflexes are preserved, so that you need not be concerned with his airway. (7) Local anaesthesia needs little equipment. (8) The patient can cooperate, for example, if you cannot find a hernial sac, you can ask him to cough. (9) Some patients prefer it.

Local anaesthesia does however have some disadvantages: (1) It is less reliable than general anaesthesia. (2) You have to learn each block separately. (3) The dose of a local anaesthetic is limited, so there is a limit to the area of the patient's body you can anaesthetize. This is one of the particular disadvantages of abdominal field blocks and of multiple intercostal blocks. (4) Although a successful local anaesthetic abolishes the sensation of pain, it does not abolish hearing, nor does it always abolish the sensations of touch and pressure. Some patients do not like to feel the operator touching them. And nobody likes to hear their bones being sawn! (5) Local anaesthesia may be more difficult if the patient is fat. (6) You cannot give a local anaesthetic through infected tissue. (7) However good your precautions are, an occasional patient collapses as a result of a local anaesthetic, so you must have resuscitation equipment ready for this. (8) Local anaesthesia is not suitable for children, or for anxious or uncooperative patients, unless you combine it with intramuscular ketamine or light general anaesthesia. Nevertheless, in spite of all these disadvantages, local anaesthesia can make a great contribution to surgery, and it is not used as often as it should be. You can also combine local anaesthesia with intravenous analgesia. So, before you do any operation, ask yourself—"Could it be done more easily or safely under local anaesthesia?"

A great help to success is to prepare the patient psychologically, to pre– or paramedicate him thoroughly (2.6, 5.2), and to start with methods that regularly work well, even in the hands of an occasional user. These are subarachnoid anaesthesia (7.4), intravenous forearm block (6.19), axillary brachial plexus block (6.18), pudendal nerve block (6.13), and digital nerve block (6.21). Success comes with practice. So practise these methods on thin patients, with a general anaesthetic available while you are learning. A battery–operated nerve stimulator is a useful learning aid.

If you do only an occasional operation under local anaesthesia, no special planning is needed. But if a whole list of patients, or most of them, are to be anaesthetized in this way, plan the list with care, so that no time is wasted waiting. If there are many short operations to be done, anaesthetize the next patient on the list, while the surgeon is preparing to scrub up for the current one. This is readily possible with a local anaesthetic, because its final stage can easily be monitored by an assistant. The operating list will probably proceed more smoothly if you try not to alternate the methods you use, so try to keep the blocks and the general anaesthetics separate as far as you can. The list will not take longer if you do a series of blocks in advance, and "stack them up" waiting for surgery.

Here is the equipment you will need.

* *NEEDLES, hypodermic. (a) 0.45×16 mm, 100 needles only (b) 0.65×30 mm, 100 needles only. (c) 1.45×60 mm, 100 needles only. (d) 0.8×100 mm, 50 needles only.* The right needles are important. They range in diameter from 0.45 mm for the smallest intradermal needles to about 3 mm for the largest intravenous ones. Needles (a) are for hypodermic injections, (b) are for subcutaneous injections, (c) are for intramuscular injections, and (d) are long needles for infiltration anaesthesia.
* *SYRINGES, plastic autoclavable, central nozzle, 'Luer-lok' mount, (a) 1 ml, 10 only. (b) 2 ml, 20 only. (c) 5 ml, 20 only. (d) 10 ml, 20 only. (e) 20 ml, 10 only. (f) 50 ml, 5 only.* 'Luer-lok' syringes are much the best ones for local anaesthesia, because they allow you to exert pressure without the needle coming off the syringe, and squirting anaesthetic solution everywhere. Some 50 ml syringes are useful because you can inject 30 ml or more of solution without refilling.
* *SYRINGES dental for 2.2 ml cartridges of anaesthetic solution, two only.* A dental cartridge syringe is much the best for anaesthetizing teeth, but you can use an ordinary one if necessary.
* *NEEDLES, dental, hypodermic, double pointed, disposable but reboilable (a) 0.5×30, (b) 0.5×42mm, one thousand only of each size.* One point on these needles goes into the patient and the other into the cartridge.

"WHY NOT DO THE OPERATION UNDER LOCAL ANAESTHESIA?"

5.2 Pre– and paramedication for local anaesthesia

The first step in any medical procedure is to *explain carefully to the patient exactly what you are going to do to him. This is especially important when you are giving him a local anaesthetic.* If he knows what is going to happen to him, he is much more likely to be still and cooperate. The next step is to pre– or paramedicate him thoroughly. Give him a modest dose of diazepam, or promethazine, to calm him and relieve his anxiety. *And,* give him pethidine or morphine to prevent him feeling any pain there might be if your block is not quite perfect. Give him these drugs intramuscularly one hour before the operation. Diazepam alone is often not enough.

Even if your block is perfect, he will probably feel touch and pressure, and he may interpret these as pain. If it is less than perfect, he will feel some pain. To prevent this some anaesthetists also give a second dose of drug intravenously at the operation. This is *paramedication;* it will sedate him further and produce general analgesia. Paramedicate him with intravenous diazepam, or ketamine, or morphine, or pethidine. A useful combination for an adult is diazepam 5 mg, with some ketamine, both intravenously (in different syringes), repeating the ketamine if necessary. Or, use inhaled trichloroethylene from a vapouriser (11.7). Don't give additional drugs blindly or without waiting for them to act, you may produce severe cardiac or respiratory complications.

Many anaesthetists don't make this distinction, and rely on premedication only. Others give nothing until the operation, and then give intravenous paramedication only. If you fail to pre– or paramedicate a patient properly, the danger is that he

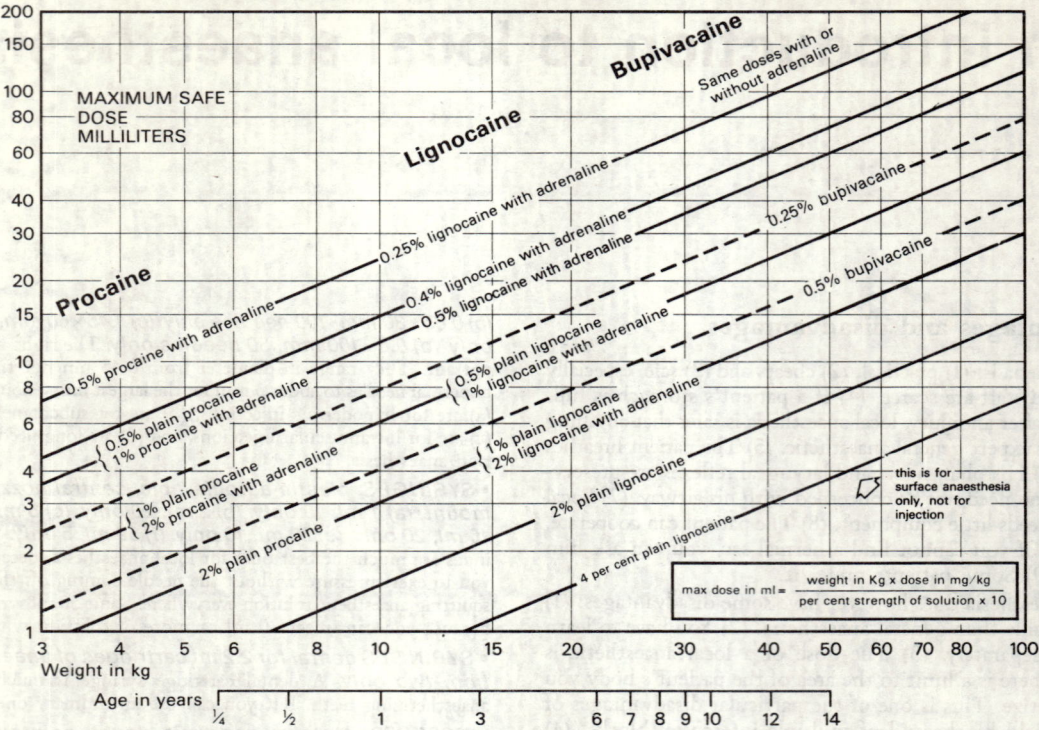

Fig. 5-1 THE MAXIMUM DOSE OF SOME LOCAL ANAESTHETICS. Find the drug you want, such as procaine, lignocaine or bupivacaine. Look underneath it for the sloping line showing the strength of the drug you are going to use. Follow that line to the vertical line showing your patient's weight, then read off the dose on the left hand scale. Note that these are MAXIMUM doses and you may need much less. Here are some examples. The answers are at the end of Section 5.9.

(1) What is the maximum dose of 1% plain lignocaine for a 50 kg patient?
(2) What is the maximum dose of 2% lignocaine with adrenaline for a 50 kg patient?
(3) What is the maximum dose of 0.5% procaine with adrenaline for a 60 kg patient?
(4) What is the maximum dose of 4% lignocaine for a 15 kg child?
(5) What is the maximum dose of 0.5% bupivacaine for a patient weighing 100 kg? *Kindly contributed by Peter Bewes.*

(or she) may become uncontrollable during the operation, like the patient Georgina below.

Mothers for Caesarean section have premedication problems of their own, see Section 6.9.

GEORGINA (55), a very large lady, was admitted for the repair of a small epigastric hernia. The doctor had done several operations like this before under infiltration anaesthesia. She was not premedicated and turned out to have a much larger hernia than he expected. She went beserk, panting, puffing, trying to get up, screaming, waving her arms in the air, and refusing to cooperate. What appeared to be the major part of the contents of her abdomen appeared from her wound. The anaesthetic assistant was summoned, whereupon he quickly and expertly induced her with thiopentone and ether. Good muscle relaxation was needed to close the wound. The suxamethonium chloride ('Scoline') in the cupboard was no longer very active, so that more than 20 vials were needed. The operation was completed uneventfully, although she did develop a wound infection. LESSONS: (1) Patients for local anaesthesia should always be premedicated, to minimise the chances of this kind of happening. (2) All patients for anaesthesia should also be starved, in case a general anaesthetic is needed. (3) Use suxamethonium as its bromide, which stores well, not as its chloride, which needs to be refrigerated. (4) Intermittent suxamethonium is not a very effective, or a very safe way of producing relaxation.

5.3 Drugs for local and regional anaesthesia

A local anaesthesic, such as bupivacaine, diffuses into a nerve from the outside. The nerve's smallest fibres, transmitting the sensation of pain and controlling the blood vessels, are blocked first, followed by the larger ones, responsible for touch and pressure, heat and cold. Vasodilation is the first sign that a block is working. This is followed by analgesia, and then by the inability to feel touch and pressure. Recovery takes place in the reverse order. A block can thus abolish pain completely, so that you can operate, but the patient may still feel touch and pressure. Warn him about this, so that he does not expect the loss of all sensation at the operation site. Sometimes, the motor fibres may be on the outside of a mixed nerve, and anaesthetized first, while the pain fibres are on the inside, and anaesthetized later. So don't think that, because the patient's limb is paralysed, he cannot feel pain. Pain is the important sensation—if he cannot feel it, you can operate.

The *latent interval* is the time between the injection of the drug, and the start of anaesthesia suitable for surgery. It varies with the drug, the kind of block, and your technique. All the latent intervals given here are for lignocaine. They are longer with procaine, and bupivacaine. Anaesthesia is almost immediate when you infiltrate into the patient's skin, and takes slightly longer when you infiltrate under it. When you block a larger nerve, such as the sciatic, the latent interval may be as long as 15 minutes. Latent intervals vary, *so don't think that a block has failed until you have waited about 15 minutes.*

When you inject local anaesthetic, some of it is fixed locally. The rest is absorbed by the patient's circulation and carried elsewhere in his body, where it may cause undesirable side effects. It can reduce his cardiac output and his peripheral resistance, and in doing so it may lower his blood pressure. An overdose can also depress his respiration. Moderate doses will sedate him and cause a general analgesia, but an overdose can cause fits, or coma, and so kill him.

In most sites you can add adrenaline to the local anaesthetic solution to constrict the patient's blood vessels, and reduce the speed at which the anaesthetic is absorbed into his circulation.

If you do this, you can safely use twice the dose of lignocaine or procaine, but you should not use twice the dose of bupivacaine.

Local anaesthetics vary in concentration. The weakest ones described here are 0.25% bupivacaine for local infiltration, and the strongest is 4% lignocaine for anaesthetizing the mucosa. Use the weaker solutions for infiltration anaesthesia, and the stronger ones for blocking larger nerves. One per cent of a drug is equivalent to 10 mg per ml, or 1 g per 100 ml. The most economical way to use these drugs is to buy them as powders and ask your pharmacy to make them up.

STRONGER SOLUTIONS ARE FOR LARGER NERVES BE PREPARED TO WAIT 15 MINUTES

Lignocaine is available as a powder, and in solutions of 1%, 1.5%, 2%, 4% and 10%, either with or without adrenaline. Two per cent is the most useful strength to order, because you can easily dilute it. Lignocaine is cheap, and you can autoclave it. It gives anaesthesia lasting 60 to 90 minutes.

In most sites the maximum dose is 3 mg/kg (200 mg for an adult dose), without adrenaline, or 6 mg/kg, (400 mg for an adult), with it.

You can use 2 or 4% lignocaine for surface anaesthesia, and to assist the passage of a tracheal tube. Four per cent is a concentrated solution, so be particularly careful not to exceed the maximum dose. For a 60 kg adult, the maximum dose of the 4% solution is about 4 ml, *but in a 15 kg child it is only 1 ml*. The danger of an overdose is less with the 2% solution.

You can also use lignocaine for isobaric (7.5) and hyperbaric (7.6) subarachnoid anaesthesia.

THE MAXIMUM ADULT DOSE OF PLAIN LIGNOCAINE is 200 mg

Bupivacaine is four times the price of an equivalent amount of lignocaine, and has a slightly longer latent interval of 15 to 25 minutes, for a large nerve and less for a small one. Its advantage is that anaesthesia lasts 3 to 6 hours, about 3 times as long as with lignocaine, so it is the best drug for regional blocks. Use it in solutions of 0.25 or 0.5%. The maximum dose of bupivacaine is 2 mg/kg and is shown in dotted lines in Fig. 5-1. The maximum adult dose of the 0.5% solution is about 30 ml. Adrenaline makes no difference to the absorbtion and duration of action of bupivacaine, which is strongly bound to the tissues anyway, so there is no point in using it.

Procaine is not the agent of choice but it is still widely available and cheap. Its latent interval is twice that of lignocaine; anaesthesia lasts only an hour; it does not anaesthetize mucous membranes, and it is useless for intravenous forearm blocks. You can however use procaine satisfactorily for infiltration anaesthesia. It is not as effective as lignocaine, or bupivacaine for regional blocks. The maximum safe dose of procaine is twice that of lignocaine—6 mg/kg without adrenaline and 12 mg/kg with it.

Adrenaline For anaesthetizing most parts of the body you can add adrenaline to a local anaesthesic to delay absorption of the anaesthetic from the tissues. The maximum safe dose of adrenaline is 0.5 mg for an adult, and its optimum concentration is one part in 200 000. Never use adrenaline on the extremities, such as the fingers, the toes, the nose or the penis, because it may constrict the end arteries in these tissues and cause gangrene. If the only local anaesthetic solution you have has adrenaline in it, you cannot do these blocks. Also, don't use solutions containing adrenaline on the ocuular nerve, or for intravenous forearm blocks. For these purposes, always use a plain solution. For all other local blocks, you can, if you wish, add adrenaline. It will prolong them, and reduce the incidence of side effects. *Make quite sure that, if you add adrenaline to a solution, it is clearly labelled!*

The maximum safe dose of solutions Each local anaesthetic has its maximum safe dose. *You can easily give too much, especially in a child.* For example, the maximum dose of plain lignocaine without adrenaline is 3 mg/kg. The maximum dose for a 70 kg adult is thus 210 mg. This is contained in 21 ml of 1% plain solution, or 10 ml of 2% plain solution. Because overdosage is so easy, this is an important dose to remember. For a 7 kg child the maximum dose of 2% lignocaine is only 1.5 ml. After you have added adrenaline to slow the absorption of the anaesthetic from the tissues, the maximum safe dose is doubled to 6 mg/kg. You can now give 21 ml of 2 per cent lignocaine with adrenaline to an adult.

The larger the nerve you wish to block, the stronger the concentration of the drug you must use, and the smaller its volume. For example, you will need 10 ml of 2% lignocaine to block the sciatic nerve. If you decide to do a Caesarean section using infiltration anaesthesia, you will need 100 ml of 0.4% lignocaine with adrenaline to anaesthetize the small nerves of a mother's abdominal wall.

Larger volumes of a weaker solution are safer than smaller volumes of a stronger ones, because they are less likely to enter the circulation rapidly. Thus 100 ml of 0.5% lignocaine is safer than 50 ml of 1% solution. It is said that 0.5% procaine is metabolised so rapidly that there is no upper limit to the safe dose (5.1).

You can use almost any local anaesthetic for almost any method, provided that: (1) You do not exceed the maximum dose. (2) You do not add adrenaline when it is contraindicated. (3) You do not use dilute solutions, or procaine, for large nerves. Subarachnoid and epidural anaesthesia are exceptions to these rules.

When you want to give a local anaesthetic, you will want to know the maximum dose in ml. Working this out from a patient's weight in kg and the dose in mg/kg can cause difficulty. Either use Fig.5-1, or the formula it contains.

DONT EXCEED THE SAFE DOSE OF A LOCAL ANAESTHETIC

5.4 Infiltration anaesthesia

This is very valuable under difficult conditions. You can use it by itself for small or large operations, or you can combine it with the appropriate nerve block, such as an axillary block. Infiltration anaesthesia is useful for suturing wounds, for circumcision, and for removing small cysts and lipomas. For larger operations, such as repairing a hernia, infiltrating the tissue planes with a local anaesthetic separates them and makes them clearer and easier to dissect. Because you need only a small dose of the drug, you can use infiltration anaesthesia for very sick patients. Infiltration anaesthesia has some disadvantages: (1) It takes time. (2) It does not relax the abdominal muscles. (3) You should not use it in areas of cellulitis, because it may spread the infection.

LOCAL ANAESTHESIA

STARVE THE PATIENT Your block may occasionally fail, and he may need a general anaesthetic.

MAKING 100 ml of 0.4% LIGNOCAINE Take 20 ml of 2% lignocaine. This is the maximum adult dose with adrenaline. Add it to 80 ml of sterile saline. If adrenaline is required, add 0.5 ml of 1:1000 solution, which will make a dilution of 1:200 000. 100 ml of this solution is a very useful volume for infiltration anaesthesia for such procedures as hernia block or

LOCAL INFILTRATION

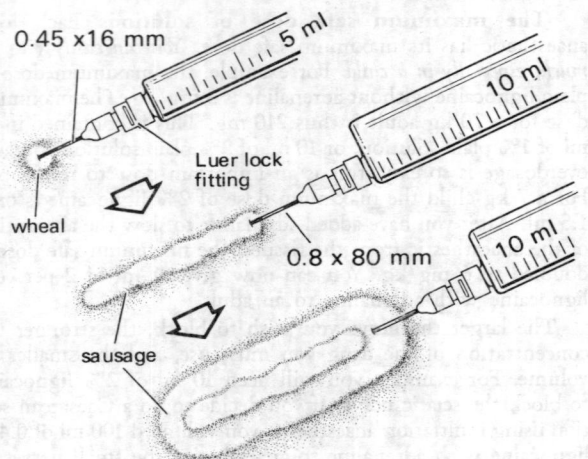

Fig. 5-2 LOCAL INFILTRATION. Raise a wheal and then insert your needle through it. *Kindly contributed by Peter Bewes.*

Caesarean section. In some hospitals this excellent fluid goes by the name of "jungle juice". You can add hyaluronidase, but is not necessary.

SYRINGES AND NEEDLES Use 'Luer-lok' syringes that fit well without sticking. Other syringes and needles are apt to come apart suddenly and spray the anaesthesic solution over everyone.

Use fine 0.45 or 0.6 mm needles for the first "prick". Use larger 0.8 or 0.9 mm needles for infiltration itself. Some needles should be 30 mm long, some 60 mm, and some 100 mm, depending on the type of anaesthesia you are doing. Keep them sharp, if they become blunt, they cause pain, which is what the anaesthetic is trying to prevent.

A useful improvement is to join the needle to the syringe with 10 cm of a fine plastic tube. This makes it easier to manipulate the syringe without moving the point of the needle away from the place where it should be.

MARKERS Sometimes, it is difficult to know how far inside a patient the point of a needle is. This may be easier if you use a marker, in the form of a short piece of sterile rubber tube, on the needle a set distance from its point, as shown in Fig. 6-9.

INFILTRATION ANAESTHESIA FOR SMALL OPERATIONS Tell the patient exactly what you are going to do. Paint his skin with an antiseptic, and fill a small syringe with anaesthetic solution. Fit a fine needle.

Inject a small wheal of solution where you intend to put in the larger needle. Wait 2 minutes for this to work. Meanwhile, fill a larger syringe with the solution, and attach a longer infiltrating needle.

Push the needle through the wheal that you have raised. Push it along the line where the incision is going to be. Keep it close to the surface of the skin (almost intradermal) as you inject the solution into the tissues. Injection may be hard, and you may need firm pressure, especially in the scalp. An 'orange skin' appearance in his skin shows that the solution is going into the right place.

Now inject more deeply into the subcutaneous tissues until you have made a sausage–shaped lump. Keep the needle moving as you inject. This will make injection into a vein unlikely, so there is no need to aspirate continually.

If you have to insert a needle in more than one place, always try to put it through a part of the skin which is already anaesthetic. *Ideally, the patient should feel one needle prick only.* Be generous with your infiltration. Inject ahead of the knife. Don't cut ahead of the anaesthetic to see if it is working there!

If you are excising a small tumour or cyst, make a barrier of anaesthetic solution all round the operation site. First, make two small wheals. Then inject through these all round the lump to make a diamond–shaped anaesthetic area which you can incise to remove the lump.

CAUTION ! Never push a needle in to the tissues up to its adaptor. If it breaks, you will have difficulty removing it.

IF POSSIBLE, THE PATIENT SHOULD ONLY FEEL ONE NEEDLE PRICK

FIELD BLOCK for excising a small lesion

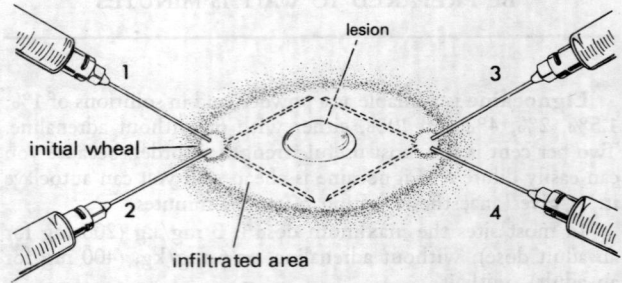

Fig. 5-3 EXCISING A SMALL LESION UNDER LOCAL ANAESTHESIA. Make wheals at either end and insert your needle through them in diverging directions. *Kindly contributed by Peter Bewes.*

5.5 Infiltrate–and–cut anaesthesia

You can inject unlimited quantities of 0.025 to 0.5% procaine *without* adrenaline into the operation site. The weak procaine solution is so widely distributed in the patient's tissues, and so readily broken down, that there is no upper limit to the dose. The method is not dangerous, provided that the needle does not enter a vein. This is unlikely to happen, if you keep the needle moving while you inject. You can, if necessary, do almost any operation by this method, but regional blocks with bupivicaine or lignocaine are usually better. This is one of the most useful methods for operating under difficult conditions, especially if you combine it with intravenous morphine carefully titrated to the patient's needs, as in Section 8.7.

This 'unlimited' method is not safe with lignocaine, or bupivacaine, because they are metabolised more slowly, but you can safely give a 60 kg adult up to 60 ml of 0.25% bupivacaine or 150 ml of 0.25% lignocaine with adrenaline.

5.6 Anaesthetizing a fracture haematoma

You can anaesthetize a fracture by injecting a local anaesthetic solution into the fracture site between the fragments of a broken bone. This provides a useful level of anaesthesia, but in the arm it is not as effective as an intravenous forearm block, or a brachial plexus block. If you do it carelessly, or the syringe and needle are not perfectly sterile, you may infect the haematoma. If possible, use a sterile disposable syringe and needle. There is also the risk of rapid absorption of the solution, and the quality of the anaesthesia is not always adequate.

INFILTRATION ANAESTHESIA FOR A FRACTURE HAEMATOMA

INDICATIONS (1) In emergencies, particularly when caring for mass casualties. (2) Extension fractures of the wrist (S 74.2). (3) Fractures of the nose (S 62.4) and some other fractures of the face.

CONTRAINDICATIONS (1) Doubtful aseptic techinque. (2) Fractures more than 24 hours old in which the haematoma will have started to organise.

METHOD Palpate the fracture and puncture the haematoma. Aspirate to make sure the needle is in the haematoma. Slowly inject 1% or 2% lignocaine without adrenaline. Rapid injection is very painful.

After 5 minutes you can reduce the fracture.

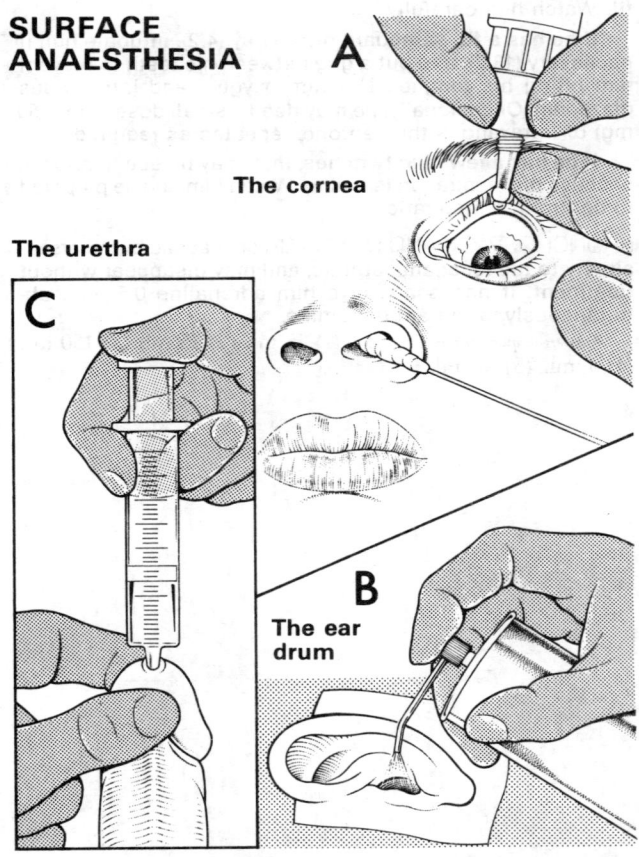

Fig. 5-4 SURFACE ANAESTHESIA. A, you may need to insert 2 eye drops 10 times during 20 minutes before you can remove sutures or foreign bodies from a patient's eye. B, direct two or three puffs towards the upper wall of his auditory canal and allow them to run down onto his drum. C, use a syringe without a needle to inject lignocaine into his urethra.

5.7 Infiltration anaesthesia for opening abscesses

Although you should not inject a local anaesthetic into an area of cellulitis, you can use it to open an abscess which is already pointing, and so is *easy to open*. Use a very fine needle to inject 0.5 ml of local anaesthetic solution slowly into the place where the pus is going to burst. Incise the abscess through the anaesthetized area. If a patient has a big abscess which needs exploring, anaesthetize him in some other way.

5.8 Surface anaesthesia

A patient's mucous membranes will absorb anaesthetic drugs and become insensitive. You can anaesthetise his conjunctiva, his ear drum, his nasal mucosa, and his urethra like this. Anaesthetizing his larynx before passing a tracheal tube is described in Section 13-5. You can use 2%, or better, 4% lignocaine for all these methods.

SURFACE ANAESTHESIA

CONJUNCTIVA Instil drops of 2 or, better, 4% lignocaine, one or two drops at a time. *The number of instillations is much more important than the number of drops you use.* You may have to instil them 20 times over 5 to 10 minutes before you can remove sutures, or foreign bodies, for example.

EAR DRUM

Direct two or three doses of a 10% lignocaine aerosol spray towards the upper wall of his auditory canal and allow them to run down onto his drum. This will minimise the discomfort of spraying cold solution onto it.

You can anaesthetize the ear drum sufficiently to incise it in 3 to 5 minutes.

NASAL MUCOSA

INDICATIONS Puncture of the maxillary antrum.

CONTRAINDICATIONS Children, especially young ones.

METHOD Soak cotton wool eye swabs on sticks in 2% or 4% lignocaine and place them under the medial and inferior concha for at least 10 minutes. Or, spray the area with 1 to 3 doses of lignocaine from a spray can.

URETHRA

INDICATIONS (1) Catheterisation. (2) Bouginage.

METHOD Using a syringe without a needle, inject 10 ml of 2% lignocaine into the patient's urethra, while holding his urinary meatus round the nozzle. Ask him to strain, as if he was passing urine, and then inject a further 10 ml. The solution should flow towards his posterior urethra.

Apply a penile clamp. His urethra will become anaesthetic in about 5 minutes.

5.9 The complications of local anaesthesia

The complications of local anaesthesia are usually caused by (1): Giving too much of the drug. If you don't exceed maximum safe dose in Fig. 5-1, this is unlikely to happen. (2) Unusual sensitivity to the drug. This you cannot anticipate, unless you find from a patient's history that it has happened before. (3) Injecting the drug into a blood vessel. Prevent this by: (a) keeping the needle moving as you inject, or, (b) if the needle is still, aspirating before you inject.

Complications may develop rapidly, so you must never give a local anaesthetic without following the "ten golden rules" in Section 3.1. You must for example, have instantly available the equipment for maintaining the patient's airway, and for controlling his ventilation (13.1). Always put up a drip, or at least an indwelling needle, whenever you do a major block.

If you are aware of mild early symptoms, you may be able to treat them before more serious later ones develop. So watch for paraesthesiae, twitching and jerking. Intravenous diazepam at this stage may prevent convulsions and perhaps cardiac arrest. Usually, convulsions are the first sign that the drug has mistakenly been given intravenously. Premedication with diazepam may make them less likely to occur.

THE COMPLICATIONS OF LOCAL ANAESTHESIA

Disorientation, nausea, and vomiting soon stop spontaneously.

IF THE PATIENT BECOMES UNCONSCIOUS, no special treatment is needed, provided his blood pressure and respiration are normal. Set up a drip, in case fits follow, and give him oxygen.

IF HIS BREATHING STOPS, start controlling his respiration immediately.

Intubate him. Connect his tracheal tube to a self-inflating bag or a bellows, and give him oxygen.

If he has had an opioid, give him a morphine antagonist, such as naloxone 100 to 200 micrograms (1.5 to 3 micrograms/kg) intravenously adjusted according to his response. Then give 100 micrograms intravenously every 2 minutes. If he is a child, give him 5 to 10 micrograms/kg. Or, give an adult nalorphine 10 mg.

IF HE SHOWS CARDIOVASCULAR COLLAPSE, it usually follows respiratory failure, except in subarachnoid and epidural anaesthesia, where the blood pressure is low, and the pulse slow. Lay him flat, give him oxygen, and give him atropine 0.6 mg intravenously; repeat this as necessary.

If his blood pressure does not improve immediately, give him a drip of saline, Ringer's lactate or plasma expander.

If necessary, add 1 mg of adrenaline or isoprenaline to 500 ml fluid. Start at 20 drops a minute, and increase the rate by 10 drops every ten minutes, provided he has no extrasystoles and his pulse does not increase above 120. His blood pressure should be normal long before this.

If he has no pulse, in his femoral or carodid arteries, and is not breathing, start immediate cardiopulmonary resuscitation (CPR), go to Section 3.6.

FITS, suspect that a patient is going to have fit if he becomes sleepy at first and then over-talkative and restless, if he rubs his nose, or if his face twitches. If any of these things happen, give him intravenous diazepam 5 mg—it may prevent a fit. Watch him carefully.

If he has a fit, safeguard his airway (4.2), intubate him if necessary (13.2), and put a gag between his teeth to prevent him biting his tongue. Give him oxygen, and intravenous diazepam. Occasionally, he may need a small dose (about 50 mg) of intravenous thiopentone, repeated as required.

If he has a few mild twitches, they may be due to anoxia, because his respiration is failing. Watch him and be prepared to control his respiration.

BRONCHOSPASM AND URTICARIA are caused by hypersensitivity to the local anaesthetic, and may disappear without treatment. If necessary, give him adrenaline 0.5 mg subcutaneously, or an antihistamine.

Answers to questions on Figure 5-1. (1) 15 ml. (2) 15 ml. (3) 150 ml. (4) 1 ml. (5) 40 ml.

6 Nerve blocks

6.1 Blocking a nerve

If necessary, you can use a nerve block to do almost any operation. But, remember that: (1) An operation through infected tissue can be very painful, and is a severe test of the efficiency of a block. To prevent the spread of infection, always do a nerve block a considerable distance above the patient's septic lesion. (2) A large nerve block can be as dangerous as a general anaesthetic, so examine the patient carefully before deciding which anaesthetic would be best for him. Severe kidney or liver disease may delay the breakdown or elimination of local anaesthetics, so, if he has either of these conditions, choose some other method. (3) Always fast the patient because the block may fail, and he may need a general anaesthetic. (4) Pre— or paramedicate him thoroughly. (5) Follow the details of each block exactly. The exact position of the patient, the position of the needle, its direction, and whether or not he should feel paraesthesiae—all these details are important.

Before you start, explain carefully to the patient what you are going to do to him. If he does not want a local anaesthetic, give him a general one. When a needle touches a nerve he may be able to feel paraesthesiae. Some anaesthetists find that this is a useful sign that they have put the needle in the right place. It is more useful in some blocks, such as a supraclavicular brachial plexus block, than in others, such as an axillary block. But the patient must know what you mean by "paraesthesiae". So start by using a fine needle to make a small skin wheal where you want to insert the needle for the block. Then, if you are doing a supraclavicular brachial plexus block, say to him, "I want you to tell me if you feel a tingling like pins and needles in your hand at any time. You will, of course, feel a prick up here, where the needle goes in. This is not what I am asking for, it is the shooting feeling in your hand. Do you understand?" *This is important, because the block may fail if he does not understand what you mean by paraesthesiae.*

FOLLOW THE DETAILS EXACTLY

By now the patient's skin wheal will be anaesthetic, so you can insert a sharp 1 mm needle in the right direction for the block. Learn to feel with the point of the needle. With practice you will be able to feel when you are going through fat, muscle, or rectus sheath, for example. As soon as the patient says—"Stop, that's it! Pins and needles in my hand!", stop, do not go any farther with the needle. It is now in a perfect position. Aspirate, then inject the local anaesthetic. Remove the needle, rub the area with a swab, go away, scrub up, and allow the latent period to elapse.

Sometimes, you will need to inject the local anaesthetic in more than one place. Do the deep part of the block first, so that its latent period can be elapsing while you do the more superficial infiltration. If you want to change the direction of the needle, withdraw it well into the subcutaneous fat, and then change its direction. If you don't withdraw it, it may bend in the tissues. Where necessary, use a rubber marker to return the tip of the needle to the required depth.

Always aspirate before injecting. If you don't, you may inject anaesthetic solution into a blood vessel, or into the lung, or into the subarachnoid space. Inject slowly. If you meet resistance, the needle may be under the periosteum, in a nerve, or in a tendon sheath. Change its position a little and try again.

Observe the patient during the latent period, and don't start operating before it is over, or you will hurt him. Distract his attention elsewhere, while you gently push a needle into some skin that you hope will be anaesthetic. If he makes no response, try several other places, until you have mapped out the anaesthetic area. Don't ask him if he feels pain, he will prabably say he does, even if it is only pressure, or movement. Some anaesthetists test for cold, instead of testing for pain with a pin. They keep a specimen bottle of cold water in the theatre refrigerator.

ALWAYS ASPIRATE BEFORE YOU INJECT

The operation When the full latent period has elapsed, drape the patient and screen the operation site so that he cannot see it, as in Fig. S 75-5. Incise him with the same confidence that you would if he were unconscious under a general anaesthetic.

Remember though that the patient is conscious. Talk to him, explaining all the time what is happening. "This is just some paint on your skin, it may feel cold... Now you are going to feel a little prick. There, the next one will not feel so bad. During the operation remember he can hear every word you say". Don't ask for a sharper knife. He may get up and run away! Find somebody who will stay close to him and talk to him about homely things, such as his job and family. Don't let anyone frighten him by asking "Can you feel the knife going in?". You can always find out if he feels pain. Watch his face. Warn him that he will feel touch and pressure, but not pain. Keep talk away from unpleasant things. If he says he feels pain, believe him and do something about it. Finally, don't put towel clips through unanaesthetized skin!

If the effects of the block wear off during an operation, repeat it.

6.2 The block has failed

What should you do? You have waited for the full latent period, and the patient can still feel pain in the area which you hoped would be anaesthetized. Don't be dismayed. Even an expert anaesthetist can rarely guarantee perfect local anaesthesia in a conscious patient. *If you have already given the full dose of local anaesthetic, don't give him any more.* For example, if an adult has already had 10 ml of 2% lignocaine without adrenaline, he cannot have any more.

If a second block would still be well within the maximum dose, repeat it. If you are not within the maximum dose, either wait 8 hours for the drug to be excreted, and then try again, or anaesthetize him in another way. Because a nerve block may fail, and a patient may need a general anaesthetic, *always starve him before you give him a regional one.* If you have used adrenaline in the block, don't give him trichloroethylene or chloroform.

You can safely give him ketamine, or ether from a vapouriser. A failed subarachnoid or epidural block will have caused widespread vasodilatation, so set up a drip, give him a low dose of thiopentone, intubate him, and give him a light anaesthetic.

Above all, don't try to operate when local anaesthesia has obviously failed. It has been well said that there are few more dangerous situations in anaesthesia, than that in which a major operation has been started under inadequate local analgesia, and has been forced unexpectedly on an unwilling and demoralized patient!

FAST PATIENTS BEFORE REGIONAL ANAESTHESIA

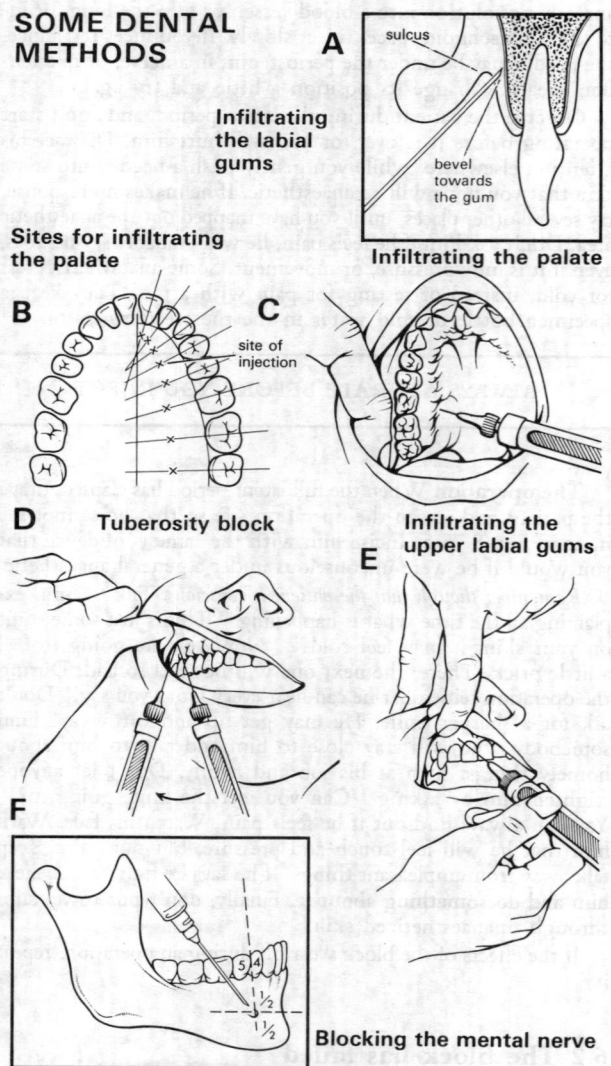

Fig. 6-1 INFILTRATION ANAESTHESIA FOR THE TEETH. A, when you infiltrate a patient's gum, put the needle into his buccal sulcus, make the bevel face his periosteum and inject just outside it. B, to anaesthetize his palatal gums inject at the point marked "X". C, infiltrating the palatal gum of his first molar. D, infiltrating the buccal aspect of his third molar (tuberosity block). E, infiltrating the gum of his lateral incisor. F, blocking his mental nerve. His mental foramen lies on a vertical line between his 4th and 5th teeth, and in a young person is half way up his mandible. *Kindly contributed by Michael Wood.*

6.3 Blocks for the mouth and teeth

Few patients are more grateful than those who have had a painful tooth removed, particularly if it was expertly anaesthetized first.

A tooth and its surrounding gum are innervated from three directions: (1) Its pulp is supplied by a nerve which passes up its root. The gum on (2) its labial and (3) its lingual sides is innervated separately. The tooth socket is partly supplied by the nerve that supplies the root and partly by those that supply the gum. If you are going to remove a patient's tooth painlessly, you will have to anaesthetize all three sets of nerves.

You can easily anaesthetize a patient's labial and lingual gums by local infiltration, but instead of blocking his palatal gums close to his teeth, it is easier to block them in his palate. Infiltrating his gums or his palate will at the same time block the nerves that supply most of the roots of his teeth. The exceptions are his lower molars and second premolars. To anaesthetize them you will have to block his inferior alveolar nerve as it enters his mandibular canal.

A patient's inferior alveolar nerve supplies all the teeth of his lower jaw, so blocking this nerve should make all his lower teeth completely anaesthetic. Unfortunately, anaesthesia is sometimes incomplete, because small accessory branches enter the bone through other foramina and so escape the block. Also, his incisors may not be completely anaesthetized by a single block, because they are innervated from both sides.

INFILTRATING THE LOWER GUMS

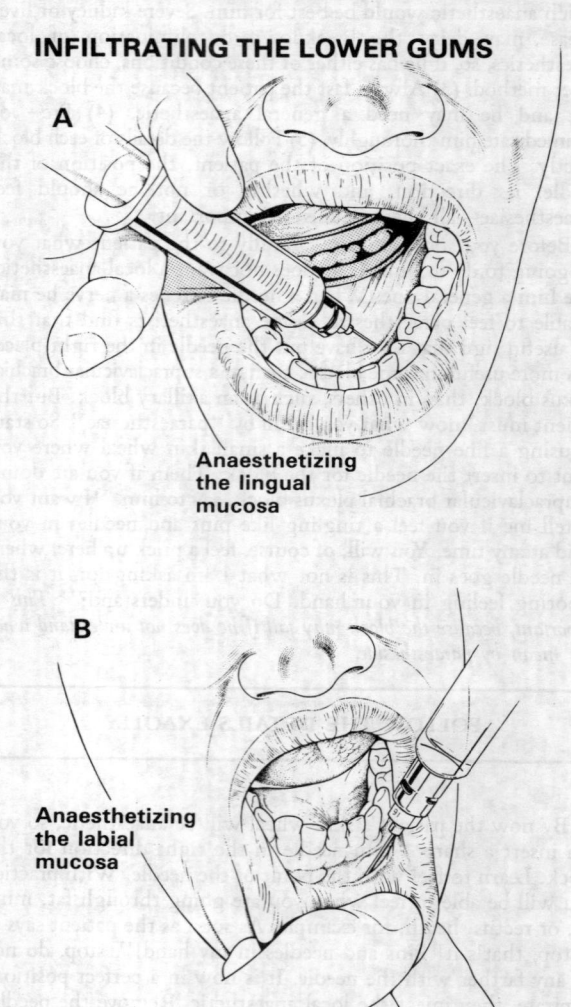

Fig. 6-2 INFILTRATING THE LOWER GUMS. A, infiltrating the lingual and B, the labial gum.

ANAESTHETIZING THE TEETH

DRUGS AND EQUIPMENT For all methods, use 0.5% bupivacaine, or 2% ligocaine with or without adrenaline, preferably in 2 ml cartridges. If possible, a 10% lignocaine spray, or 5%

lignocaine paste. A dental cartridge type syringe. If necessary, you can use an ordinary one, preferably one with a "Luer-lok". Use thin needles—0.3×23 and 42 mm. A spirit lamp to flame the end of the cartridge which has to be pierced. A pair of straight-nosed pliers, or artery forceps, to remove the broken end of a needle. A decontaminant, such as 0.5% chlorhexidine. Forceps and some pledgets of cotton wool.

GENERAL METHOD

Sedate the patient with diazepam 10 to 20 mg. Explain to him what you are going to do. Clean his mucosa with the decontaminant. If possible, spray his mucosa with 10% lignocaine, or apply it as a 5% paste.

After a few seconds put his mucous membrane at the site of the injection on the stretch and quickly pierce it with the bevel of the needle parallel to the bone. Inject quickly—there is nothing more painful than a local dental anaesthetic given slowly.

Once you are through his mucosa, you can pause a little while you find the landmarks. When your needle is in the right position, inject. You cannot aspirate with a dental cartridge.

Test for analgesia. If you are going to fill a patient's tooth, drill its exposed dentine. Before pulling it out, test the sensitivity of the gum around it.

LOCAL INFILTRATION

FOR ALL UPPER TEETH, THE LOWER INCISORS AND CANINES, AND ALL DECIDUOUS TEETH Infiltrate the solution outside the periosteum, near the apex of the tooth. This is where its nerves enter the bone, so this is your target.

Labially in his upper jaw. Inject at the reflection of the mucous membrane where it forms the base of the sulcus, as in A, Fig. 6-1. Inject 1-2 ml of solution, or about half a cartridge. The tip of your needle should come to lie opposite the tip of the root of the tooth you are going to extract. For front teeth insert the needle in line with the tooth. This is impossible with molars, so, if you want to anaesthetize a patient's third molar, insert the needle over his second molar, and aim it obliquely so that its point comes to lie over the root of his third. If you move the point of the needle fanwise, as in D, very carefully, you can anaesthetize 2 or 3 teeth without removing it.

When you inject his upper molars (D), feel the gum on the outer surface of his upper back teeth. The crest of bone jutting down from above is his infrazygomatic crest. Insert your needle immediately behind this crest, distal to his second molar.

Push your needle in 2 cm, as far as it will go, and inject 2 ml of solution. Move it as fanwise as you inject. This is also called a tuberosity block.

Palatally in his upper jaw Inject at the points marked "X" about 1 cm from the tooth half way between the edge of the gum, and the mid line, as in B, Fig. 6-1. This is a shallow injection because his palate lies close below a patient's mucous membrane. Inject just enough solution to make his gum go white. You will not be able to inject much, and you will have to press quite hard.

Labially in a patient's lower jaw. Hold his lip out of the way so that you can see the sulcus clearly. Insert the needle next the chosen tooth, so that its point lies against the outside of his mandible, level with the tip of the root. Inject half a cartridge.

Lingually in his lower jaw. Insert the needle a short distance at the point where the mucosa is reflected off the lingual side of his alveolus, as in A, Fig. 6-2. You may have to hold his tongue out of the way to see the floor of his mouth. Inject about a quarter of a cartridge. There will be a small swelling, which will quickly disappear.

THE LOWER PREMOLARS Labially do a mental block like this:

Pull down the patient's lower lip. Use the tip of your index finger to feel the labial surface of his gum as it turns upwards to join his cheek just posterior to his first premolar tooth. You should be able to feel his mental nerve as it comes out of the mental foramen in his mandible.

Inject from behind, as in F, Fig. 6-1. Pull the corner of the patient's mouth out of the way. Tilt the needle mesially between his first and second premolars. Aim to place the needle just outside his mental foramen. This is half way between his gingival margin and the lower border of his mandible. As a person gets older, his mandible is absorbed, so that his mental foramen comes to lie nearer the upper border of his mandible. Inject 2 ml of solution. If necessary, repeat the procedure on the other side.

Try not to enter his mental foramen, because you may injure the vessels that come out of it, and so cause a large haematoma.

Lingually inject his premolars in the same way as for his lower incisors and canines.

LOWER MOLARS Do an inferior alveolar and lingual nerve block, as described below.

BLOCKS FOR THE LOWER JAW

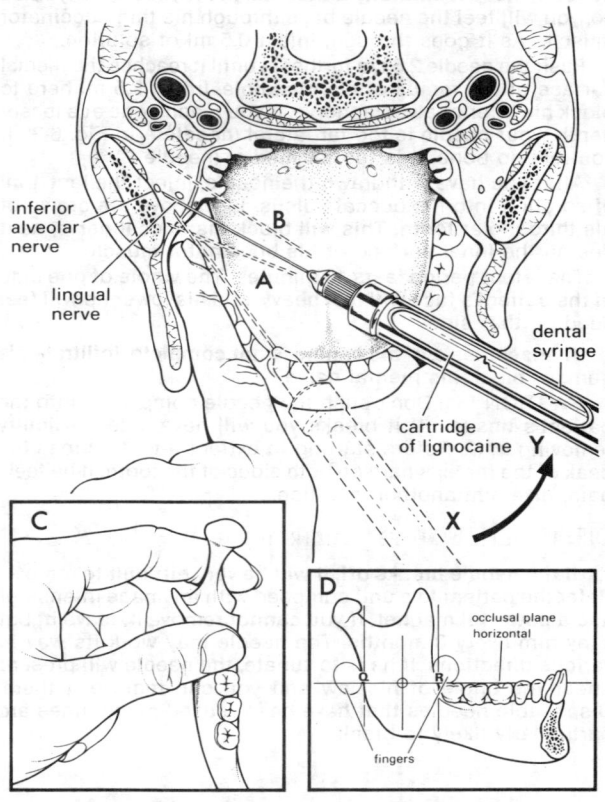

Fig. 6-3 BLOCKING THE LINGUAL AND INFERIOR ALVEOLAR NERVES. A, is an injection which is too lateral and B is one which is too medial. X, is the initial position for the syringe, and Y, its final position. C, is the position of your fingers feeling the ascending ramus of the patient's mandible. D, is the position to aim for, midway between your two fingers. *Kindly contributed by Keith Birkenshaw.*

RIGHT INFERIOR ALVEOLAR AND LINGUAL NERVE BLOCK

Landmarks The secret of success is to visualize where the patient's mandibular foramen is, and to aim the tip of a 42 mm needle at it. As usual, the details are all important.

Adjust the headrest, so that when the patient's mouth is wide open, the occlusal plane of his mandible is horizontal, as in D, Fig. 6-3. When you are learning, use a dental stick dipped in gentian violet to draw a line QR on the mucous membrane of the inside of his cheek in the line of the occlusal surfaces of his lower teeth. If he has a denture, draw it with this in place. If marking it makes him retch, anaesthetize his mucosa first.

Feel the anterior and posterior borders of the ascending ramus of his mandible between the thumb and index finger of your left hand, as in C. Make sure that your index finger is as far up his mandible as it will go. The tips of your fingers should lie at either end of line QR. Aim at the mid point between them—usually 2 cm behind point R. Rest the syringe on the occlusal surfaces of his teeth.

The block Now that you know the landmarks, put your left index finger into the patient's mouth, above his lower third molar, as in the upper diagram in Fig. 6-3, you will feel a depression in the bone immediately above and behind it (his retromolar fossa). Behind this you will find a ridge (the oblique line), on the inner surface of his mandible.

Ask him to open his mouth even wider.

Insert the needle, as described above, immediately medial to the oblique line, 1 cm above the patient's third molar. At first, place the syringe in the line of the body of his mandible. This is position "X". As you push the needle in 2 cm, move the barrel of the syringe across his teeth, so that it lies over his opposite premolar. This is position "Y". As you move the needle, keep it in contact with his teeth all the time. If he has no teeth, keep it carefully horizontal in his mouth. As you do so, you will feel the needle pass through his thin buccinator muscle. As it goes through, inject 0.5 ml of solution.

Push the needle 2.5 cm further in until it reaches the medial surface of the ramus of his mandible. Inject 2.5 ml here to block his inferior alveolar nerve. If you reach bone at a lesser depth, your needle is too far lateral (needle A in Fig. 6-3). If you feel no bone, it is too far medial (needle B).

After you have withdrawn the needle, inject the last 1 ml of solution into his buccal sulcus, just above the crown of his third molar tooth. This will block his buccal nerve, as it lies on the inner surface of his buccinator muscle.

The latent period lasts 10 minutes. The whole of one side of the patient's face will feel heavy, and his lower lip will feel dead on that side.

If anaesthesia of his canine is not complete, infiltrate his gum, or block his mental nerve.

CAUTION ! (1) Don't push the needle completely into the patient's tissues, if it breaks you will have great difficulty removing it. (2) Before starting to extract a tooth, press the beak of the forceps hard on both sides of the tooth. If he feels pain, give him another injection.

DIFFICULTIES ANAESTHETIZING THE TEETH

If the needle breaks off, it will be very difficult to remove. Refer the patient to a unit equipped with an image intensifier and a powerful magnet. If you cannot remove it, leave it, but x-ray him every 3 months. The needle may work its way in various directions. If he is fortunate, the needle will present under the angle of his jaw and you can remove it there. Disposable needles that have been reused many times are particularly likely to break.

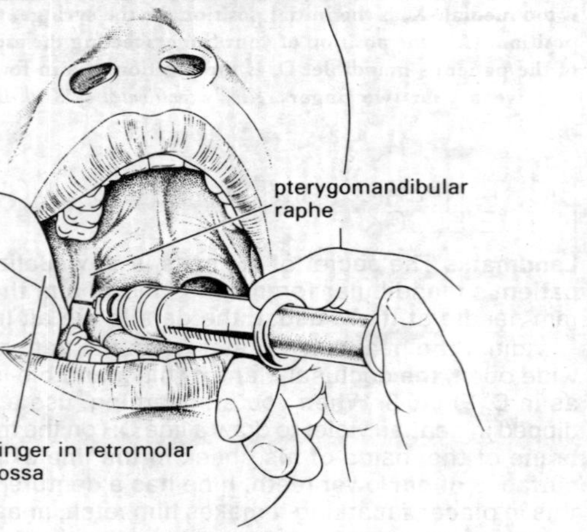

INSERTING THE NEEDLE

Fig. 6-4 INSERTING THE NEEDLE TO BLOCK THE INFERIOR ALVEOLAR NERVE. Notice the position of the point of the needle.

6.4 Pterygopalatine (sphenopalatine) block

This block is easier than it looks. Use it on both sides if necessary, for operations on a patient's upper lip and nose, especially those following trauma. If he is bleeding from the back of his nose, and his stomach is full, this block will be safer than general anaesthesia. Aim to pass the needle posterior to his maxilla, into his pterygopalatine fossa, so as to block his maxillary nerve on its way to supply his upper jaw and nose.

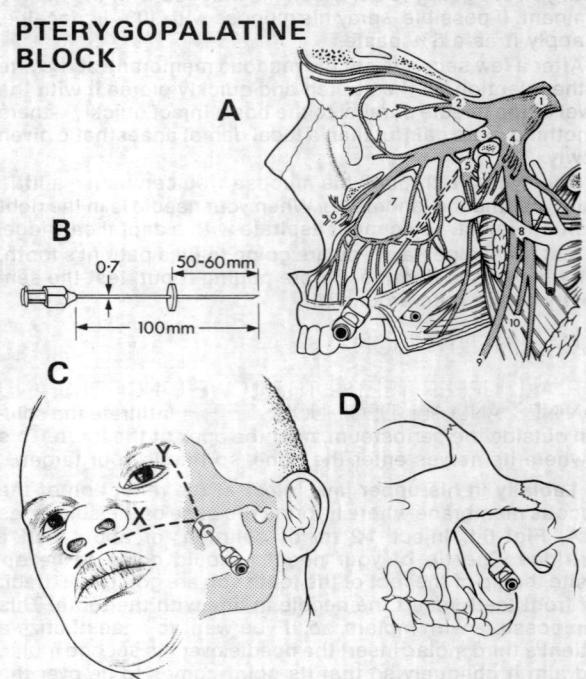

Fig. 6-5 PTERYGOPALATINE BLOCK. A, shows the anatomy of a patient's pterygopalatine fossa, with (1), his trigeminal nerve, (2), his ophthalmic nerve. (3), his maxillary nerve. (4), his mandibular nerve. (5), his pterygopalatine ganglion. (6), his infraorbital nerve, (7), his superior alveolar nerves, (8), his maxillary artery, (9), his lingual nerve, and (10), his inferior alveolar nerve. B, use a 100 mm needle, and place a marker as shown. C, shows the site of insertion of the needle, and D where you are placing the needle in relation to the patient's skull. *After Gray, and Peyman, Sanders and Goldberg, Principles and Practice of Ophthalmology, 1980 WB Saunders Co. The method is that of Frank Prior.*

PTERYGOPALATINE BLOCK

INDICATIONS (1) Injuries to a patient's upper lip and nose. (2) Maxillofacial injuries, bilaterally if necessary. (3) Caldwell Luc's operation. It is seldom necessary for dentistry.

EQUIPMENT A 0.7 × 100 mm needle. Fix a small piece of corrugated rubber drain on it at 5-6 cm, to act as a marker. Another fine needle to raise a skin wheal. 5 ml of 0.25% bupivacaine, or 1% lignocaine.

METHOD Explain to the patient what you are going to do to him. Mark the injection point at the intersection of a line (X) drawn laterally from mid-way between his upper lip and his nose, and another line (Y) dropped vertically from his outer canthus, as in C Fig. 6-5. Feel his maxilla carefully.

If his maxilla extends more laterally than normal, shift the injection point a little laterally.

Pierce his skin, which is often tough at this point, and aim the needle upwards and inwards in the direction of his pupil with his eyes looking forwards.

If you reach bone at 2 to 3 cm, you have hit the anterior surface of his maxilla. Inject a few drops of anaesthetic solution, and redirect the needle so as to pass it.

If the needle advances up to the marker, or you hit bone at 5 cm, you are probably in the right place. Inject 5 ml of solution. It will spread in the loose tissue of his pterygopalatine fossa and block the nerves passing through it.

If you are going to do Caldwell Luc's operation, use a fine needle to infiltrate the line where his gum joins his lip at the place where you will make the incision.

If nasal polyps are to be treated at the same time, instil 5 ml of 4% lignocaine into the patient's nose, with his nostrils facing the ceiling.

6.5 Blocks for the eye

The muscles of a patient's eyelid are supplied by his 7th nerve, and the extrinsic muscles of his eye by his 3rd, 4th and 6th nerves. His 5th nerve supplies sensation. If you want to operate on his eye or his eyelid, neither should move, and both should be anaesthetic. To achieve all this you will need more than one block.

You can block the patient's facial nerve: (a) as it passes over the neck of his mandible, or (b) at the outer side of his eye. A block here also blocks the branches of his 5th nerve. Neither block may be completely effective so, to be on the safe side, you may have to use both. You can block (c) the supraorbital and (d) the infraorbital branches of his 5th nerve. (e) You can block his 3rd, 4th and 6th nerve and the sensory branches of his 5th nerve to his sclera and cornea by passing a needle under his globe, and injecting solution behind it (retrobulbar block). Unfortunately, this block sometimes misses his 4th nerve to his superior rectus muscle, so you may have to block that separately. (f) You can anaesthetize his conjunctiva with a topical anaesthetic, such as amethocaine (also called decicaine or pontocaine) 1% or cocaine 4 to 10% (5.8).

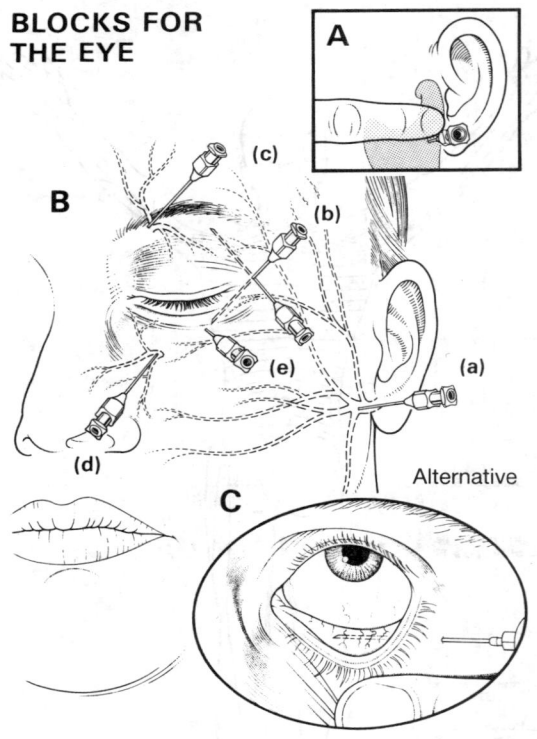

Fig. 6-6 BLOCKS FOR THE EYE. A, finding a patient's facial nerve at the neck of his mandible. B, the main blocks for his eye. (a) Blocking his facial nerve at the neck of his mandible. (b) Blocking his facial nerve peripherally. (c) Blocking his supraorbital nerve. (d) Blocking his infraorbital nerve. (e) A retrobulbar block. C, an alternative method for the eyelid, injecting under the conjunctiva. *Partly from Peyman et al. with the kind permission of the W.B Saunders Company.*

BLOCKS FOR THE EYE

INDICATIONS If necessary, you can do most eye operations in adults under local anaesthesia.

PREMEDICATION Do this thoroughly. If the patient is restless and bronchitic and thus liable to cough during the operation, consider giving him ketamine.

FACIAL NERVE BLOCK

DOSE 10 ml of 0.5 per cent bupivacaine with adrenaline or 2% lignocaine.

(a) AT THE NECK OF THE MANDIBLE Explain the procedure to the patient. Feel for the head and neck of his mandible as you ask him to open and close his mouth.

Lay your index finger across the neck of his mandible. Push the needle perpendicularly into his skin at the lower border of your finger until it touches the neck of his mandible.

Inject 2 ml of solution, withdraw the needle 3 mm and inject another 3 ml. Rub the area vigorously for 2 minutes with a swab.

(b) PERIPHERALLY Push the needle into the patient's skin 2 cm behind the outer margin of his orbit, level with his outer canthus.

Pass the needle underneath his skin towards the middle of his upper eyebrow. Inject 2.5 ml as you withdraw it.

Withdraw the needle almost to the skin and then pass it subcutaneously towards the middle of his lower eyelid. Inject another 2.5 ml as you withdraw.

Massage the skin of his eyelids to spread the anaesthetic.

The latent period lasts 10 minutes. Check that the block has worked by asking him to close his eyes. There should be no movement of his eyelids. If there is, repeat the block at the neck of his mandible.

Alternative. The tarsal plate limits the spread of the solution. So, if it is important that his conjunctivae be anaesthetic, use separate injections for his upper and lower lids.

Pass a 15 mm needle through his skin at the lower lateral margin of his tarsal plate. Infiltrate 3 ml of anaesthetic solution with adrenaline subcutaneously.

Evert his eyelid over the needle, and then push its point in until you can see it under his conjunctiva. Then infiltrate another 3 ml.

(c) SUPRAORBITAL BLOCK

Feel for his supraorbital nerve at the upper border of his orbit. Using a fine short needle, search for the nerve, until you obtain paraesthesiae. Inject 1 to 8 ml of solution with adrenaline.

(d) INFRAORBITAL BLOCK

Use the middle finger of one hand to feel for the midpoint of the lower border of his orbit. Then feel 1 cm lower down. You will probably be able to feel his neurovascular bundle. Aim your needle at it obliquely by entering his skin 1 cm lower down. He will probably feel paraesthesiae. Aspirate, and then inject 1.3 ml of solution.

(e) RETROBULBAR BLOCK

INDICATIONS Most eye operations in adults.

CONTRAINDICATIONS Perforating eye injuries. If the block should happen to bleed, an increase in the pressure in the patient's orbit may cause the tissues of his eye to extrude from the perforation in his globe. For these use general anaesthesia.

EQUIPMENT Either use a needle exactly 35 mm long, or use a longer needle with a marker at this point. If the needle is too long, or has burrs on it, you may puncture the blood vessels at the apex of his orbit.

CAUTION! Don't add adrenaline to the solution when you do a retrobulbar block.

Lay the patient flat. Ask him to look upwards and medially. This puts his eye into the best position for the injection.

Feel for the lower outer angle of his orbit, and inject 0.5 ml of plain 2% lignocaine without adrenaline into the skin over this point.

Push the needle slowly through his skin. You will feel resistance as the needle goes through his skin and again as it goes through his orbital septum. The point of the needle is now inside his orbit. Angle the needle medially and slightly upwards towards the apex of his orbit, injecting 0.5 ml of solution as you do so. You will feel a slight resistance as it passes through the cone of muscles that move his eye. Push the needle up to the level of the marker.

Aspirate. If you don't withdraw any blood, inject 2 ml of solution slowly over 10 seconds. If you want complete paralysis of the extrinsic muscles of his eye, inject 4 ml. For enucleation, always inject 4 ml. If there is resistance to injection, alter the position of the needle slightly, and inject again. Don't waggle the needle; this is the chief cause of retrobulbar haemorrhage.

The latent period lasts about 5 minutes.

DIFFICULTIES ANAESTHETIZING THE EYE

If the patient's eye is pushed forwards and its lids become swollen and tense, a retrobulbar haematoma is forming. Fortunately, this is rare, unless you insert the needle more than 3.5 cm. If a haematoma is going to form, it does so within 5 minutes. Apply a pressure dressing and defer the operation for at least 5 days until his exophthalmos has gone down.

If, when you have done a retrobulbar block, he can still move his eye upwards, the nerve to his superior rectus muscle has not been blocked. This can be a nuisance. Retract his upper eyelid, and ask him to look downwards. Insert a 2 cm needle into the lateral edge of his superior rectus muscle. Inject 1 ml of anaesthetic solution with adrenaline into it just posterior to the equator of his globe.

ANAESTHETIZING THE SCALP

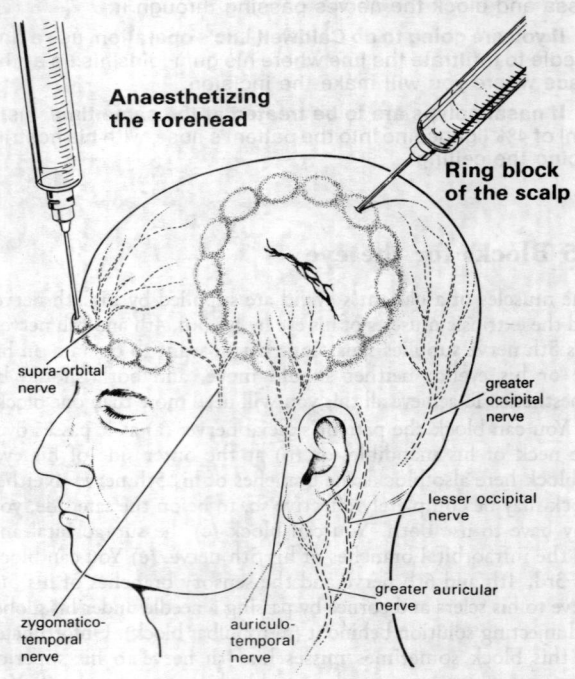

Fig. 6-7 ANAESTHESIA FOR THE SCALP AND FOREHEAD.
Kindly contributed by Keith Birkenshaw.

THE SPINAL DERMATOMES

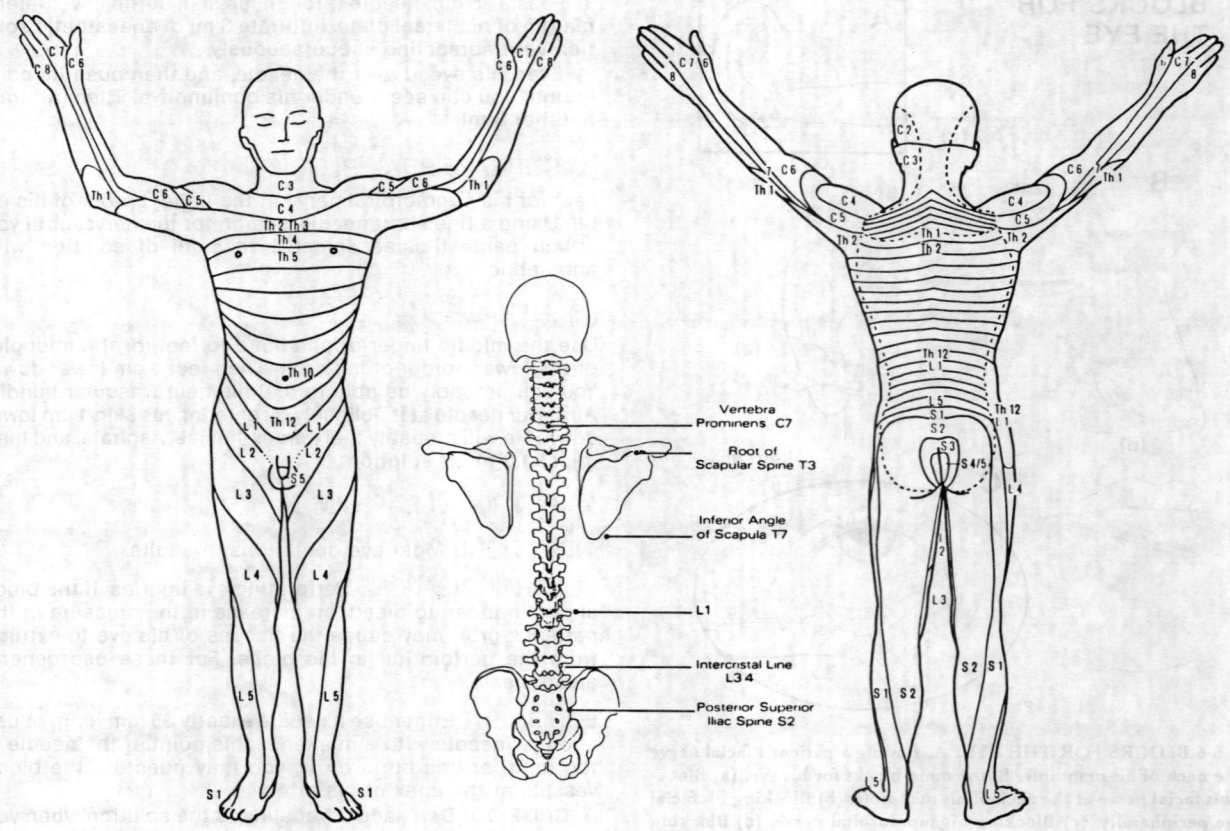

Fig. 6-8 THE SPINAL DERMATOMES. Futher views of these are to be found in Fig. S 64-2. *From Ciba–Geigy with kind permission.*

34

6.6 Anaesthetizing the scalp

Use this method for scalp wounds (S 63.6). Infiltrate anaesthetic solution into the patient's scalp to block the nerves as they ascend over his head. Don't try to aim for any particular nerve. On top of his head you will need a complete ring of solution, but on the sides, you will only need the lower part of the ring. If necessary, you can make a ring all round the head to anaesthetize his whole scalp.

ANAESTHESIA FOR THE SCALP AND FOREHEAD
For most purposes, local infiltration of the patient's scalp is enough. If necessary, make a ring block like this.

DOSE Up to 60 ml of 0.25% bupivacaine, or 80 ml of 0.5% lignocaine, with adrenaline.

METHOD Explain to the patient what you are going to do. First inject the anaesthetic solution into the fibro-fatty tissue of his scalp between his skin and his galea. This needs considerable force, so use a 'Luer-lok' needle. Most of the nerves and vessels are in this layer, so this is the most important layer to anaesthetize. Then, if necessary, infiltrate the space under his galea.

6.7 Local anaesthesia for abdominal operations (intercostal nerve block)

The use of local anaesthesia to produce abdominal relaxation has been known for many years, but it has been neglected since the introduction of relaxants. Nevertheless, some anaesthetists consider that it is a very useful method if you are working single-handed. The alternatives when good muscle relaxation is needed are: (1) surgical anaesthesia with ether (11.2), or (2) a long-acting relaxant, such as alcuronium (14.3). Ether is not ideal in a very sick patient, and long-acting relaxants need special skill, so local anaesthesia is a useful alternative.

There are however other anaesthetists who doubt that local anaesthesia has *any* part to play in abdominal surgery, and consider the methods described here to be complex, risky, and difficult. They would advise you, the novice, to use the standard "crash induction (16.5)" with either a subarachnoid or epidural anaesthetic as second best, but these latter need fair skill.

So you can take your choice! Much will depend on your equipment and experience. If you decide to use local anaesthesia, you need to know that three structures in a patient's anterior abdominal wall hurt when you cut them, and so need to be anaesthetized—his skin, his rectus sheath, and his parietal peritoneum. His visceral peritoneum is much less sensitive, but it is usually wise to anaesthetize it before you incise a woman's uterus. There are three methods, which you can use either alone, or combined: (1) You can infiltrate the sensitive structures immediately before you cut them. (2) You can block a patient's lower six intercostal nerves under his ribs. This should be easy, but many beginners find it difficult. The danger with this method is that it can cause a pneumothorax, which can be fatal if it is bilateral and you do not notice it. (3) You can pool local anaesthetic solution in the rectus sheath.

Local anaesthesia has three important limitations: (1) Although it anaesthetizes and relaxes the patient's abdominal wall, it does not anaesthetize his gut. This can be done by blocking his coeliac plexus and the root of his mesentery, but neither of the approaches for doing this are sufficiently easy or safe to be included here. Fortunately, a coeliac plexus block is not absolutely necessary if you handle the gut gently. (2) Local anaesthesia is slow, so it is contraindicated if a mother needs a Caesarean section in a hurry. (3) You may approach the maximum safe dose of the drug. This is particulararly important, especially with intercostal blocks. (4) If the patient's gut is obstructed, he is likely to vomit, and you may also have difficulty closing his abdomen.

You can combine any of the above three kinds of local anaesthesia, with either of these two:

(1) Ketamine by any convenient route (8.1). This is very useful for a shocked or sick patient. Because ketamine does not relax the abdominal muscles, whereas a rectus block does, these two methods make a useful combination.

(2) You can induce the patient, intubate him, connect him to a vapouriser, give him light ether, halothane or trichloroethylene, and let an assistant observe him while you do the intercostal blocks and the surgery. This is useful method if you are single-handed and have a totally unskilled assistant, because all the assistant needs do is adjust the control lever of the vapouriser. This method does however have the disadvantages of the large volume of anaesthetic solution needed for bilateral intercostal blocks, and the risk of pneumothoraces. If you have suxamethonium, you will probably find that multiple doses of it with atropine will be a better way of producing muscle relaxation (14.2).

The main danger of intercostal blocks (apart from exceeding the dose) is the possibility of a pneumothorax from puncturing his lung, perhaps on both sides. So you should be aware that this can happen and be able to treat it (S 65.5).

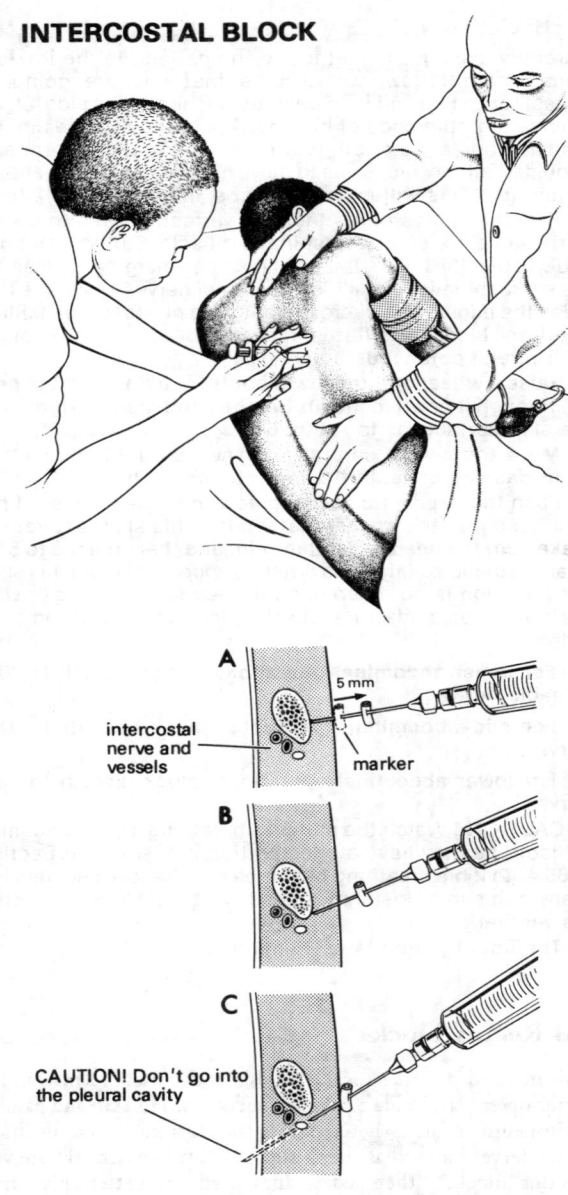

Fig. 6-9 INTERCOSTAL NERVE BLOCK *After Keith Birkenshaw with kind permission.*

INTERCOSTAL BLOCK

INDICATIONS (1) Minor operations on the chest wall. (2) Major upper or lower abdominal surgery, especially if the patient is not fit, or you are single-handed. You can usefully combine it with ketamine. (3) An intercostal block with bupivacaine lasts several hours, so you can use it for relieving pain in severe chest wounds and fractured ribs (S 65.3).

CONTRAINDICTIONS (1) The need for speed. (2) Intestinal obstruction.

PREMEDICATION See Section 5.2.

EQUIPMENT AND DOSE Push an intramuscular needle through a small piece of sterile rubber tube or sheet. This rubber acts as a depth gauge. For each nerve use 4 ml (in a large patient 5 ml) of 1% lignocaine, or use 2 ml of 0.5% bupivacaine. To both of them add adrenaline, except when you are also using halothane or trichloroethylene.

CAUTION ! (1) Keep the needle attached to the syringe. If you don't, and it is in the patient's pleural cavity, you may give him a pneumothorax. (2) This can also happen if the patient takes a sudden deep breath when the needle is in his chest, and so tears his lung. (3) Don't exceed the maximum safe dose (Fig. 5-1).

METHOD OF INTERCOSTAL BLOCK

Carefully explain the method to the patient. In the instructions which follow, we assume that you are going to anaesthetize him and then operate. Lay him on his side. Stand a nurse the other side of his bed. Ask her to put one arm on his shoulder, and her other arm on his hip. Let his arm and shoulder fall forward, so as to move his scapula off the angles of his ribs. This will expose his ribs, including the 12th.

Feel the spines of his thoracic vertebrae. On either side of these lie his soft sacrospinalis muscle. Further laterally, you will feel the hard sufaces of his ribs emerging from under his sacrospinalis. Block his intercostal nerves anywhere between the edge of his sacrospinalis, and his posterior axillary line. Don't block them further forwards, or you will fail to block their lateral cutaneous branches.

Raise a wheal over the lower border of a rib. Push the needle through it down to the rib. Set the depth gauge 5 mm from the skin surface, as in A Fig. 6-9.

Move the needle carefully downwards until you feel its point passing beneath the lower border of his rib (B).

Push the needle point just below the lower border of his rib (C), so that the marker just touches his skin. Aspirate to make sure the needle is not in vein, and then inject 3 to 5 ml of anaesthetic solution. If a swelling appears beneath his skin, the injection is not deep enough. Repeat the process with the other ribs, and, if necessary, block the nerves on both sides.

For upper abdominal operations, block his 6th to 10th thoracic nerves.

For mid-abdominal operations, block his 7th to 11th nerves.

For lower abdominal operations, block his 8th to 12th nerves.

CAUTION ! Watch the patient's breathing: (1) If it becomes difficult, he may have a pneumothorax. If so, go to Section S. 65.4. (2) If his breathing becomes too shallow, because too many of his intercostal muscles have been blocked, control his ventilation.

The latent period lasts 10 minutes.

6.8 Rectus block

This method provides local analgesia and muscle relaxation for minor operations inside a patient's abdomen. His skin and parietal peritoneum are anaesthetized by local infiltration, and his intercostal nerves blocked as they enter his rectus sheath. Before you do this block, either sedate him well or, better, give him ketamine. The combination of ketamine and a rectus block is particularly useful for very sick patients and children.

RECTUS BLOCK

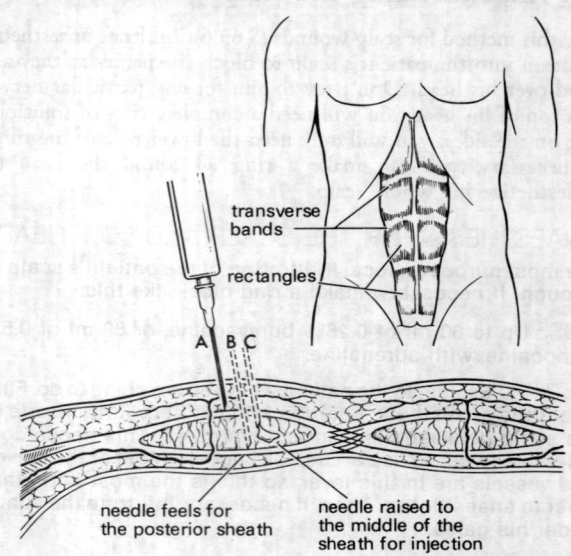

FIG. 6-10 RECTUS BLOCK. *Kindly contributed by Michael Wood*

RECTUS BLOCK

INDICATIONS (1) Midline and paramedian incisions only. (2) Abdominal operations needing only moderate muscular relaxation, or small incisions needing little abdominal traction. (3) Epigastric and umbilical herniorrhaphy. (4) Transverse colostomy and its closure. (5) Tubal ligation.

CONTRAINDICATIONS (1) Any operation requiring good muscular relaxation, a large incision, or much traction on the viscera. (2) A distended abdomen. (3) A laparotomy for intestinal obstruction.

DOSE Six to 8 portions of 5 ml of 0.5% lignocaine or 0.25% bupivacaine with adrenaline. This provides some solution for each segment of the rectus sheath.

METHOD OF RECTUS BLOCK

Explain the method to the patient. Define his rectus sheath, and feel for the transverse bands which cross it and divide his rectus muscle into a series of rectangles.

Raise a wheal of lignocaine in the centre of each rectangle. Push the needle vertically through the wheal until you feel his anterior sheath. Hold the syringe lightly in your hand, bounce it up and down on the anterior sheath, to help define it, and then push it through into the muscle.

Push the needle onwards for about 0.5 cm until you feel the increased resistance of the posterior sheath. You will not feel this in his lower abdomen, because the posterior sheath ends at the arcuate line, half way between his umbilicus and his pubis. If you feel the posterior sheath, withdraw the needle a few millimetres, so that its point is in the middle of the muscle. Aspirate, and then inject 5 ml of anaesthetic solution.

Do the same with all the other rectangles of his rectus muscle. Finally, infiltrate his skin and subcutaneous tissues in the line of the incision.

The latent period lasts about 5 minutes.

Alternatively, because it is so easy to inject his peritoneal cavity by mistake, you can inject and incise his skin and subcutaneous tissue, and then inject his rectus under direct vision.

DIFFICULTIES Puncture of the peritoneal cavity, or bowel is the most common complication. This is more likely to happen if the patient has a distended abdomen. Fortunately, peritoneal puncture is unlikely to be serious.

6.9 Local anaesthesia for Caesarean section

This is a safe, inexpensive way of anaesthetizing a mother for Caesarean section. It reduces bleeding, it does not usually aggravate hypotension, and it is easy for a single-handed operator. If a mother's general condition is very poor, for example from antepartum haemorrhage or eclampsia, it may be the safest way to anaethetize her. Provided she has not been oversedated, her baby's respiration is not depressed. Not suprisingly, local anaesthesia for Caesarean section is growing in popularity. The baby is usually delivered kicking and screaming and his mother has the joy of hearing his first cry. The method does however have some disadvantages: (1) She feels considerable discomfort as you lift his deeply engaged head from her pelvis. A saddle block avoids this, which is why it is much the best local or regional method. (2) Local anaesthesia takes a little longer unless you are expert, and exposure is more limited. When you are expert you can do it fast enough, even for such operations as cord prolapse.

You have several methods to choose from; they all assume that you are going to make a midline incision. Method (6) and after that method (4) are probably the best.

(1) You can premedicate a mother and infiltrate the incision site alone, as in Fig. 6-11.

(2) You can use local infiltration, without giving her any pethidine until the cord is cut.

(3) You can combine local anaesthesia with blocking her intercostal nerves or her rectus sheath. With this method she is not completely comfortable while you are working in her pelvis. Handling her uterus, intestines, or mesentery can be painful. Delivering the baby's head also causes severe discomfort, so does suturing a tear in her lower segment.

(4) You can use local infiltration, ketamine and diazepam. As we point out later (8.1) ketamine and diazepam are not ideal drugs for Caesarean section.

(5) You can use pethidine and diazepam, but you need to be quick with this method, so it is not for the inexperienced operator.

(6) You can use an augmented saddle block, as described in Section 7-7. This is a combination of local infiltration of a mother's abdominal wall with a hyperbaric subarachnoid anaesthesia of the lower part of her spinal cord. This is the best method—she is completely comfortable and is in no risk of hypotension.

Provided you do not give more the maximum safe dose (5-1), it seems to matter little which agent you use. For all these methods (except a saddle block), add adrenaline.

Premedication for Caesarean section is difficult because a mother's needs and those of her baby conflict. Any kind of premedication will depress him, so he is most likely to breathe normally and have a good Apgar score if she has no premedication, as in method (3) below. But if she is conscious and you try to deliver her upremedicated under local anaesthesia, she may struggle and be difficult to control, so you may have to premedicate her, especially if your local analgesia is imperfect. Ketamine crosses the placental barrier, so if you are going to use it as premedication, use it in low dose (0.25 mg/kg). One of the advantages of pethidine is that you can reliably reverse its effect on the baby by giving him the opiod antagonist naloxone (nalorphine is less satisfactory). If you don't have naloxaone or nalorphine, problems will arise with pethidine, and to a lesser extent with diazepam and promethazine, all of which may depress his Apgar score and make him difficult to resuscitate. So: (1) Try not to give any premedication until you actually need it, then to give it in small doses intravenously. If possible, delay giving part of the dose until the baby's cord has been cut, or just before, so that the drugs do not have time to reach his circulation. Once his cord is cut, you can give her much as she needs. Warn her that she may feel pain when you lift out the baby's head, and then give her a further dose of pethidine into the drip. (2) When he has been born, give him the opioid antagonist naloxone, or if you don't have it nalorphine.

LOCAL ANAESTHESIA FOR CAESAREAN SECTION

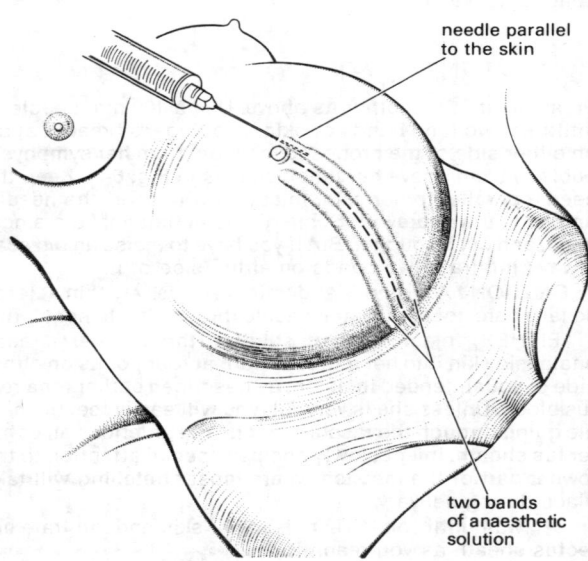

Fig. 6-11 ANAESTHESIA FOR CAESAREAN SECTION. Using a 100 mm needle, infiltrate two bands of skin, two fingers breadth on either side of your proposed incision.

LOCAL ANAESTHESIA FOR CAESAREAN SECTION

INDICATIONS (1) Elective or emergency Caesarean section. Local anaesthesia is more suitable for mothers in labour than for elective surgery, because mothers with some degree of fatigue appear to tolerate local anaesthesia better.

CONTRAINDICATIONS (1) Known hypersensitivity to local anaesthesia. (2) Gross obesity. (3) Intrauterine sepsis (because you cannot pack off the uterine cavity). (4) An uncooperative patient, although you may be able to sedate and reassure her. (5) Caesarean section when you are learning to do it.

EXPLANATION Explain to the mother exactly what you are going to do to her. If she does not want a local anaesthetic, give her a general one.

DRIP With all methods, set up an intravenous drip.

PREMEDICATION This varies with the different methods. Method (2) gives her nothing until the cord is cut. For the others, give her pethidine 50 mg and promethazine 50 mg intravenously, into the drip at the operation, or, less satisfactorily, orally an hour before. Alternatively, substitute the promethazine for the diazepam. If necessary, give her a second dose as the cord is cut.

Give the pethidine and diazepam in different syringes. Ketamine in analgesic doses of 0.25 mg/kg is a useful addition to all methods of local anaesthesia.

DOSE OF LOCAL ANAESTHETIC This also varies with the method. If necessary, you can use up to 60 ml of 0.25% bupivacaine, or up to 100 ml of 0.4% lignocaine, or up to or up to 80 ml of 1% procaine—all with adrenaline. Adrenaline is unnecessary with bupivacaine, but is essential with the others.

LEFT LATERAL TILT Tilt the table 15° to the mother's left to avoid the supine hypotensive syndrome (16.6).

OXYGEN Give her oxygen while her uterus is being opened, until her baby's cord is clamped.

ERGOMETRINE Intravenous ergometrine and its derivatives make a concious patient vomit. Preferably, give her an oxytocin drip, of 10 to 20 units per litre, at 2 to 3 ml a minute when the baby has been delivered. Or, give her 5 units of oxytocin intravenously instead. If you are giving intravenous ergometrine, give it slowly, or give it into the drip as the baby's head is delivered.

(1) LOCAL INFILTRATION FOR CAESAREAN SECTION

Premedicate the mother as above. Use a 100 mm needle to infiltrate two long bands of skin, two finger's breadth apart on either side of the proposed incision, from her symphysis pubis to 5 cm above her umbilicus, as in Fig. 6-11. Keep the needle parallel to her skin. Inject as you insert the needle, and as you withdraw it. Some anaesthetists make a single band, and cut through it. But if you have to incise an old scar, always infiltrate two bands on either side of it.

CAUTION ! A mother's abdominal wall is very thin at term, so take care not to push the needle through it into her uterus.

EITHER, inject 5 ml of solution through her already analgesic skin into her rectus sheath at four points on either side of your intended incision, as described earlier for a rectus block. Unless she is very fat, you will easily feel the needle going through the fascia covering the anterior wall of her rectus sheath. Inject slowly and pay special attention to the lowest part of the incision where most stretching will take place during delivery.

OR, wait until you have incised her skin and infiltrate her rectus sheath as you reach it.

Except in emergencies, allow 5 minutes for the anaesthetic solution to act, then make a midline skin incision, down to her linea alba.

When you have reached her linea alba, inject 10 ml of solution immediately underneath it, so as to anaesthetize her parietal peritoneum. When you reach her uterus, inject 5 ml of solution under the loose visceral peritoneum where you are going to incise her lower segment. Don't use packs. The rest of her peritoneum is not anaesthetized, and she will find packs very uncomfortable.

If sewing up her abdominal wall is painful, give her pethidine 50 mg intravenously, or infiltrate her abdominal wall with more solution.

(2) LOCAL INFILTRATION FOR CAESAREAN SECTION WITH NO PETHIDINE UNTIL THE CORD IS CUT

Without any premedication whatever, infiltrate 15 to 20 ml of 0.25% bupivacaine or 1% lignocaine into the site of the incision from a mother's umbilicus to her symphysis pubis. Infiltrate first her skin and subcutaneous tissue, and then her rectus sheath and peritoneum.

When her abdomen is open, infiltrate her uterovesical folds and her lower uterine segment over the site where you will be making the incision.

Deliver her baby and give her intravenous oxytocin as usual. As soon as his cord is clamped and divided, give her pethidine 50 mg, and diazepam 5 mg intravenously.

If necessary, give her a second dose of pethidine 50 mg before closing her abdominal wound in layers. She may need more local anaesthetic solution as you do this.

(3) USING INTERCOSTAL BLOCKS FOR CAESAREAN SECTION

Premedicate the mother as above. Lay her first on one side and then on the other. Use a 25 mm needle to block her 9th, 10th, 11th and 12th thoracic nerves on both sides, each with 2.5 ml of solution, as in Section 6.7.

CAUTION ! Take care not to exceed the safe dose.

Raise a skin wheal over her symphysis pubis. With a 50 mm needle infiltrate 20 ml of solution behind her pubis, along both her pubic rami, and at the insertion of her rectus muscles.

Raise a skin wheal in the midline below her umbilicus. With a 100 mm needle, infiltrate 20 ml of solution intradermally and subcutaneously along the line of the skin incision. Keep the rest of the solution until you have opened her abdomen. Use it to infiltrate the peritoneum between her uterus and her bladder. This also helps dissection.

(4) LOCAL INFILTRATION, KETAMINE AND DIAZEPAM FOR CAESAREAN SECTION

Infiltrate the mother's skin with local anaesthetic solution as above. When you are through it and about to cut her perietal peritoneum, give her diazepam 5 mg and ketamine 50 mg intravenously. If this is not enough, repeat the dose later in the operation.

(5) LOCAL INFILTRATION, PETHIDINE AND DIAZEPAM FOR CAESAREAN SECTION

INDICATIONS This is a method for the experienced operator who can do a Caesarean section quickly.

Get everything ready, with all the instruments set out, the mother's skin cleaned and towels applied. Immediately before injecting the local anaesthetic solution, give her the first dose of pethidine 50 mg, and diazepam 10 mg into the drip. She will then be in no discomfort while you do the infiltration. There is no need to wait for the latent interval; start operating immediately. If you are a quick operator, the baby is usually ready for delivery through a lower segment incision in about 3 minutes.

At this point you will have to do some heavy manipulating to get him out, and she may feel some discomfort. So, alert your assistant to give her the second dose of pethidine 50 mg and diazepam 10 mg into the drip. Little if any of the second dose will reach his circulaion. He will probably come out crying vigorously, as his cord is cut. The deep analgesia from the pethidine and the local infiltration will allow you to repair her abdominal wall.

BONDING—ALL METHODS One of the great advantages of local anaesthesia is that a mother remains awake and conscious, so give her baby to her as soon as he is delivered. This will help to establish the bond between them.

DIFFICULTIES WITH CAESAREAN SECTION

If you don't have pethidine and diazepam, don't be tempted to give a mother thiopentone while you do the infiltration, and more when you are struggling to get the baby out. This is very dangerous (12.1).

If you need to tie her tubes, infiltrate her mesosalpinx.

6.10 Field block for the breast

Use this for breast abscesses and biopsies. It combines blocking some spinal nerves with local infiltration.

FIELD BLOCK FOR THE BREAST

DOSE 80 ml of 0.25% bupivacaine, or 0.5% lignocaine both with adrenaline.

METHOD Explain to the patient what you are going to do to her. Lay her down with her arm extended. Block her 3rd, 4th, 5th and 6th intercostal nerves in her posterior axillary line using 2.5 ml of solution for each nerve, as already described (6.7).

Raise a wheal at the lateral border of her pectoralis major. Use a 100 mm needle to infiltrate 40 ml of solution into the skin and subcutaneous tissue over the muscle. Reinsert the needle and extend the infiltration to her sterno–clavicular joint.

6.11 Field block for inguinal operations

You can use this block for a variety of inguinal operations, but it needs slightly more skill than the special hernia block that follows. If you have difficulty finding the patient's pubic tubercle, remember that his adductor longus tendon, which runs up the medial side of his thigh, is inserted into it.

FIELD BLOCK FOR INGUINAL OPERATIONS

INDICATIONS Operations for hydrocoele, smaller inguinal hernias, orchidectomy, inguinal node biopsy, and vasectomy.

CONTRAINDICATIONS (1) For very large inguinoscrotal hernias, or for strangulated or bilateral hernias, extradural, subarachnoid or general anaesthesia is better. (2) Obesity. (3) Femoral hernias.

DOSE Use two solutions, the stronger one can be 0.5% bupivacaine or 1% lignocaine. Make the weaker one half this strength, and add adrenaline to both.

Use 10 ml of the stronger solution for the patient's first lumbar nerve, and another 10 ml for his spermatic cord.

Use 20 ml of the weaker solution for his skin, and 5 ml for his pubic tubercle.

BLOCKING HIS FIRST LUMBAR NERVE Raise a skin wheal 2 cm medial to his anterior superior iliac spine. Push the needle downwards and outwards through the wheal until you touch his ilium. Withdraw the needle 5 mm and inject 5 ml of the stronger solution. Inject the other 5 ml as you slowly withdraw the needle through the muscle layers.

BLOCKING HIS SPERMATIC CORD Push your little finger from the patient's scrotum, up his inguinal canal as far as his deep inguinal ring. It will act as a depth gauge and also reduce any hernia that might otherwise be punctured.

Raise a skin wheal at his mid-inguinal point and push the needle as far as the aponeurosis of his external oblique muscle.

Hold the syringe gently and "bounce it through the aporeurosis with a click", so that it lies in his inguinal canal within half a centimetre of your little finger. Inject 10 ml of the stronger solution here and around the area.

INFILTRATING AROUND HIS PUBIC TUBERCLE If you are repairing his hernia, infiltrate 5 ml of the weaker solution around his pubic tubercle. Later, you will have to insert some stitches here.

INGUINAL SKIN Infiltrate 10 to 20 ml of the weaker solution into his skin along the line of the incision.

The latent period lasts about 10 minutes.

6.12 Hernia block

This is the best anaesthetic for an easy hernia. There is little blood loss, it is pleasant for the patient who usually sleeps through the operation, and it shows up the tissue planes beautifully. He can show you the sac, any time you want, by coughing. Dissecting with a knife is kinder than hard scraping with a guaze swab.

HERNIA BLOCK

INDICATIONS Easy hernias.

DOSE 100 ml of 0.25% bupivacaine, or 0.5% lignocaine both with adrenaline.

METHOD Explain to the patient what you are going to do to him. Clean his skin, but do not paint it. Find his anterior superior iliac spine and his pubic tubercle. Mark out the incision 1 cm above the medial part of his inguinal ligament. Make a wheal with a fine needle at the lateral end of the incision.

Wait 2 to 3 minutes.

Infiltrate the whole length of the incision as in A Fig. 6-12, intradermally first, then subcutaneously quite widely to make a 'sausage' of solution under his skin. When you have done this, infiltrate more deeply down onto the aponeurosis of his external oblique muscle.

Now raise a wheal 2 cm above and medial to his anterior superior iliac spine. Inject fanwise just deep to the muscle aponeurosis. You can feel the needle 'click' through it quite easily.

Do the same thing over his external inguinal ring, to anaesthetize any nerves crossing from the other side.

By now you should have 15 ml of solution left for the neck of the sac, so leave the patient for the latent period of five minutes while you scrub up. Paint and drape him.

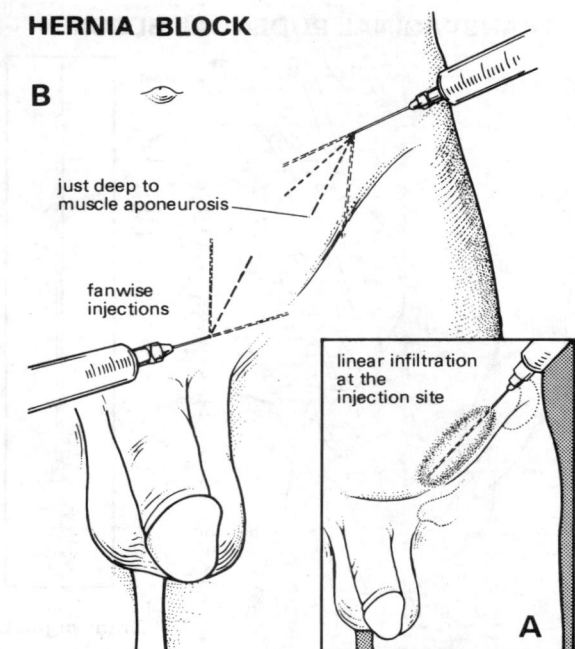

Fig. 6-12 HERNIA BLOCK. You can use this for unstrangulated and strangulated inguinal hernias, and for a femoral hernia. For a femoral hernia you will also have to infiltrate the neck of the sac.
Kindly contributed by Peter Bewes.

When you reach the neck of the sac, infiltrate 15 ml of solution around it. Wait a little before you tie it, because this is a very sensitive area.

6.13 Transvaginal pudendal block

This is an easy and cheap alternative to general anaesthesia, and is suitable for most patients whose vaginal delivery has to be assisted. It anaesthetizes a patient's vagina, her perineum and the inner part of her labia. Anaesthesia is rapid, and she remains conscious throughout her delivery. There is no danger of hypotension or vomiting, her baby's respirations are not depressed, and she does not need to be nursed while she is unconscious in the ward afterwards, as she would be if she had a general anaesthetic. But, her mons veneris and the anterior half of her labia majora are not anaesthetized. Also, good analgesia is more difficult than with a saddle block.

You can approach her pudendal nerve through her perineum, but it is better to approach it through her vagina, and block it as it crosses her sacrospinous ligament close to her ischial spine. Here, you can anaesthetize all its branches simultaneously; there is no trauma to her perineum; a wider area of anaesthesia is produced; her levator ani muscles are more relaxed; and you will need less local anaesthetic.

• *NEEDLE, with bulbous guard, for transvaginal pudendal block, Luer fitting, 140 mm, 4 only.* The bulbous guard on the end of this needle prevents it penetrating too far and missing the pudendal nerve.

TRANSVAGINAL PUDENDAL BLOCK

INDICATIONS Normal deliveries, episiotomies, low forceps extraction, vacuum extraction, breech delivery.

CONTRAINDICATIONS Intraterine procedures such as a manual removal of the placenta, high forceps extraction etc.

EQUIPMENT Use either an ordinary strong flexible 1.4×150 mm spinal needle, or a special needle with a small bulbous guard (6.13).

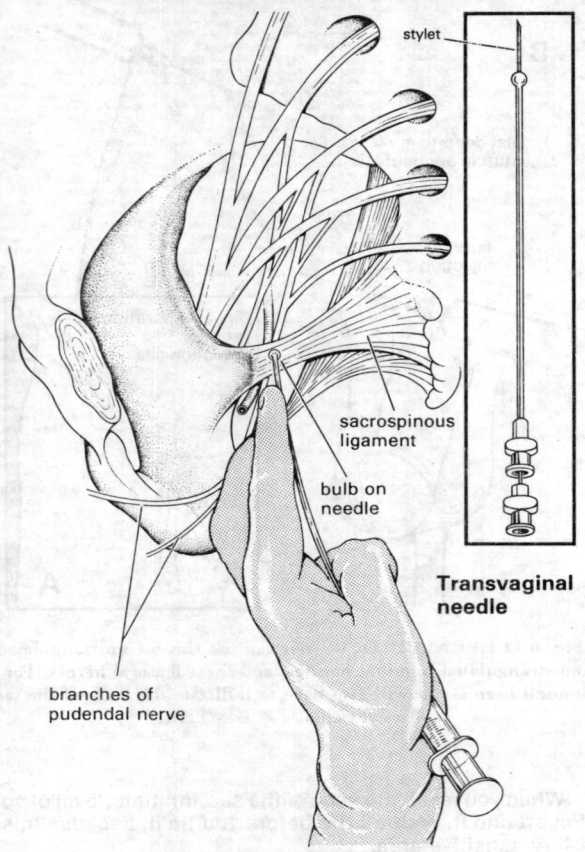

Fig. 6-13 TRANSVAGINAL PUDENDAL BLOCK. This is an easy and cheap alternative to general anaesthesia and is suitable for most patients who need an assisted delivery.

DOSE Use 0.5% bupivacaine, 1% lignocaine, or 1.5% procaine, all with adrenaline. Fill a 20 ml syringe and use 10 ml for each pudendal nerve.

METHOD Explain to the mother what you are going to do, put her into the lithotomy position, swab, drape and catheterize her.

To block her right pudendal nerve, hold the barrel of the syringe in your left hand. Use your left index finger to guide the end of the needle into her vagina up to the tip of the right ischial spine. Put your left thumb round the needle and make it arch upwards.

Feel for the tip of her ischial spine with the end of your left index finger. If it is difficult to find, feel for the upper border of her sacrospinous ligament, and follow it to the spine. Push the needle through her vaginal wall into her sacrospinous ligament, about 5 mm beyond the tip of her ischial spine. Only occasionally will she feel any pain as you do this.

Now, push the needle through her sacrospinous ligament until resistance starts to give (about 1 cm). This shows that the needle must now be through the ligament close to the nerve. If you are using the special needle, advance it up to the limit of this guard. Aspirate, and then, if you don't aspirate blood, inject 10 ml of solution. If you do aspirate blood, change the position of the needle.

Change hands and block her left pudendal nerve.

Prick her perineum with a needle and ask her if she can feel it. Ask her to draw in her anus. If anaesthesia is satisfactory, she can do neither of these things. When the block is effective, her introitus will gape open.

Anaesthesia starts in about 2 minutes, and lasts 30 minutes. You can repeat the block if necessary.

If necessary, infiltrate the site of the episiotomy.

If you are doing a symphysiotomy, use additional local infiltration.

6.14 Paracervical block

The autonomic nerve fibres which supply a patient's uterus and vagina form a plexus in her parametrium. Anaesthetizing them will minimise the pain of the first stage of labour, but not that from the second stage. If you want to make this painless, combine a paracervical block with a pudendal block. But: (1) a woman's parametrium is difficult to get at during labour; (2) because her parametrium is so vascular there is a danger that the drug will be absorbed too quickly and affect the fetus; (3) with lignocaine, analgesia is short, about 2 hours at the most.

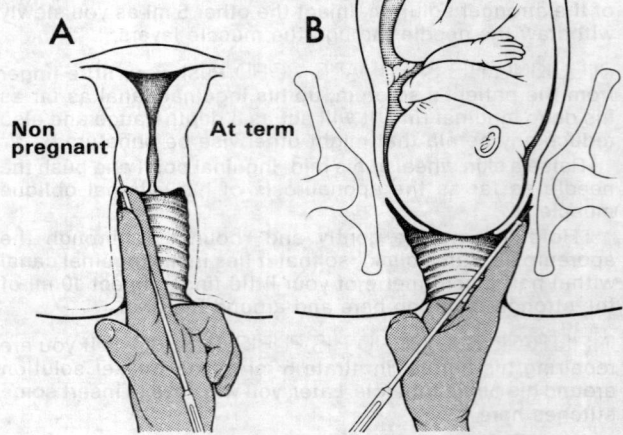

Fig. 6-14 PARACERVICAL BLOCK. A, a non–pregnant uterus. B, a uterus at term.

INDICATIONS (1) Analgesia during the first stage of labour, if necessary combined with a pudendal block during the second stage. (2) Dilatation and curettage. (3) Hysterotomy.

DRUGS AND EQUIPMENT Ten to 15 ml of 1% lignocaine. Or, 8 to 10 ml of 0.125% or 0.25% bupivacaine. If you are adding adrenaline, make it weaker than usual—1:300 000 or 1:400 000. Make this by making the usual concentration of 1:200,000 (5.4) and then adding it to plain solution in a proportion of 2:1 or 1:1 respectively. Adrenaline in the standard 1:200 000 concentration is particularly necessary for hysterotomy, because it minimises the severe bleeding that may occur.

If possible, use a special guarded (Kobak) needle, if not use a spinal needle.

METHOD Place the patient in the lithotomy position and prepare her vagina and surrounding skin. If she is a primip do the block when she is 3 cm dilated; if she is a multip do it when she is 5 cm.

Using your index and middle fingers, guide the needle into the lateral fornix of her vagina in the 3 o'clock position, pointing it cranially, laterally and dorsally. Push the needle about 5 mm through her vaginal fornix, aspirate and inject 10 to 15 ml of solution.

Wait a few minutes, for any excess drug to be absorbed and repeat the block on the other side in the 9 o'clock position.

CAUTION! (1) If you also do a pudendal block, be careful not to exceed the safe dose for both blocks combined. (2) Be sure to aspirate before you inject. (3) Be prepared to control her ventilation if necessary.

6.15 Ring block for the penis

You can use infiltration anaesthesia to do most minor operations on a patient's penis. His foreskin is supplied by two dorsal cutaneous nerves which traverse his penis in the one o'clock and 11 o'clock positions. If you infiltrate these areas at the base of

RING BLOCK OF THE PENIS

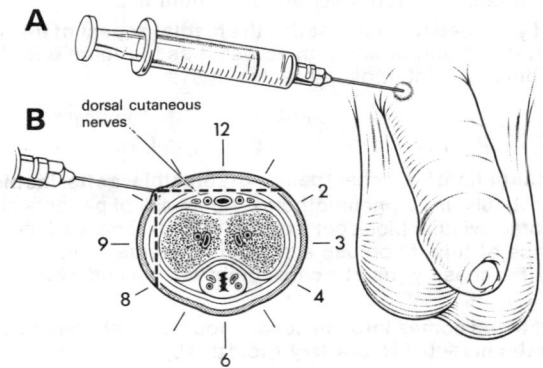

Fig. 6-15 RING BLOCK OF THE PENIS. *After G.J. Hill II, with kind permission.*

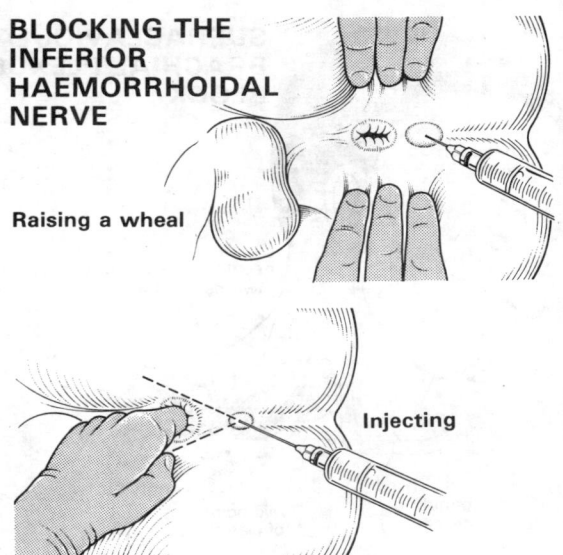

Fig. 6-16 BLOCKING THE INFERIOR HAEMORRHOIDAL NERVES. A, raising the wheal. B, doing the injection. *Kindly contributed by J. C. Goliger.*

his penis, it will usually become completely anaesthetic. To make quite sure, most surgeons make a ring block all round it. *Don't add adrenaline to the anaesthetic solution. If you do his penis may become gangrenous!* If you use bupivacaine, this method is as effective and long—lasting as a caudal block. Another method is described in 'Primary Surgery' using local infiltration along the lines of the incision, and is said to be more effective in unskilled hands.

RING BLOCK FOR THE PENIS

INDICATIONS (1) Circumcision. (2) Dorsal preputial slit. (3) Meatotomy. (4) Cutaneous biopsy. (5) Reduction of paraphimosis.

DRUGS 0.25% bupivacaine or 0.5% plain lignocaine, both *without* adrenaline!

METHOD Make a subcutaneous skin wheal. Then advance the needle subcutaneously across the patient's penis, as in B, Fig. 6-15. Aspirate to make sure you have not entered his corpora cavernosa, and then inject 3 to 5 ml of solution in the 2 o'clock position. Do the same thing for the 8 o'clock position. Then take the needle out and do the same thing on the other side, until you have anaesthetized all four quadrants.

6.16 Anaesthetizing the anus

If you want to do a minor operation on a patient's anus, you will find that local infiltration anaesthesia is very convenient. If you need to divide his internal sphincter to relieve a fissure, you can block his inferior rectal nerves and with them the fourth branch of his sacral nerve on both sides. In about 5 minutes this will paralyse his external sphincter, and provide a varying but usually considerable degree of anaesthesia of his anus.

LOCAL INFILTRATION OF THE ANUS

INDICATIONS (1) Evacuation of an anal haematoma. (2) Excision of a skin tag. (3) Hypertrophied anal papilla. (4) Piles can be done by this method. (5) Division of the internal sphincter for fissure–in–ano.

Infiltrate the patient's tissues with 1% lignocaine or procaine in the site where you are going to operate.

INFERIOR HAEMORRHOIDAL NERVE BLOCK

INDICATIONS Internal sphincterotomy.

METHOD
If you are right handed, you will find that you can do this block more conveniently if you lay the patient on his *right side*, and then turn him over to do the operation.

Separate his buttocks and clean the skin behind his anus with an antiseptic solution. Using a fine needle, raise a wheal 2.5 cm behind his anal verge in the midline.

Attach a 75 mm needle to the syringe. Put the index finger of your left hand into his anus. Using this as a guide, inject 15 to 20 ml of 2% lignocaine with adrenaline beside his anal canal on either side.

CAUTION ! (1) Keep the needle deep, so that there is no visible swelling of his perianal tissues. (2) 20 ml of 2% lignocaine with adrenaline is the maximum adult dose, so don't exceed it.

If anaesthesia is not complete, infiltrate the subcutaneous tissues all round his anus, or merely the lesion you are going to deal with.

6.17 Supraclavicular brachial plexus block

You can block a patient's brachial plexus, either: (1) above his clavicle, as its cords pass over his first rib, or (2) in his axilla, where its nerves lie close to his axillary artery. The aim of both methods is to inject the drug inside the fibrous sheath that covers the plexus from its exit from his spine to several centimetres beyond his axilla. An axillary block is easier, and there is less danger of complications, but it will not anaesthetize his shoulder. Operations on a patient's hand and forearm are so much more common that those on his forearm and shoulder, that some surgeons and anaesthetists consider that a supraclavicular brachial plexus blocks is obsolete. It is a certainly *not* a method for the careless operator!

If you block the patient's brachial plexus above his clavicle, his intercosto—brachial nerve will not be anaesthetized. This nerve may supply skin near his elbow, so block it separately for operations on his elbow.

SUPRACLAVICULAR BRACHIAL PLEXUS BLOCK

INDICATIONS (1) Dislocation of a patient's shoulder. (2) All operations below his shoulder. (3) Fractures of his arm. You can use it for an amputation, but this is not kind.

CONTRAINDICATIONS (1) Operations on both arms. You will exceed the safe dose, and if you cause pneumothoraces on both sides they may be dangerous. You can also block the

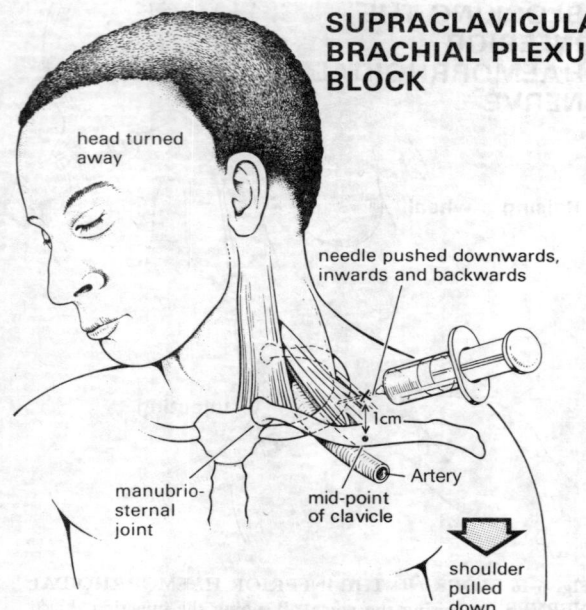

Fig. 6-17 BLOCKING A PATIENT'S BRACHIAL PLEXUS above his clavicle as its cords pass over the first rib. This is not such an easy or such a useful block as an axillary brachial plexus block. There is also the danger that you may cause a pneumo– or a haemothorax. Its advantage is that anaesthesia extends higher in a patient's arm. *Kindly contributed by Keith Birkenshaw.*

phrenic nerve by mistake. (2) The block will be difficult if the patient has a fat neck.

EQUIPMENT Use a needle that is not longer than 2 cm, and is 0.8 mm or smaller, so that, if you accidentally puncture the subclavian artery, no harm will be done.

PREMEDICATION See Section 5.2.

DOSE 15 to 20 ml of 0.5% bupivacaine, or 2% lignocaine, both with adrenaline. This approaches the maximum safe dose for an adult.

LANDMARKS Put a rolled up towel under the middle of the patient's back. Turn his head away from the arm to be anaesthetized. Put his arm by his side. Push his shoulder down, so as to stretch his brachial plexus over his first rib.

Define a point "X" 1 cm above the mid point of his clavicle. Feel for his subclavian artery. The point should be just lateral to it. Mark it and raise a wheal there. Palpate it carefully; you will feel the trunks and divisions of his brachial plexus. They are inside a firm sheath and pass over something which feels very hard—his first rib.

Find his manubrio–sternal joint. Directly behind it lies his fourth thoracic vertebra.

INJECTION Insert the needle through the wheal 1 cm above the midpoint of the patient's clavicle. Hold the syringe like a spear and push the needle downwards, inwards, and backwards towards his fourth thoracic vertebra. Push his subclavian artery medially while you do this. If you have pushed his shoulder well downwards, the needle should hit the first rib within 2 cm. When you hit his rib, aspirate to make sure the needle is not in his subclavian artery, and inject 10 ml. Then, palpating his first rib with the point of the needle, direct the needle slightly more anteriorly and inject 5 ml more, to anaesthetize the lower trunk of his brachial plexus.

If the needle travels on past the first rib, it will soon be in his pleura. A warning sign may be a cough. If you do not hit his first rib, withdraw the needle slightly, change its direction, and push it in again.

CAUTION ! Don't push the needle up and down while you are searching, or you will fill the patient's pleura with holes.

If possible the patient should feel paraesthesiae. If he does not feel them, withdraw the needle and try again. If you can obtain paraesthesiae, the block will be more certain and work more quickly.

The latent period lasts about 20 minutes.

If you need to anaesthetize the medial aspect of his arm, infiltrate a band of solution across it as in Figure 6-18. This will block his intercosto–brachial nerve.

DIFFICULTIES WITH A SUPRACLAVICULAR BLOCK

If the patient feels chest pain and is breathless after the block he probably has a pneumothorax. About 4% of patients given a supraclavicular block get a pneumothorax. There will be less chance of this if you use a short fine needle. Take an x-ray, and, if necessary, insert a chest drain with an underwater seal (S 65.2).

If blood comes into the needle, you have entered a vessel, probably his subclavian artery. Avoid this by pushing the subclavian artery medially when you push in the needle. In any nerve block, *always aspirate before you inject.*

If you have blocked other nerves by mistake, you have not placed the needle correctly. If the patient is only able to whisper, his recurrent nerve is blocked. If his pupil is smaller on the side of the block, and his face is warm, pink, and without sweat, you have blocked his stellate ganglion. These signs are not important, except that they show anaesthesia may be inadequate, because the solution is in the wrong place.

ALTERNATIVE METHOD FOR A SUPRACLAVICULAR BLOCK

Use 30 ml of 1.5% lignocaine. Push the needle (unconnected to the syringe) through the skin. Then fill the needle with a few drops of solution, leaving a drop of solution on the adaptor. Advance the needle downwards, inwards and backwards, asking for paraesthesiae. If you get them, connect the syringe and inject all 30 ml. If the needle strikes his first rib, draw it back 5 mm and inject 10 ml. Then come back to his skin and advance the needle at a slightly different angle, trying again to elicit paraesthesiae. If you get them inject the rest of the solution. If you don't get them, inject above his rib.

If blood comes out of the needle, you are too medial. Draw back and advance the needle to the same depth a little laterally. Aspirate again. If now you get no blood, inject all 30 ml. If you enter his subclavian artery, you know where you are, because his brachial plexus is immediately lateral to it.

If the drop of fluid on the adaptor of the needle is sucked into it, withdraw the needle quickly—it is in the pleural cavity! Don't abandon the procedure; check your landmarks, and try again.

6.18 Axillary block

This is a very useful block. You can use it for any operation on a patient's arm, distal to and including his elbow. It is particularly useful for hand surgery. The same fibrous sheath that encloses his brachial plexus and its associated structures in his neck also extends into his axilla. Try to inject anaesthetic solution into this sheath as high in his axilla as you can, so that the nerves that arise from his brachial plexus are blocked before they leave it. Unfortunately, the intercosto–brachial nerve runs outside the brachial plexus, immediately superficial to the axillary artery, so it is always missed. It supplies the medial side of the upper arm. If you are going to operate on his elbow, you will have to block his intercosto–brachial nerve separately.

Sometimes, you will also miss his musculocutaneous nerve, which supplies the lateral side of his forearm. If necessary, you can block that too, low in his arm.

In the method described below, a rubber tube round the patient's arm is used to compress the axillary sheath, and encourage the solution to move proximally. Some anaesthetists rely on pressing the sheath against the head of the patient's humerus. They grasp his upper arm firmly during and after injection.

AXILLARY BLOCK

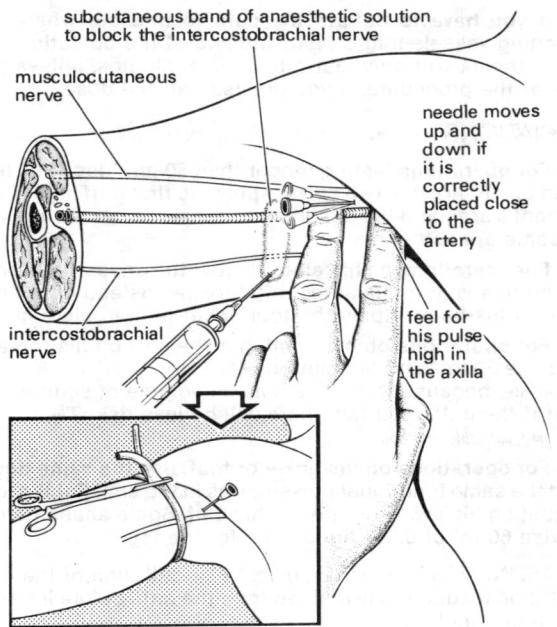

Fig. 6-18 AXILLARY BLOCK. This is a very useful block, especially for hand surgery. *Kindly contributed by Keith Birkenshaw.*

AXILLARY BLOCK

INDICATIONS Operations distal to and including a patient's elbow, especially those on his hand.

CONTRAINDICATIONS (1) Dislocated shoulder. (2) Enlarged axillary lymph nodes. (3) Obesity.

PREMEDICATION See Section. 5.2.

DOSE 30 ml of 0.5% bupivacaine or 2% lingnocaine both with adrenaline. In large patients use 40 ml.

EQUIPMENT Use a 0.8×40 mm needle.

METHOD Explain to the patient exactly what you are going to do. Abduct his arm to a right angle, and place it on the table so that his hand is beside his head.

Feel for his axillary pulse with your fingers as high in his axilla as you can under his pectoralis major.

Keep your finger on his axillary pulse and raise a small wheal above it. Now, put a rubber tube around his arm just below the wheal, to act as a tourniquet, and clamp it with a haemostat to hold the tube tightly in place.

Push the needle, without a syringe, through the wheal. It will immediately fall over, as it is not supported by fat.

Pick up the needle again and push it towards his arterial pulse. You will feel resistance, followed by a "give" as you go through the fibrous sheath that protects his axillary nerves and vessels. The needle should lie almost parallel to the artery. It will now stick out, held by skin and fascia. Meanwhile, compress the neurovascular bundle and depress it slightly downwards with your index finger.

If the needle is in the right place, it will jerk up and down because of its closeness to the artery, or he may feel paraesthesiae. When you think the needle is in the right place, aspirate, and inject. Aspirate several times as you inject all but 3 ml of the solution. As you remove the needle, inject the last 3 ml of solution subcutaneously over the artery. This will usually block the intercosto-brachial nerve.

If there is no anaesthesia on the inner side of the patient's upper arm, you have missed his intercosto-brachial nerve. If you are operating above his elbow, inject a subcutaneous band of solution, as shown in Fig. 6-18. If you are operating on or below his elbow, there is no need to block this nerve.

CAUTION ! Be sure to aspirate repeatedly, before and during the injection, or you may inject the solution into a vein.

Leave the patient with his arm aside during the latent period of 20 minutes, then remove the tourniquet.

If the block fails, do an intravenous forearm block as an alternative.

6.19 Intravenous regional anaesthesia (forearm block, Bier's block)

This is the most useful block in the arm. First, most of the blood in the patient's forearm is drained by raising it, and pressing on his brachial artery. Or, if you want to operate in a completely bloodless field, you can use an Esmarch bandage (S 3.7). Then, you seal his arm from the rest of his circulation by applying a syphygmomanometer and inflating it. Next, you inject a large volume (40 ml in an adult) of dilute anaesthetic solution into one of the veins of his forearm while it is still sealed off. The drug will diffuse from his capillaries and anaesthetize his whole forearm below the cuff.

The great danger with this method is that, if the cuff slips off before the anaesthetic solution has been fixed by his tissues, the solution will suddenly be released into the circulation, causing fits or sudden cardiac arrest. So: (1) *You must use a reliable blood pressure cuff.* (2) You must not remove the cuff for at least 20 minutes after you have injected the drug. This will allow time for most of the drug to enter the patient's tissues and be metabolized. (3) You must have the equipment to treat complications instantly ready (5.9). This is *not* a method for the careless operator!

Prilocaine is the drug of choice, because the results of cuff failure are less severe. Lignocaine and particularly bupivacaine, are effective, but if the cuff fails, the effects of their release are more severe, especially with bupivacaine. Most anaesthetists consider that lignocaine but *not* bupivacaine is sufficiently safe—*if you are careful! There have been several deaths from cardiac arrest following the sudden release of bupivacaine into the circulation when a cuff has failed with this block, or when the drug has been absorbed into the circulation through the bony sinuses, that have been opened by a fracture.*

Never, add adrenaline, to *any* drug you use for an intravenous forearm block, or the patient's arm may become gangrenous.

INTRAVENOUS REGIONAL ANALGESIA - ONE

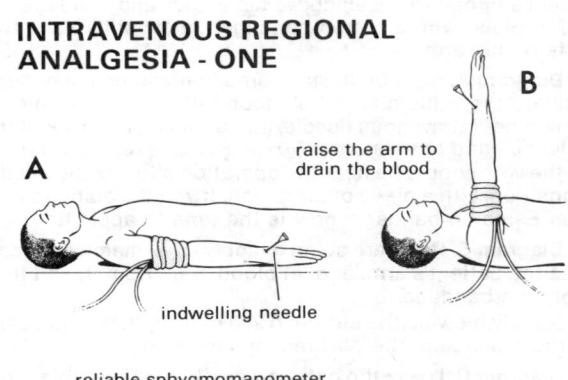

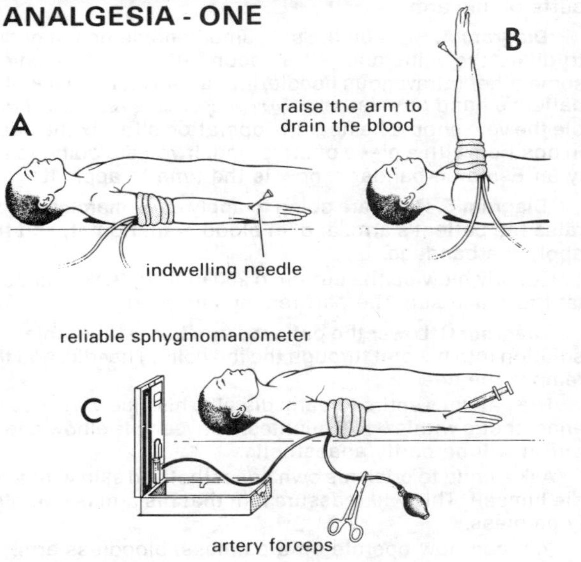

FIG. 6-19 INTRAVENOUS REGIONAL ANAESTHESIA—One. A, insert an indwelling needle and apply a sphygmomanometer cuff. B, Raise the patient's arm, let the blood drain from and it and blow up the cuff. C, lower his arm to the table and inject the solution. *Kindly contributed by Peter Bewes.*

Although bupivacaine and lignocaine produce satisfactory analgesia, they do not cause perfect muscular relaxation. If you want to improve this, you can add 10 mg of gallamine or 2 mg of alcuronium to the anaesthetic solution.

Sometimes, the cuff becomes very uncomfortable. You can avoid this by using two cuffs, and blowing up the distal one as soon as the skin under it is anaesthetized. You then remove the upper cuff.

INTRAVENOUS FOREARM BLOCK

INDICATIONS (1) Operations on a patient's forearm and hand. (2) Reducing fractures below his elbow. (3) This method is only moderately effective for operations on his elbow, including reducing a dislocation.

CONTRAINDICATIONS (1) Any fracture in which the cuff would prevent plaster being applied above the elbow. (2) Operations extending above the elbow. (3) Operations lasting longer than 60 minutes. (4) Cellulitis, because the block may spread it. (5) Vascular disease of the arm. (6) Hypersensitivity. (7) Sickle cell disease or trait. (8) Inadequate equipment. *Don't use this method if the only cuff you have leaks.* (9) Children under 7.

FASTING, PREMEDICATION Neither of these are strictly necessary, but they are advisable.

ASSISTANT *Find a reliable assistant who will take charge of the sphygmomanometer* and watch the patient for abnormal reactions.

EQUIPMENT A reliable sphygmomanometer, or better, two of them, a 40 or 50 ml syringe, or, two 20 ml syringes, and two intravenous needles. Two diaphragm needles, or less satisfactorily, two ordinary intravenous needles.

CAUTION ! Resuscitation equipment must be available.

DOSE Prilocaine 0.5%, 3 mg/kg. Or, lignocaine 0.5% in the following doses.
Adults, 40 ml.
Adolescents 14 to 17 years, 30 ml.
Children 11 to 13 years, 20 ml.
Children 7 to 10 years, 15 ml.

CAUTION ! Don't add adrenaline to any of these drugs.

Put a diaphragm needle into the patient's *normal* arm. If he collapses later, you may need it in a hurry.

Fully expose the upper part of the arm you are going to operate on. Apply a blood pressure cuff over padding, to the patient's upper arm, well above his elbow, and bandage the cuff in place with a cotton bandage. Better still, place two cuffs on his arm.

Diagram A. Blow up the sphygmomanometer just enough to dilate the veins and put a second diaphragm needle, or some other intravenous needle, into a vein on the back of the patient's hand or wrist. *An accurate venepuncture is essential.* If possible the vein should be near the operation site. Fix the needle in position with a piece of strapping. If you are going to apply an Esmarch bandage, now is the time to apply it.

Diagram B. If you are going to apply an Esmarch bandage, raise the patient's arm, and let blood drain from it, and then apply the bandage.

Quickly blow up the cuff(s) to 250 mm/Hg. Ask your assistant to make sure the cuff remains inflated.

Diagram C. Lower the patient's arm to the table. Inject the solution into his arm through the indwelling needle, and then remove the needle.

The patient's entire forearm distal to his elbow will become anaesthetic within 6 to 8 minutes. Between his elbow and the cuff it will be partly anaesthetic.

Ask a child to prick his own anaesthetized skin with a needle himself. This will reassure him that his arm is completely painless.

You can now operate on a painless, bloodless arm.

CAUTION! (1) Don't leave the cuff on for more than an hour, or an ischaemic contracture may develop. (2) Don't leave it on for less than 20 minutes, or too little anaesthetic will have diffused into the tissues. (3) Watch the cuffs carefully.

At the end of the operation, deflate the cuff, and then immediately reflate it. Leave it inflated for 2 minutes. Do this twice to slow the release of solution into his circulation. Sensation will return in about 10 minutes.

If you have to deflate the cuff, to find out where the bleeding vessels might be at the end of the operation, the anaesthesia will only last a few more minutes, unless you repeat the procedure. If you do, use half the dose.

VARIATIONS FOR INTRAVENOUS REGIONAL ANAESTHESIA

For operations lasting longer than 30 minutes, (and less than one hour), use two cuffs. Apply the first cuff high in the patient's arm, and the second one below it after his arm has become anaesthetic.

For operations on his elbow, inject the anaesthetic solution into a vein in his antecubital fossa, instead of the dorsum of his hand. Apply the tourniquet high in his arm.

For operations on his hand, put the cuff on his forearm and use 20 to 25 ml of solution. *Always put the cuff on his forearm if you can,* because you use a smaller volume of solution, so that if the cuff does fail, there will be less risk. *This is a particularly valuable method.*

For operations on his ankle or foot, use the same doses and the same tourniquet pressures as in the arm. Put the tourniquet on his lower leg, not on his calf. Some anaesthetists advise 60 ml of 0.5% lignocaine for the leg

REASONS FOR FAILURE (1) Leaks or deflation of the cuff. (2) Blood inadequately drained from the arm, before inflating the tourniquet.

SIDE EFFECTS The minor ones are ringing in the ears, a metallic taste in the mouth, and slight drowsiness. Convul-

INTRAVENOUS REGIONAL ANAESTHESIA — TWO

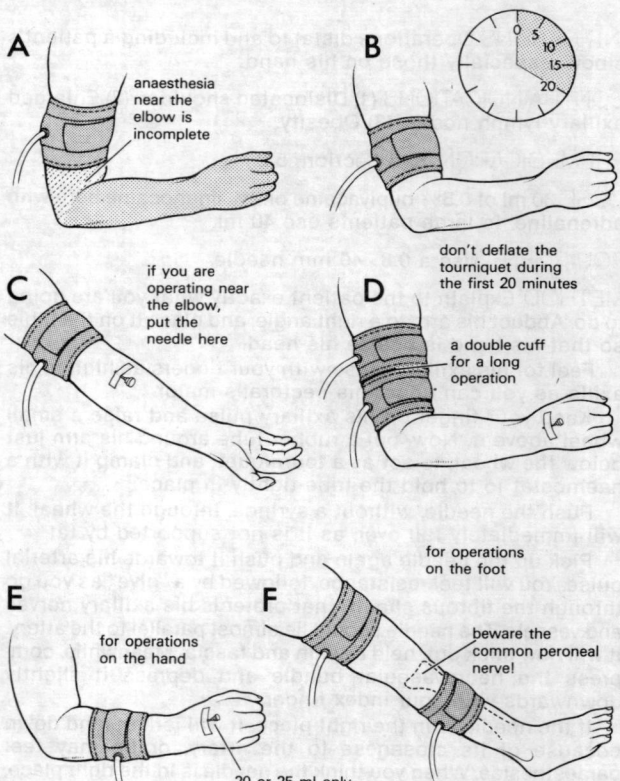

Fig. 6-20 INTRAVENOUS REGIONAL ANAESTHESIA–TWO. A, anaesthesia near the patient's elbow may be incomplete. **B,** don't deflate the tourniquet during the first 20 minutes. **C,** if you are operating near his elbow, put the needle there. **D,** for a long operation, use a double cuff. **E,** if you are operating on his hand, put the cuff on his forearm and use only 20 or 25ml of solution. Hand injuries are common, so this is a particularly useful method. **F,** you can use this method in the leg. *After William Wallace, Riccardo Guardini, and Sue Ellis.*

sions are very rare. If necessary give the patient a bolus injection of 5 mg diazepam, and further doses as required.

DONT USE THIS METHOD WITH A FAULTY TOURNIQUET

6.20 Blocks for the wrist

You can use a partial or complete wrist block for minor surgery. This is especially useful when you want a patient to be able to move his wrist during the operation. The palmar branch of his ulnar nerve passes between the tendons of his flexor carpi ulnaris and his ulnar artery, as in Fig. 6-21. The flexor carpi ulnaris tendon is the most medial one on his wrist. You can usually feel his ulnar artery, especially if his wrist is flexed. His median nerve runs between the tendons of his superficial and deep flexor muscles. At his proximal wrist crease his median nerve lies immediately lateral to the tendon of his palmaris longus. If this tendon is missing, it lies between his superficial flexor tendons and the tendon of flexor carpi radialis. Several superficial branches of the radial nerve run down the radial aspect of the back of the wrist.

A patient can tolerate an Esmarch bandage only for short period with these blocks. An intravenous forearm block or an axillary block is often more convenient.

BLOCKING THE MEDIAN AND ULNAR NERVES

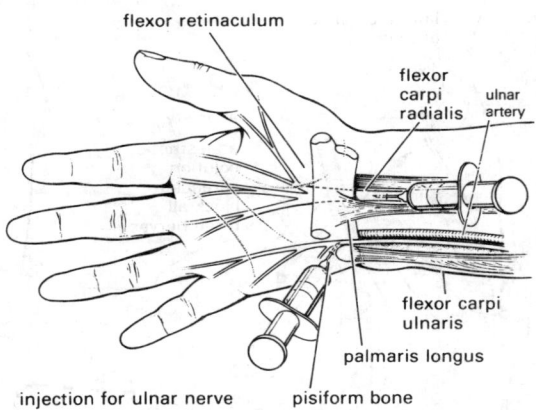

Fig. 6-21 BLOCKING THE NERVES AT THE FRONT OF THE WRIST. Kindly contributed by Keith Birkenshaw, with the kind permission of the editor of 'Tropical Doctor'.

ULNAR NERVE BLOCK

THE PALMAR BRANCH Insert a 0.5 mm needle between the patient's flexor carpi ulnaris, and his ulnar artery, at the level of his ulnar styloid.

If you can elicit paraesthesiae, inject 2 to 4 ml of 1% lignocaine, with or without adrenaline.

If you cannot elicit paraesthesiae, lift the needle a little from the bone and inject 5 to 10 ml of the same solution.

THE DORSAL BRANCH Use 5 ml of 1% lignocaine to infiltrate a subcutaneous band of solution round the ulnar aspect of his wrist dorsally from the tendon of his flexor carpi ulnaris.

MEDIAN NERVE BLOCK

Place a rolled up towel under the patient's wrist. Insert a fine needle between the tendons of palmaris longus, and flexor carpi radialis perpendicular to his skin, at his proximal wrist crease. Move the needle up and down fanwise in a plane at right angles to the long axis of his forearm, until you obtain paraesthesiae. Inject 2 to 5 ml of 1% lignocaine with or without adrenaline. Withdraw the needle and inject a further 2 ml subcutaneously.

RADIAL NERVE BLOCK

SUPERFICIAL BRANCH Use 5 ml of 1% lignocaine with adrenaline to infiltrate a subcutaneous band of solution around the radial border of the patient's wrist. Start it over his flexor carpi radialis, and lead it dorsally over the styloid process of his radius.

CUTANEOUS NERVES OF THE FOREARM

These may supply the proximal part of the skin of the patient's hand. Block them with a subcutaneous ring of infiltration round part of the wrist.

CAUTION! Don't take the band of infiltration all round the his wrist, and don't injure his subcutaneous veins, or you will cause an unpleasant bruise.

BLOCKING THE NERVES ON THE BACK OF THE WRIST

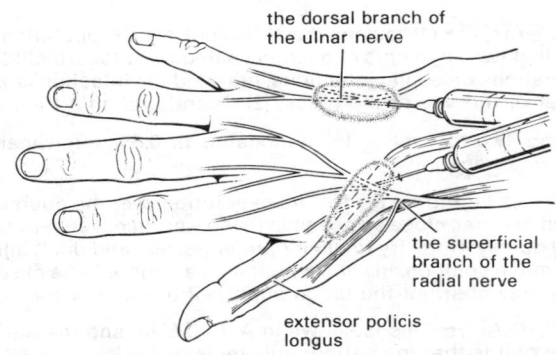

Fig. 6-22 BLOCKING THE NERVES AT THE BACK OF THE WRIST. Kindly contributed by Keith Birkenshaw.

6.21 Blocks for the fingers and toes

Each finger or toe is supplied by four nerves, two on the front, and two on the back. You can anaesthetize these nerves by injecting a ring of anaesthetic solution all round a patient's finger, or better, you can block each nerve separately. If you want to anaesthetize two or more of his fingers, you can block his digital nerves in the palm of his hand. Most hand surgeons prefer this to blocking individual fingers. You will need more solution, but the injection is less painful. Alternatively, a more proximal block may be better, such as an axillary block (6.18), or an intravenous forearm block (6.19).

BLOCKING SEVERAL DIGITAL NERVES IN THE PALM

Inject 2.5 ml of 0.5% bupivacaine, or 1% lignocaine *without adrenaline* in the areas marked with crosses in Fig. 6-23. Feel for the heads of the patient's metacarpals, the injection sites are at the level of his distal palmar crease opposite his web spaces. Sites, 2, 3 and 4 block the adjacent sides of two fingers. Site 1 is more difficult to find, it lies almost over the metacarpal head and nearly in the midline of his finger. Site 5 is similar. Inject about 3 mm deep. If you inject between the metacarpal heads, you are too deep.

To anaesthetize the back of his fingers, inject the dorsal branch of the ulnar nerve and the superficial branch of his radial nerve as described above.

BLOCKING SEVERAL DIGITAL NERVES IN THE PALM

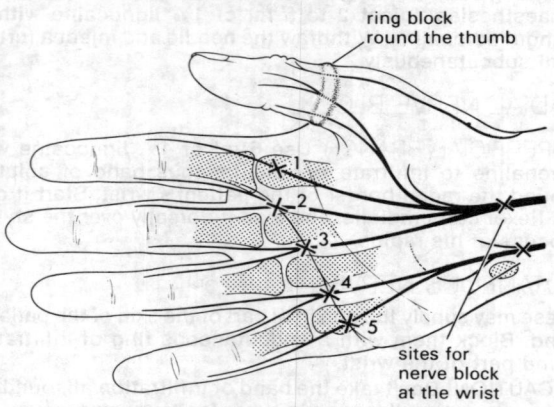

Fig. 6-23 BLOCKING SEVERAL DIGITAL NERVES IN THE PALM. This is better than trying to block several fingers separately. *Kindly contributed by Peter Bewes.*

FINGER OR TOE BLOCK

INDICATIONS (1) You can use this block for any operation on the last two segments of a patient's fingers or toes, including operations on septic infections, provided the infection is well clear of the site of the block. (2) Operations on a toe nail.

DOSE Two to 4 ml of 1% lignocaine, or 0.5% bupivacaine, *without* adrenaline.

METHOD Infiltrate 0.5 to 1 ml of solution over the course of each nerve as close as possible to the web. Inject superfically and deeply. Don't try to elicit paraesthesiae, and don't inject too much solution. In such a tight area a large volume of solution may obstruct the blood supply of a finger or toe.

ALTERNATIVE This is shown in A, Fig. 6-23, and the advantage of it is that the patient only feels one prick. Inject 1 ml on the dorsolateral side of his finger (1), then advance the needle over the bone towards his palm, until you feel the needle under his skin. Draw back 2 mm, inject 2 ml slowly, then withdraw the needle and inject the last 1 ml under your entry point. Now turn the needle horizontally (2) and advance it across the dorsum of his finger. Inject the dorsal nerves on the other side, and the skin over them. Then take the needle out and advance it through the anaesthetic skin (3) to anaesthetize the palmar nerve on the other side.

The thumb. Make a ring block as shown in Fig. 6-23.

CAUTION! *Never* use adrenaline in blocks for the fingers or toes, or gangrene may result.

6.22 "Three-in-one block"

Because the nerves of a patient's legs are not so conveniently arranged as those of his arms, most anaesthetists prefer subarachnoid anaesthesia to a combination of nerve blocks. But you can anaesthetize his whole leg with only two injections, one for his sciatic nerve, and another that will block his femoral nerve, his obturator nerve and the lateral cutaneous nerve of his thigh simultaneously. This block is sometimes called the "Three-in-one block". Success depends on using a large volume of solution (30 ml) and preventing it spreading distally by pressing below the injection site. This is the easiest way of blocking the obturator nerve, which is otherwise difficult to block. Leg blocks may be useful when there is some contraindication to subarachnoid anaesthesia, such as deformity or sepsis on a patient's back.

THE THREE IN ONE BLOCK

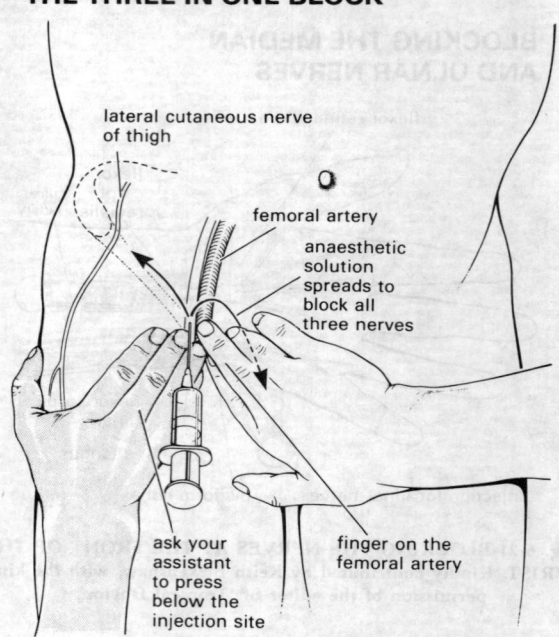

Fig. 6-25 "THREE-IN-ONE BLOCK". This will block a patient's femoral nerve, his obturator nerve, and the lateral cutaneous nerve of his thigh simultaneously. *Kindly contributed by Eugene Egan.*

INDICATIONS Taking a skin graft from the medial side of the front of a patient's thigh. (2) If you block his sciatic nerve also, you can do almost any operation on his leg. (3) Manipulating a closed fracture of the femur. (4) Setting up skin traction.

DOSE 30 ml of 1% lignocaine with adrenaline. Smaller volumes of solution will block his femoral nerve only.

METHOD Explain to the patient what you are going to do to him. Lay him flat, and paint the skin of his groin.

Find his femoral pulse. This lies exactly midway between his pubic tubercle, and his anterior superior iliac spine. Ask your assistant to press below it firmly.

Preferably use a needle on the end of a plastic tube (5.4). Push it through his inguinal ligament just lateral to his femoral

FINGER BLOCK

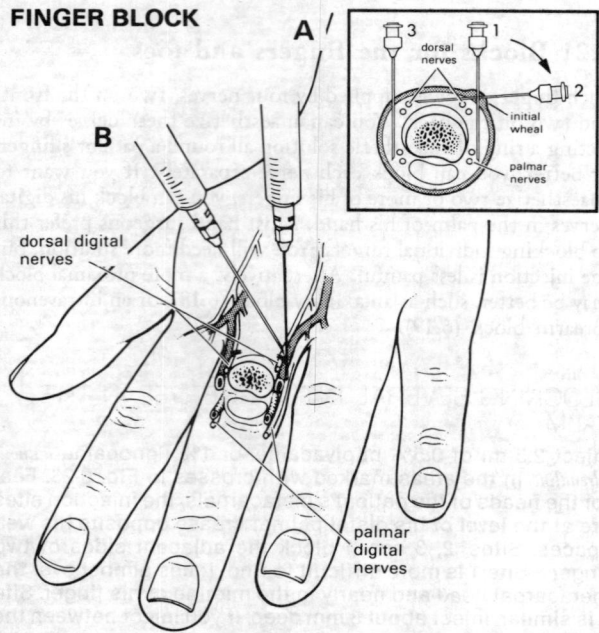

Fig. 6-24 FINGER BLOCK. A, shows how you can inject all four nerves while the patient only feels one "prick". B, shows the more usual method.

46

artery. You should feel it "bounce" through the ligament onto his femoral nerve. Check for paraesthesiae.

As soon as you obtain paraesthesiae, inject. Maintain pressure below the injection site for a few minutes and then massage the solution firmly up and down into his tissues. The latent period lasts 10 minutes.

BLOCKING THE LATERAL COUTANEOUS NERVE OF THIGH ONLY The "Three-in-one" method occasionally misses this nerve. If only a small donor area is wanted for skin grafting, blocking this nerve alone may be enough.

Raise a wheal at a point just medial to the anterior superior iliac spine. Infiltrate the lateral 1.5 cm of his inguinal ligament with 5 to 8 ml of 1% lignocaine, or 0.5% bupivacaine.

6.23 Sciatic nerve block

This is one of the more difficult blocks. The supine position described below may be easier than the clasical posterior approach.

Winnie, AP, "Regional Anaesthesia" Surgical Clinics of North America, 1975; 54, 4: 861-891.

SUPINE SCIATIC NERVE BLOCK

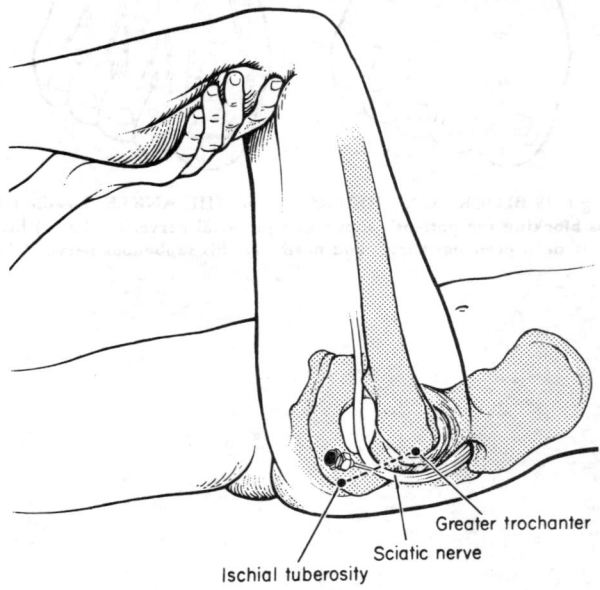

Fig. 6-26 SUPINE SCIATIC NERVE BLOCK After Alon P. Winnie, with kind permission.

SUPINE SCIATIC BLOCK

INDICATIONS Operations on the leg.

DOSE 15 to 20 ml of 0.5% bupivacaine, or 2% lignocaine, both with adrenaline. Use a 0.8×90 mm spinal needle.

METHOD Lay the patient on his back. Ask an assistant to bend the patient's knee to 90°, to flex his hip to 90°, to abduct it slightly, and to hold his leg in this position.

Palpate his ischial tuberosity, and his greater trochanter. Insert the needle at the centre of a line joining these two points.

Push in the needle horizontally, towards the patient's head, parallel to the table, and perpendicular to his skin in each plane while inclining the needle slightly towards the midline. It will meet his sciatic nerve in the hollow between the greater trochanter and his ischial tuberosity.

As soon as he feels paraesthesiae, inject while maintaining digital pressure distal to the injection site.

The latent period lasts 5 minutes.

BLOCKS ON THE BACK OF THE ANKLE

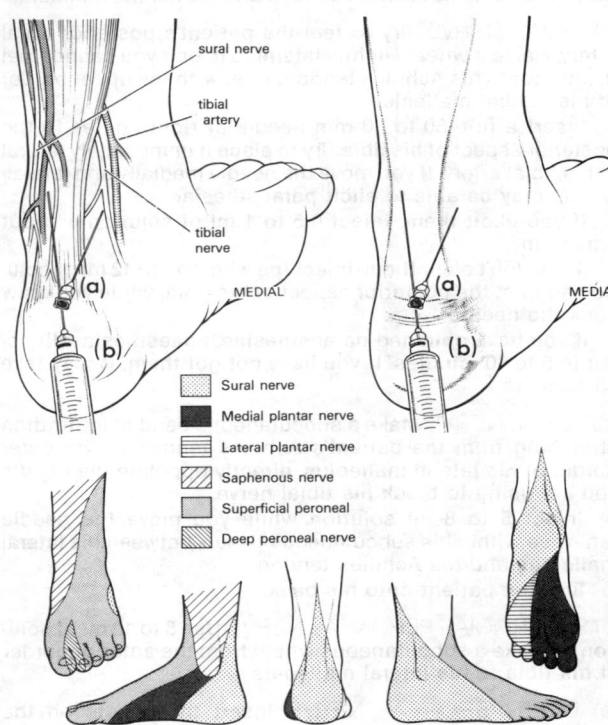

Fig. 6-27 BLOCKS ON THE BACK OF THE ANKLE. Needle (a) is blocking the patient's tibial nerve, and needle (b) his sural nerve.

6.24 Blocks for the ankle

Infiltration anaesthesia is impracticable on the sole of a patient's foot, because his skin is so thick, especially if he walks barefoot, but you can block the nerves at his ankle quite easily. The nuisance is that there are 5 of them, and you may need to block more than one. Decide which ones you need to block by studying Figures 6-27 and 6-28 carefully. Avoid blocking all of them because, it is bad practice to place a band of anaesthetic solution subcutaneously all round a limb.

(a) The tibial nerve lies underneath the flexor retinaculum, close to the medial side of the Achilles tendon behind the tibial artery, and between the tendons of flexor digitorum longus and flexor hallucis longus. Soon afterwards it divides into the medial and lateral plantar nerves. The tibial nerve supplies the whole of the sole of the foot, except for its most proximal and lateral parts.

(b) The sural nerve lies with the short saphenous vein, behind and below the lateral malleolus.

(c) The superficial peroneal nerve runs subcutaneously down the anterolateral side of the ankle.

(d) The deep peroneal nerve runs down the anterior surface of the ankle joint between tibialis anterior and extensor hallucis longus under the superior and inferior extensor retinaculae.

(e) The saphenous nerve runs with the long saphenous vein in front of the medial malleolus.

ANKLE BLOCK

INDICATIONS (1) Operations on a patient's foot. (2) Amputations.

DRUGS AND EQUIPMENT 0.5 or 1% lignocaine with adrenaline or 0.25 or 0.5% bupivacaine. If the patient has vascular disease, don't add adrenaline.

METHOD Lay him face down, with a pillow under his ankles. Clean his heel, his Achilles tendon and his medial malleolus.

(a) TIBIAL NERVE. Try to feel the patient's posterior tibial artery. Raise a wheal slightly lateral to it, or if you cannot feel it, anterior to his Achilles tendon, level with the upper border of his medial malleolus.

Insert a fine 60 to 80 mm needle at right angles to the posterior aspect of his tibia. Try to place it immediately lateral to his tibial artery. If you move the needle medially and laterally, you may be able to elicit paraesthesiae.

If you elicit them, inject 0.5 to 1 ml of solution without adranaline.

If you don't elicit them, inject the whole 10 to 12 ml of solution against the posterior aspect of his tibia, while you draw back the needle 1 cm.

If you have obtained paraesthesiae, anaesthesia will occur in 5 to 10 minutes. If you have not got them, it may take 30 minutes.

(b) SURAL NERVE Make a subcutaneous band of infiltration stretching from the patient's Achilles tendon to the outer border of his lateral malleolus, directly opposite the needle you are using to block his tibial nerve.

Inject 5 to 8 ml solution while you move the needle fan–wise within his subcutaneous tissue, between his lateral malleolus and his Achilles tendon.

Turn the patient onto his back.

(c) SUPERFICIAL PERONEAL NERVE Use 5 to 10 ml of solution to make a subcutaneous wheal from the anterior border of his tibia to his lateral malleolus.

(d) DEEP PERONEAL NERVE Insert the needle on the anterior surface of his ankle slightly towards his tibia, between the tendons of his tibialis anterior and his extensor hallucis longus. Inject 5 to 10 ml of solution.

(e) SAPHENOUS NERVE Infiltrate subcutaneusly immediately above his medial malleolus with 5 to 10 ml of solution.

CAUTION ! There is a risk that you might inject the solution into his saphenous vein, so make sure that you aspirate first.

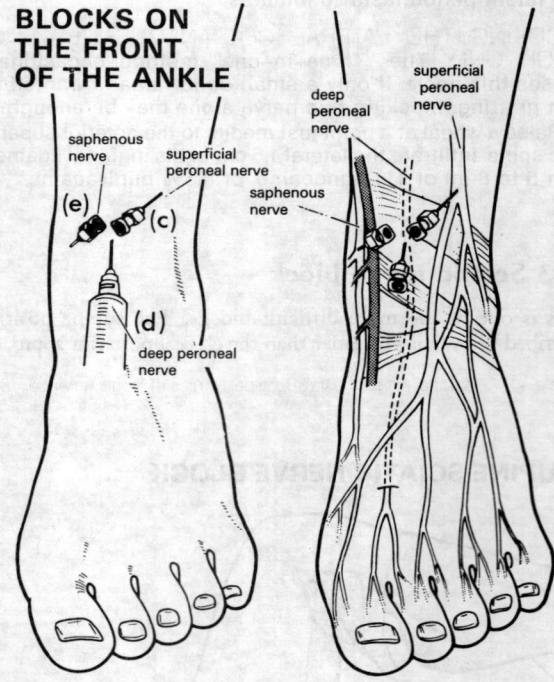

Fig 6-28 BLOCKS ON THE FRONT OF THE ANKLE. Needle (c) is blocking the patient's superficial peroneal nerve, needle (d) his deep peroneal nerve, and needle (e) his saphenous nerve.

7 Epidural and subarachnoid anaesthesia

7.1 Advantages and disadvantages

In subarachnoid (spinal) anaesthesia you inject a drug into the CSF of the patient's subarachnoid space to anaesthetize his spinal nerve roots as they run through it. In epidural anaesthesia you inject *a dose which is 5 to 10 times larger* outside his dura to anaesthetize his spinal nerves as they pass through his epidural space. You can inject by two routes— the lumbar route using lumbar puncture, and the caudal route up his sacral canal. Through a lumbar puncture you can give the patient an epidural or a subarachnoid anaesthetic. Through his sacral canal you can only give him an epidural anaesthetic. Both subarachnoid and epidural anaesthetics are cheap and need little equipment; they allow you to give the anaesthetic and then operate. But they both need careful patient monitoring and *the strictest aseptic precautions. If possible, use disposable equipment.*

Caudal (sacral) epidural anaesthesia is easy and safe. It is well suited to the beginner, and is not used as often as it should be. Unfortunately, even in expert hands, it has a failure rate of about 10%.

Subarachnoid anaesthesia is: (1) Easier than lumbar epidural anaesthesia. (2) More consistent in the segments it blocks. (3) Better suited to a long operating list, because its latent interval is half as long as for epidural anaesthesia—about 10 minutes instead of 20 minutes. Its main disadvantage is its comparatively short duration of action—about two hours with cinchocaine and 3–4 hours with bupivacaine. Fortunately, this is enough for most operations.

Epidural anaesthesia has one great advantage—it lasts longer—3 or 4 hours with bupivacaine, and you can prolong it indefinitely by using a catheter. But: (1) It is more difficult. (2) It is less reliable than subarachnoid anaesthesia, because one or more segments may occasionally be missed, so that you may fail to get a complete block. In expert hands it has a failure rate of about 2%. (3) It is somewhat inconvenient because of its long latent interval. Its use thus requires good planning if you are going to use it routinely in a long list. (4) It is potentially dangerous, because there is a greater danger of a "total spinal", if you manage it badly.

Nevertheless, when you are familiar with epidural anaesthesia, you will find it invaluable, especially for obstetrics. In some hospitals it has become the method of choice for almost all operations on the lower part of the body. In some countries it is routinely used by anaesthetic assistants. But, it is not suitable for the single-handed operator doing an emergency operation for the first time. Don't try it unless: (1) you have the patience to master it, (2) you intend to use it regularly, and (3) you are already expert at lumbar punctures. You will have to become very good at knowing where the tip of your needle is. So, whenever you do a lumbar puncture practise going into the epidural space, and then into the spinal theca, in two stages. This needs skill and some anaesthetists never learn it. Both methods require lumbar puncture, and are easier in young, thin, flexible patients.

Both subarachnoid and epidural anaesthesia have one big disadvantage. They paralyse a patient's sympathetic nerves, thus increasing the size of his vascular bed, and so lowering his blood pressure. If this hypotension is severe, and you manage it badly, it can be fatal. But provided the patient is not hypovolaemic before you anaesthetize him, you can prevent serious hypotension by "preloading" him with some cystalloid solution just before you do the block. If all patients were preloaded with 500 or 1000 ml of saline or Ringer's lactate (the volume depending on the height of the block) before anaesthesia began, "unexplained" deaths under subarachnoid anaesthesia would be rarer than they are. Because of the danger of hypotension, never use either of these methods if: (1) a patient is hypovolaemic or hypotensive before the operation, or (2) you have no intravenous fluids.

Sterility is critical. The equipment for subarachnoid and epidural anaesthesia must be sterile, so use disposable equipment if you can. Chemical sterilisation is dangerous, and has caused meningitis. Never use needles or syringes which have been stored in spirit, or any other antiseptic solution. Besides not being very effective, injecting even a little sterilising fluid into the subarachnoid space can cause permanent neurological damage. If you cannot autoclave the needles, boil them. But you can only do this safely below an altitude of about 1000 metres. If your hospital is higher than this, or your autoclave or the staff who operate it are unreliable, use some other anaesthetic method. Repeated autoclaving, or autoclaving at high temperatures, chars the glucose in hyperbaric anaesthetic solutions and turns them slightly brown, but you can still use them.

TAKE THE STRICTEST ASEPTIC PRECAUTIONS

With both methods, don't forget these rules—:

(1) Look at the patient's back, and if there are septic lesions on it, anaesthetize him in some other way. If you push a needle through an infected lesion, you may cause meningitis. (2) Explain the procedure to the patient. (3) Preload him with saline or some other crystalloid solution, and sedate him beforehand. (5) Follow the procedures we give as to doses and positions exactly and consistently. If you don't do this, you will not know whether some unexpected happening is due to a variation in your method or to some peculiarity of the patient. (6) Don't give him a subarachnoid or an epidural anaesthetic if he has a spinal or a neurological abnormality. (7) Sterilise the equipment with great care. (8) Monitor his blood pressure, pulse and respirations carefully. And (9), most important, have resuscitation equipment instantly ready and know how to use it.

MARY (25 years) was in labour and was being given an epidural block by an anaesthetist at a London teaching hospital. He withdrew CSF. Instead of abandoning epidural anaesthesia and giving her a subarachnoid anaesthetic or trying in another space, he injected the phenol he was using as an antiseptic, mistaking it for lignocaine. She became quadriplegic and was awarded a million pounds in damages. LESSONS You must have a system. Take the anaesthetic solution straight out of the ampoule and don't tip it into a galipot, as this anaesthetist did.

• NEEDLE, spinal, Pitkin, Luer, 0.6×83 mm, 4 only. This is the standard fine spinal needle for patients of all ages and is used with a Sise introducer.

• INTRODUCER, Sise, for spinal needle, 4 only. This allows you to use a thin spinal needle, which will make a smaller hole in the patient's dura and reduce the chance that enough CSF will escape to lower the CSF pressure and cause a headache later. Push it into the patient's back and then push a thin spinal needle down through it. If you don't have one, use a stout intramuscular needle, and push a fine spinal needle down that. A Sise introducer is only to help a spinal needle go through the interspinous ligament. The introducer does not go through into the subarachnoid space. You will not need a Sise introducer for a spinal needle larger than 0.7 mm. Also, it is larger than is needed for a really thin (0.5 mm) spinal needle.

• NEEDLE, spinal, Pannet, Luer, 0.9×100 mm, 4 only. This is an extra long spinal needle for large, fat patients with deep backs. Use it without an introducer.

• NEEDLE, epidural, Tuohy, Huber point, keyed stylet, Luer fitting, 1.6×76 mm, 2 only. This is the standard needle for epidural anaesthesia. Its curved point enables you to direct an epidural catheter up the epidural space, and reduces the risk of puncturing the dura.

• CATHETER, EPIDURAL, Either, CATHETER, epidural disposable, 50 catheters only. Or, CATHETER TUBING epidural, 1 mm outside diameter, autoclavable, to fit 1.6 mm ext. diameter, Tuohy needle, 5 metre roll, one roll only. This is a fine plastic tube used for epidural anaesthesia in lengths of one metre. You can autoclave it and reuse it about 5 times.

• ALTERNATIVELY, purchase all the above equipment in disposable form. If money to buy disposable equipment is limited, disposable epidural catheters are one of the best ways to spend it.

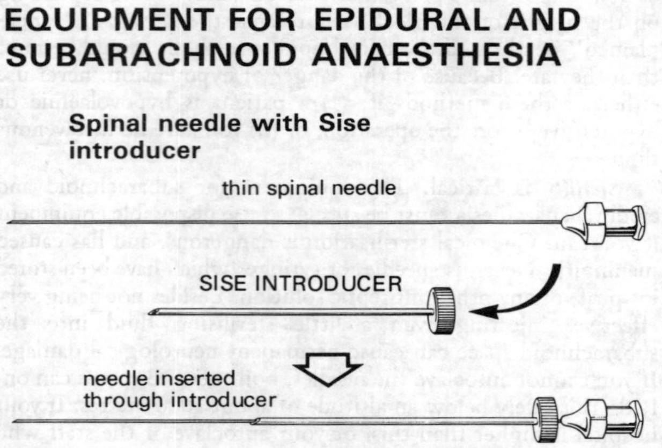

7.2 Lumbar epidural anaesthesia

In this method you inject the anaesthetic solution into the patient's extradural space between the dura covering his spinal cord, and the bones and ligaments of his spinal canal. This space runs from his foramen magnum to the hiatus of his sacrum, and is filled with fat, vessels, and nerve roots. You need a much larger dose of the anaesthetic solution for epidural anaesthesia than you do for subarachnoid anaesthesia. So take great care not to inject it into the subarachnoid space by mistake! This is the great danger of the method.

If you inject an anaesthetic solution into the patient's fourth lumbar space, you will produce anaesthesia which is suitable for lower abdominal, pelvic, and lower limb operations. The patient cannot feel pain, but he is usually not quite so insensitive as he is with subarachnoid anaesthesia. He will have been well sedated, he breathes quietly, and he usually has a slightly low blood pressure. So he bleeds little and is a good subject for surgery. Don't use epidural anaesthesia if the patient is shocked, or if he is a child.

EQUIPMENT FOR EPIDURAL AND SUBARACHNOID ANAESTHESIA

Spinal needle with Sise introducer

thin spinal needle

SISE INTRODUCER

needle inserted through introducer

Making a Huber point on an epidural needle

ordinary spinal needle bent

tip of needle ground off

Epidural needle and spinal catheter

Fig. 7-1 EQUIPMENT FOR EPIDURAL AND SUBARACHNOID ANAESTHESIA. If you don't have a Sise introducer, you can use a thick intramuscular needle. If you don't have an epidural needle with a Huber point, you can bend an ordinary spinal needle, grind it down and make one. 1.2 mm is the practical gauge for an epidural needle, and you may not have one which is so large.

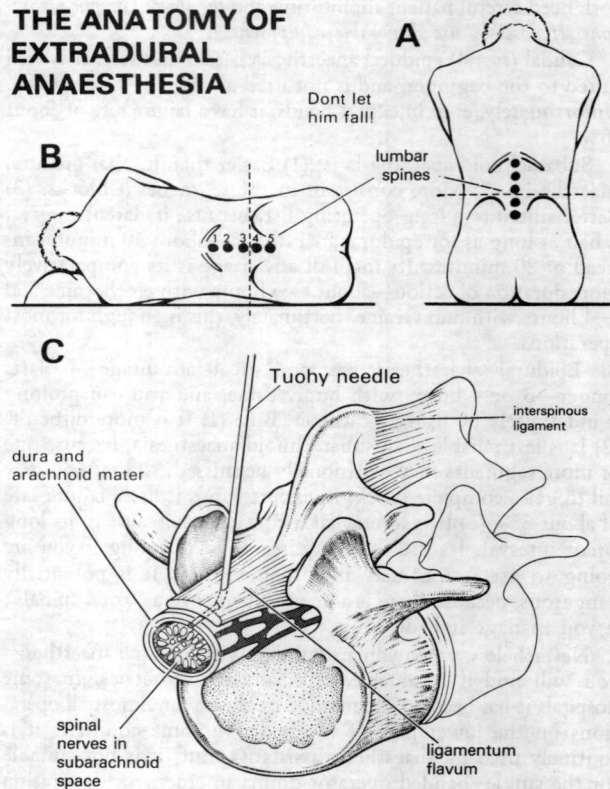

Fig. 7-2 THE ANATOMY OF EPIDURAL AND SUBARACHNOID ANAESTHESIA. A, the anatomy for lumbar puncture with a patient in the sitting position. B, with the patient in the lying position. The line between his iliac crests passes between his 3rd and 4th lumbar spines. C, an epidural needle goes first through his interspinous ligament and then through his ligamentum flavum before it reaches his extradural space. In this figure his interspinous ligament has been dissected away in the segment through which the needle is passing. For subarachnoid anaesthesia the needle goes further on through his dura and arachnoid mater into his subarachnoid space, which is filled with CSF.

There are potential complications.

(1) Transient hypotension is common, but only when the patient's diastolic pressure falls below 70 mm need you speed up the drip, or give him a vasopressor drug. He will usually respond to these measures quickly, provided he is not hypovolaemic, in septic shock, or you have not made a serious mistake in the dose.

(2) The most dangerous complication is mistakenly injecting the large dose of drug, which you had hoped would go into his epidural space, into his subarachnoid space. Fortunately, this error is rare. If it does occur, the patient will suddenly stop breathing, and his blood pressure will fall severely; but if you ventilate him adequately, he will start to breathe normally again some hours later when he has metabolized the drug.

(3) You may mistakenly inject the anaesthetic solution into one of the patient's vertebral veins. This causes fits, hypotension and collapse. This is more common than injecting the solution into his subarachnoid space. If no blood comes back down the catheter, the catheter is unlikely to be in a vein. Pulling back on the plunger of the syringe before injecting, to see if you aspirate blood, is some help in preventing inadvertent injection of drug into a vein. But even if no blood appears in the syringe, the tip of the needle can still be in a vein. A further safeguard is to add adrenaline to the anaesthetic solution and to count the patient's pulse rate after giving a test dose. If his pulse rises within a few seconds, the needle may be in a vein. Unfortunately, there are other causes of tachycardia, such as hypovolaemia.

Some anaesthetists give a test dose of 3 ml of anaesthetic solution. This is only a little larger than the correct dose for a subarachnoid anaesthetic, so if the drug has gone intrathecally, little harm has been done. If the block has reached T10 5 minutes after 3 ml of bupivacaine, the drug is intrathecal, so don't give more. Unfortunately a test dose is not infallible, and its value is disputed, so it is not described in the method below.

LUMBAR EXTRADURAL ANAESTHESIA

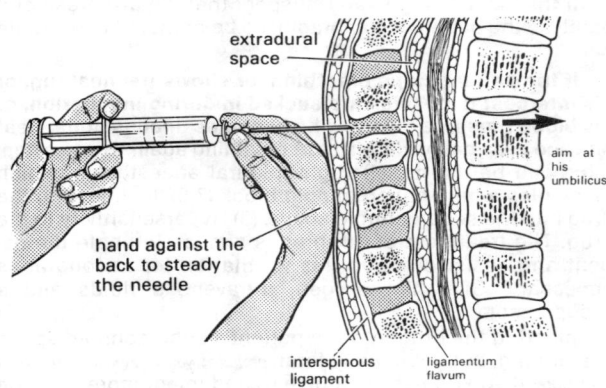

Fig. 7-3 LUMBAR EPIDURAL ANAESTHESIA. Notice how the anaesthetist's right hand rests against the patient's back to support the needle. *Kindly contributed by John Farman.*

LUMBAR EPIDURAL ANAESTHESIA

INDICATIONS (1) Abdominal, pelvic, and lower limb surgery. You can obtain anaesthesia from L5 to T4. (2) Caesarean section, provided the patient is not shocked and the operation is not needed urgently. (3) Normal delivery. (4) Continuous analgesia. (5) Patients in cardiac or renal failure who need surgery. (6) Patients with bronchial asthma and chronic bronchitis who need surgery.

CONTRAINDICATIONS Most of these are the same as for subarachnoid anaesthesia. (1) Any patient who will not cooperate. (2) Hypovolaemic shock. (3) Children. (4) Sepsis anywhere on the back. (5) Intestinal obstruction or peritonitis. (6) Diabetic neuropathy, but not diabetes itself. (7) Lack of intravenous fluids. (8) Equipment which cannot be guaranteed sterile. (9) Old arthritic patients who cannot bend their spines are a relative contraindication. (10) Intervertebral disc lesions, or any other spinal abnormality. (11) The absence of facilities for emergency intubation and controlled ventilation. (12) Bleeding disorders. (13) Any operation on the thorax or above. (14) Epidural anaesthesia is less suited to the inexperienced operator than is subarachnoid anaesthesia.

Additional obstetric contraindications include (15) antepartum haemorrhage, (16) abruptio placentae with coagulopathy, and (17) PIH (pregnancy induced hypertension or pre-eclamptic toxaemia).

EXPLANATION Explain to the patient what is going to happen to him.

PRELOADING If the block is to go to T10, give him 500 ml of some crystalloid solution such as 0.9% saline, Ringer's lactate or 5% dextrose intravenously. If it is to go to T4, give him 1000 ml. Give this immediately before you do the block, and leave the drip up. Don't give the fluid load too long before the block, or the patient will have excreted it before the operation starts.

CAUTION ! An intravenous drip is absolutely essential.

PREMEDICATION Premedicate the patient with diazepam 10 mg and pethidine 50 mg, both orally. If you are doing a Caesarean section, try to avoid sedating a mother, but you may have to.

OTHER MEASURES FOR CAESAREAN SECTION Give the mother oral antacids (16.3), tilt the table (16.5), and avoid ergometrine (6.9).

NEEDLE This depends on whether or not you are inserting a catheter.

If you are not inserting a catheter, use a 1 to 1.2 mm needle with a short bevel. If the bevel is too long it can easily penetrate the subarachnoid space.

If you are going to insert a catheter, use a 1.6 or 1.8 mm Tuohy needle with a Huber point. This is a specially rounded point which directs the catheter up the epidural space. Ideally, the needle should be fairly thick and not too sharp. If necessary, you can put a Huber point onto an ordinary spinal needle. Bend its tip, and then grind away the bent part of the tip, finally, rub it flat with an oilstone, as shown in Fig. 7-1.

DRUGS AND SYRINGES (1) 0.5% bupivacaine will anaesthetize the patient for 2 to 4 hours. (2) 1.5% or 2% lignocaine will only anaesthetize him for 1½ to 2 hours. If possible use single-dose containers without preservative. The doses are given below. Weaker solutions than these may provide only a sensory block. If you are using lignocaine, add adrenaline 1:200 000. To make this, add 0.5 ml of adrenaline 1:1000 to every 100 ml of anaesthetic solution. This is desirable but not essential. If you are using bupivacaine, there is even less indication for adding it.

You will need a 20 ml syringe for the drug, and a 5 or 10 ml glass or plastic syringe filled with saline to test for loss of resistance as you enter the extradural space. The plunger of this syringe must slide easily. Some anaesthetists use a hanging drop on the adaptor of the needle, which is usually sucked in as the needle enters the patient's epidural space.

CAUTION ! (1) Take great care that your equipment is sterile, and take strict aseptic precautions, especially when using the catheter. Scrub up, wear gloves and use a mask and gown. (2) Apply a blood pressure cuff to the the patient so that you will be readily able to monitor his blood pressure.

METHOD USING A TUOHY NEEDLE ONLY

Measure the patient's blood pressure before you start. Turn him onto his side, and draw his knees up to his chin. Alternatively, sit him up, ask him to bend forwards, and ask an assistant to support him.

CAUTION ! If you sit the patient up, make sure he is always supported, because he may faint and fall to the floor.

Prepare a wide area of his back and drape him. Find his iliac crests. A line joining them crosses his vertebral column between the spines of L3 and L4.

Choose an appropriate intervertebral space. For pelvic and lower abdominal operations, use the space between L3 and L4. For upper abdominal operations use the space between L2 and L3.

Raise a wheal in the patient's skin with local anaesthetic solution at the site where the needle is to go. With a scalpel, make a small full–depth incision through the skin, or punch a hole with a big hypodermic needle.

Turn the needle so that the Huber point faces laterally. Like this, it will part the fibres of the interspinous ligament rather than cutting them. Push the needle through the skin cut, well into the interspinous ligament. Make sure the needle is central in this ligament and aim it at the patient's umbilicus.

When the needle is part of the way into his interspinous ligament, remove the sylet. Withdraw the plunger of the empty glass syringe half way up the barrel, and connect it to the needle. Some anaesthetists fill this syringe with saline.

Press the needle slowly but steadily farther into the interspinous ligament. As you do this, put the back of your hand against the patient's back, and steady the hub of the needle with your fingers as in Fig. 7-3. With your other hand push the needle steadily into the ligament, while you try to inject at the same time.

At a depth of about 4 to 5 cm the needle will emerge from the ligamentum flavum, and there will be a sudden loss of resistance to injection. The point of the needle is now in the fat of the extradural space, and the air or saline in the syringe will enter easily. The saline will also help to push the dura away from the needle.

Disconnect the syringe, and turn the needle so that its Huber point faces the patient's head.

If CSF comes out, the needle has punctured the dura. You can now: (1) Abandon epidural anaesthesia in that space, and give him a subarachnoid anaesthetic instead. Or, (2) try epidural anaesthesia in another space. Or, (3) give him a general anaesthetic.

CAUTION ! If CSF appears, don't inject the dose of solution for epidural anaesthesia!

If all is well, and CSF does not appear, proceed:

DOSE Withdraw the plunger so as to aspirate through the needle and help make sure that it is not in a vein. If all is well, give him (or her):

For pelvic operations, 7 to 10 ml.

For a pregnant woman, or a woman in labour (not having a Caesarean section) give less than the usual adult dose. In labour 8 ml of bupivacaine will give a block to T10.

For Caesarean section, 15 to 22 ml. Don't inject during a contraction. Supplement the block by local infiltration of the upper part of the incision as in Section 7.7.

For lower abdominal operations, 15 to 20 ml.

For upper abdominal operations, 25 to 30 ml.

If you are using a catheter, you can, if necessary, give up to three more doses later through it.

LATENT PERIOD FOR LUMBAR EPIDURAL ANAESTHESIA

This lasts 10 to 15 minutes with lignocaine. Pain may have gone after 3 minutes with bupivacaine. Sufficient analgesia for surgery may not appear for 10 minutes and you may occasionally have to wait for 20 minutes. Be prepared to wait for the necessary time. Check the patient's pulse, blood pressure (and the fetal heart during Caesarean section) every 5 minutes. If a patient is going to become hypotensive, he will usually do so in the first 15 minutes. The zone of analgesia will spread up and down from the segment of injection, and reach a maximum in about 45 minutes.

The spread of the anaesthetic solution will be more certain if the patient sits up for about a minute (to encourage sacral spread), and then lies down with the table in a 5° head–down tilt.

If you are doing a Caesarean section, remember to put a wedge under the mother's right buttock.

ALTERNATIVE METHOD USING A CATHETER

This is seldom necessary. Only use a catheter if you expect the operation to last more than 3 hours with bupivicaine, or 2 hours with lignocaine.

Insert a Tuohy needle with its bevel pointing laterally, exactly as described above. Then turn it so that its bevel faces the patient's head. If the catheter is provided with lateral openings cut them off. Use only the terminal opening. Thread the catheter into the needle until about 10 cm are inside the patient. Then remove the needle and carefully feed the catheter through it as you do so. Adjust the catheter so that 2 or 3 cm are inside the epidural space, and about a metre are outside. The length of catheter lying free inside the epidural space is important, so record it. If it is too long the incidence of unilateral blocks or missed segments increases. A Tuohy needle is marked in centimetres, so is the catheter.

CAUTION ! (1) Coil the catheter to make it less likely to be pulled out, and fix the coil to the patient's skin with strapping, as in Fig. 7-4. Bring the free end up over his shoulder and tape it in place without kinking. (2) Leave the syringe firmly attached to the catheter to avoid introducing infection, or use one of the special stoppers. (3) Change the syringe only with full aseptic precautions. (4) Never try to pull the catheter back through the needle, or a piece may break off inside the extradural space. This is a common error. If you want to remove the catheter, do so at the end of the operation and take the needle out with it.

Blood staining of the fluid in the catheter is a potentially dangerous sign, because it indicates that the end of the catheter may be in a vein. So watch for it by leaving a length of tubing exposed, as in Fig. 7-4. If the fluid in the catheter is only stained with blood, leave the catheter in, but start by giving a 3 ml test dose. If pure blood appears in the catheter, take it out.

ALTERNATIVES FOR LUMBAR EPIDURAL ANAESTHESIA

If a mother is being delivered other than by Caesarean section, you can give her 4 to 10 ml of 0.25% bupivacaine, and top it up with 10 ml of 0.5% bupivacaine when the baby's head reaches her pelvic floor.

DIFFICULTIES WITH LUMBAR EPIDURAL ANAESTHESIA

The patient may have any of the complications of local anaesthesia, especially convulsions, described in Section 5.9.

If the block is high early, suspect that it may spread and paralyse the patient's diaphragm, so be prepared to ventilate him.

If the patient stops breathing, or shows tracheal tug, or his intercostal muscles are sucked in during inspiration, or his blood pressure falls and he becomes unconscious, treat him and keep calm! He will start breathing again. These symptoms can be due to: (1) High epidural anaesthesia, which resembles a high subarachnoid block (7.5). (2) Injecting the drug into the subarachnoid space. (3) Hypersensitivity to the drug. The treatment of all three is similar. Intubate the patient and assist or conrol his ventilation for as long as is necessary. Give him oxygen, intravenous fluids and a vasopressor.

Injecting the drug into the patient's subarachnoid space is alarming, but not usually fatal, *provided you recognise it and treat it in time*. If you do not recognise it, and inject more solution after the test dose, total spinal anaesthesia results. The patient becomes suddenly or gradually unconscious and his pupils dilate.

If the patient has twitches you may have injected the drug intravenously, or he may be anoxic due to intercostal paralysis. Try controlling his ventilation.

If he has convulsions, give him intravenous diazepam, or a small dose of thiopentone, 50 to 100 mg. Oxygenate him, intubate him and assist his respiration if necessary. If his heart has stopped, apply sternal compression (3.6).

If anaesthesia is incomplete, the solution may have failed to reach particular segments, or have blocked only half his body. One reason is that the catheter may be in too far. If necessary, extend the area of anaesthesia with local blocks.

If the patient complains of a severe headache postoperatively, reassure him. Headache can occasionally follow extradural anaesthesia, even in the absence of accidental puncture of the dura, and take weeks to go.

If an epidural block for Caesarean section fails, you cannot proceed with local infiltration (which you can with subarachnoid anaesthesia), because you will exceed the safe dose, so change to general anaesthesia. Or, give the mother diazepam 10 mg combined with ketamine 0.25 mg/kg or pethidine 50 mg, but this is not so safe.

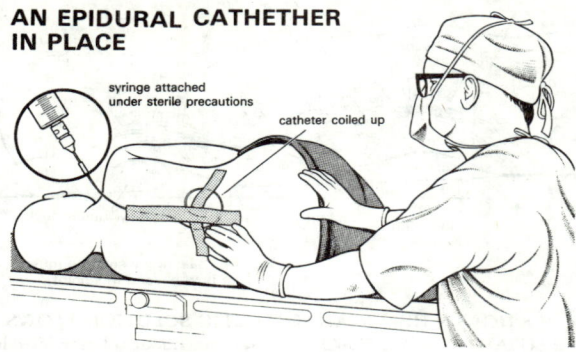

Fig. 7-4 AN EPIDURAL CATHETER IN PLACE. Note that it is coiled so that it is less likely to come out if it is accidentally pulled on. *Kindly contributed by Nigel Pereira.*

7.3 Caudal (sacral) epidural anaesthesia

This is an excellent method for perineal operations. The latent period is short, about 5 minutes, so that by the time you have scrubbed up the patient is ready for you to start operating. There are few complications and no risk of hypotension, so there is no need for a drip. You inject the drug into the patient's sacral extradural space through the membrane covering his sacral hiatus. This is much easier than pushing a needle between the spines of his lumbar vertebrae, and there is less danger of injecting the drug into his subarachnoid space. However, the subarachnoid space does occasionally come down to the second sacral segment, so before injecting, aspirate to make sure that your needle does not withdraw CSF. The sacral hiatus varies considerably: (1) It is sometimes at a much higher level, so that the risk of injecting into the subarachnoid space is greater. (2) Sometimes you cannot find the sacral hiatus. In about one patient in ten you will fail to get adequate anaesthesia. When this happens, you will have to use some other method.

Try the method in thin young patients first.

CAUDAL EPIDURAL ANAESTHESIA

INDICATIONS (1) Anal, perineal, urological, gynaecological and obstetric operations that do not involve the anterior abdominal wall, particulary in outpatients. (2) Dilation and curettage, Lord's anal stretch haemorrhoidectomy, cystoscopy, circumcision in adults and older children, bouginage, and anal fistulae.

CONTRAINDICATIONS (1) Infants. (2) An uncooperative patient. (3) Anatomical abnormalities. (4) Caesarean section. (5) Local infection over the sacrum.

EQUIPMENT AND DRUGS FOR CAUDAL EPIDURAL ANAESTHESIA

A 1×35 mm needle. An ordinary 0.8 mm "green", disposable intravenous needle is satisfactory, or a 0.5 mm blue one in children. 30 ml of 0.5 % bupivacaine, or 1.5% lignocaine. If possible, use single-dose containers without preservative. Add 0.25 ml of adrenaline to 30 ml of local anaesthetic solution. Inject 1 ml solution for every 3 kg body weight. Children can have up to 0.5 ml/kg.

METHOD FOR CAUDAL EPIDURAL ANAESTHESIA

The following method describes the use of a fine needle to begin with, followed by a thicker one, but you can do it with only one needle.

CAUDAL EPIDURAL ANAESTHESIA

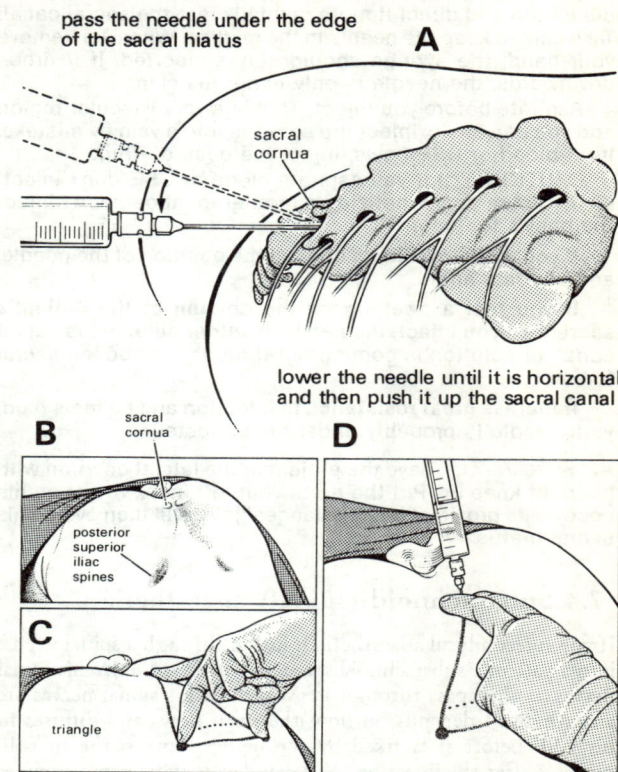

Fig. 7-5 CAUDAL EPIDURAL ANAESTHESIA. A, the position of the needle in relation to the sacrum. B, the patient ready for the anaesthetic with a pillow under his pubis. C, making a triangle with the anatomical landmarks. D, injecting.

Lay the patient on his abdomen with a pillow under his pubis, his legs apart and his toes turned inwards. This will relax his gluteal muscles. If this is not convenient, turn him onto his left side with his legs bent, or into the knee–elbow position.

Feel for the anatomical landmarks in B, Fig. 7-5. If you cannot easily find them, try another method. A pad of fat sometimes forms over the sacral hiatus at the end of pregnancy, which makes finding the hiatus difficult.

Clean the skin over the area of the sacral patient's hiatus, and infiltrate anaesthetic solution into his skin and subcutaneous tissue.

While you are learning to do the block, mark the posterior superior iliac spines, as in C, Fig. 7-5, and draw an equilateral triangle. The caudal angle of this should be over the sacral hiatus. Feel for the sacral cornua. These are two knobs of bone on either side of the sacral hiatus. Find the sacral cornua by putting your thumb and middle finger on the posterior superior iliac spines, and moving your index finger caudually so as to make an equilateral triangle, as in C in this figure. Feel for the cornua with your index finger.

Put the tips of your fingers on the cornua, and insert a fine (0.5 mm) needle slightly cranially between them. You can usually feel the needle piercing the caudal membrane.

When the needle reaches the ventral wall of the sacral canal, withdraw the needle slightly and inject 4 ml of anaesthetic solution.

Remove the fine needle and push a 1 mm needle cranially and ventrally along the same track as you inserted the fine one.

Hold the needle and syringe at 45° to the horizontal and pass it under the posterior margin of the sacral hiatus. You will feel a sudden loss of resistance as the needle goes through the caudal membrane. Try to recognise the structures through which the needle passes, because this is the best guide to where it is.

Lower the point of the needle until it is horizontal, then push it further up the sacral canal. It will pass quite easily if it is in the right place. If you touch bone, withdraw the needle a little and direct it more cranially into the sacral canal. Take care to keep the needle in the midline. When you remove your hand, the syringe should stay supported. If it drops downwards, the needle is only under his skin.

Aspirate before you inject. This is a very vascular region and you can easily inject the solution into a vein by mistake. If no blood or CSF flows, inject the dose of drug.

CAUTION! (1) If you aspirate blood or CSF, don't inject. (2) If you are anaesthetizing a mother in labour, don't inject the baby's fontanelle!

If you withdraw blood, change the position of the needle, and aspirate again.

If you feel a swelling on the dorsum of the patient's sacrum as you inject, the needle is either outside his sacral canal, or solution is coming out through his second sacral foramen.

If there is great resistance to injection and he feels pain, your needle is probably under his periosteum.

ALTERNATIVELY, have the patient in the lateral position with his right knee up. Put the tip of your left index finger on his coccyx. Its proximal interphalangeal joint will then overlie his sacral hiatus.

7.4 Subarachnoid (spinal) anaesthesia

If you inject a local anaesthetic solution through a spinal needle into a patient's subarachnoid space, it will anaesthetize his spinal nerves as they pass through it. Which of his spinal nerves are anaesthetized depends on how the drug flows and diffuses in his CSF before it is fixed by the nerves, during the first 10 minutes after the injection. You can decide which spinal nerves you want to anaesthetize in two ways.

(1) You can use a local anaesthetic solution made up in 6% dextrose. This solution is heavy (hyperbaric) and falls like syrup through the CSF. By varying the patient's position you can vary the extent of the block.

(2) You can use 0.5% bupivacaine solution of nearly the same specific gravity as his CSF (isobaric). It will diffuse regardless of gravity, so that his position immediatley after the injection is not important.

Hyperbaric subarachnoid anaesthesia is the most consistently reliable of all methods of local anaesthesia. It provides good conditions for surgery in a fit patient. The operative field is remarkably bloodless, his gut is well contracted, and the muscles in the lower part of his body are perfectly relaxed. Unfortunately, if complications do arise, they can be serious. Subarachnoid anaesthesia can kill a patient if he is shocked and is maintaining his blood pressure by constricting his blood vessels. This is much less likely to happen if you have already preloaded him with saline (7.1).

One of the disadvantages of subarachnoid anaesthesia is that CSF may leak out of the hole that the needle has made in the dura and give the patient a severe postoperative headache. So use a fine spinal needle, which will only make a small hole. Less CSF will leak, and the patient will have less chance of a headache. The difficulty with a fine needle is that it easily bends and is more difficult to insert. So push down the needle through a thicker introducer needle. You can use an ordinary thick intramuscular needle, or you can use a special Sise introducer. Either of these will help to prevent the bacteria on the patient's skin reaching his subarachnoid space.

Although bupivacaine is the drug of choice for isobaric anaesthesia, you can use lignocaine, as described below.

IS SUBARACHNOID (SPINAL) ANAESTHESIA APPROPRIATE?

The indications are the same for both the hyperbaric and the isobaric methods.

HOW A HEAVY ANAESTHETIC SOLUTION FLOWS IN THE CSF

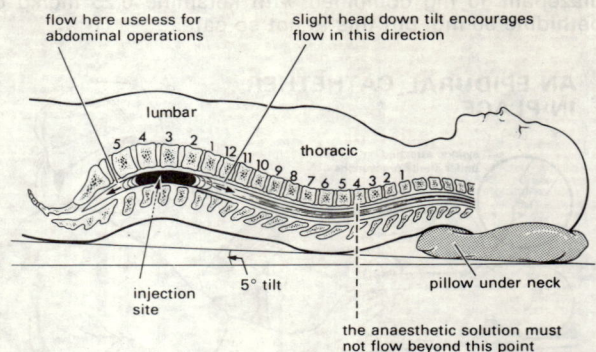

Fig. 7-6 HOW A HEAVY ANAESTHETIC SOLUTION FLOWS IN THE SUBARACHNOID SPACE. A heavy anaesthetic solution introduced at the summit of the lumbar curve will fall towards the patient's sacrum and his thorax. For abdominal operations the flow towards the sacrum is useless, so the table is given a slight head down tilt.

INDICATIONS (1) A fit patient requiring lower abdominal, pelvic, anal, or leg operations. (2) A patient having some relative contraindication to general anaesthesia, such as a respiratory infection, asthma, or a deformed airway. (3) Operations, such as some methods for the reduction of a dislocated hip, or amputation of the lower leg in which it is useful to be able to turn the patient onto his abdomen. (4) A patient in cardiac or renal failure who requires lower abdominal pelvic, or lower extremity surgery.

You can do a Caesarean section using subarachnoid anaesthesia, if you give the patient a saddle block, as in Section 7.7. A standard subarachnoid anaesthetic, however, is contraindicated.

CONTRAINDICATIONS (1) Any patient who will not cooperate. (2) Operations lasting more than two hours. (3) Hypovolaemic shock. (4) Children of any age, unless you are expert. (5) Sepsis anywhere on the back is an absolute contraindication. (6) Diabetic neuropathy, but not diabetes itself. (7) Lack of intravenous fluids. (8) Equipment which you cannot guarantee sterile. (9) Any operation on the thorax or above.

Intestinal obstruction is normally considered a contraindication, but you can, if necessary, use subarachnoid anaesthesia for an obstructed inguinal hernia, if you have rehydrated the patient thoroughly before the operation.

7.5 Subarachnoid (spinal) anaesthesia with isobaric bupivacaine

The use of isobaric bupivacaine is a recent method of subarachnoid anaesthesia, which has several important advantages: (1) It avoids the need to position a patient during the period immediatly after the injection to achieve the desired level of the block. As soon as you have injected the bupivacaine you can turn him in any position you like. If necessary, you can tip him head down to increase his venous return and raise his blood pressure, without raising the level of the block. (2) You can reautoclave the solution as often as you wish without it charring.

Subarachnoid anaesthesia with isobaric bupivacaine has some disadvantages: (1) You cannot use it for for unilateral blocks or saddle blocks. (2) It is not so predictable as hyperbaric subarachnoid anaesthesia, particularly for abdominal surgery, because it sometimes fails to block segments below the upper level. Its reputation for occasionally failing probably comes from using too small doses. Here we advise you to use 3 ml for a block to T10, and 4 ml for a block to T6. Less than 3 ml will cause a patchy block.

You can make isobaric anaesthesia more predictable if: (1) You use a fine needle and an introducer. (2) You use the method of barbotage. To do this you aspirate a little CSF, and mix it with the bupivacaine in the syringe. You then inject the mixture and repeat the process. Barbotage: (a) makes quite sure that the needle is in the patient's subarachnoid space, and (b) mixes the drug with his CSF more evenly. You can do it in various ways, and the method described below is merely one of them. Many anaesthetists don't use it. It can cause a very high block.

Isobaric bupivacaine provides 2 to 4 hours of surgical analgesia combined with good muscle relaxation below the level of about T8, with up to 8 hours of postoperative analgesia. Occasionally, the block ascends as high as T4.

Decide with care the volume of the drug you inject, because drug volume is the main factor in determining how high the block will spread.

Although bupivacaine is the drug of choice for isobaric anaethesia, you can use lignocaine as described below.

SUBARACHNOID ANAESTHESIA WITH ISOBARIC BUPIVACAINE

The indications and contraindications are same as for any form of subarachnoid anaesthesia (7.4).

EQUIPMENT Use a fine (0.5 mm) spinal needle with a Sise introducer, or a thicker needle without one. If you have no Sise introducer, use a 1 mm intramuscular needle.

Make a roll with pockets to hold the equipment. This should contain 2 spinal needles, and an introducer, all with their correct stylets. Also a 2 ml syringe, a 5 ml syringe, a 0.9 mm needle, an ampoule file, two ampuoles of the drugs, a pair of Lane's tissue forceps, a gallipot and some swabs. Put the roll and a towel in a drum. Autoclave the drum, seal it, and mark the date on the seal. Reautoclave the drum each week.

If you do subarachnoid or epidural anaesthesia routinely, you may find it practical to have a special trolley to contain the equipment. Don't use Cheatle forceps kept in antiseptic fluid for laying it out.

CAUTION ! (1) Take the drug solution from a single dose ampoule, not from a rubber-capped multidose vial, which may contain preservatives that should not be injected into the subarachnoid space. Also, the solution might be contaminated in spite of its preservatives. (2) Don't add adrenaline.

PRELOADING Set up a drip with a large bore needle. If the block is to go to T10 the patient will need 500 ml of a crystalloid solution. If it is to go to T4, he will need 1000 ml. Be prepared to give more if necessary. The anaesthetic will dilate his blood vessels and increase the volume of his vascular bed. The fluid you give before operation will help to fill the vascular bed; keep the drip running throughout the operation.

PREMEDICATION Premedicate the patient with diazepam 10 mg and pethidine 50 mg, both orally.

EXPLANATION Explain to the patient exactly what is going to happen. If he will not co-operate, don't give him a subarachnoid anaesthetic.

PREPARATION Wrap a sphygmomanometer cuff and a stethoscope round one of his arms. Measure and record his blood pressure.

LUMBAR PUNCTURE FOR SUBARACHNOID ANAESTHESIA

Here we describe lumbar puncture with the patient on his left side as in B, Fig. 7-2, but you can do it while he sits, as in A in this figure.

Scrub up. Take the gallipot from the trolley and ask the nurse to fill it with iodine. This will prevent it being spilt on the trolley. Use an iodine swab to draw a vertical line across the patient's back at the level of his iliac crest as in Fig. 7-2. This line will cross his vertebral column between the spines of L3 and L4, and make it easier to identify the correct injection site later.

Swab his lumbar region twice with iodine, using a fresh swab each time.

Fill the small syringe with a little anaesthetic solution. Fit a fine needle to it and use it to anaesthetize the patient's skin. Fill the other syringe with the full dose needed for the anaesthetic.

Sit on a low stool, so that the puncture site is level with your eyes.

Ask your assistant to place one hand behind the patient's neck, and the other behind his knees. Ask the patient to relax as much as possible. Your assistant should then arch the patient's back as much as he can so as to open up the intervertebral spaces. Choose the space between L3 and L4, but any space will do, provided it is L2 or below.

Use a fine needle to raise a wheal over the space you have chosen, in the midline midway between two spines. Push the Sise introducer through this wheal. Keep the needle strictly at right angles to the skin in the vertical plane. Direct it slightly towards the patient's head while aiming at his umbilicus.

CAUTION! Be sure to insert the needle in the midline of the vertebral column. The median skin of a fat patient may sag 2.5 cm.

The Sise introducer should reach as far as the ligamentun flavum at about 2 cm, but should not go through it into the subarachnoid space, so that CSF comes out of it. Pass the spinal needle through the introducer, holding the needle by its hub. You will usually feel a distinct loss of resistance as the spinal needle goes through the ligament flavum.

If you are using a fine needle, and you don't have a Sise introducer, push it through a thick (1 mm) hypodermic needle.

CAUTION ! Sterility is critical. Never touch the point or shaft of a spinal needle with your hand. If you do have to hold it, support it with a sterile swab. Your gloves might be contaminated.

Once the needle is through the ligamentum flavum, remove the stylet and push the spinal needle slowly through the dura. You will feel another slight loss of resistance as it goes through this. CSF should flow out of the needle. As soon as CSF flows freely, put back the stylet and leave the needle and the introducer in.

CAUTION ! CSF must flow freely. If it does not flow freely, reinsert the stylet and rotate it.

If CSF does not come out of the needle, rotate the needle once, put the stylet back, and remove it again, holding the hub firmly with your other hand meanwhile. If you are still unsuccessful, ask the patient to strain to raise his CSF pressure.

If you hit bone, withdraw the needle into the introducer. Check the direction of the introducer. It may not be in the midline, it may be pointing too high or too low, or the patient's back may not be flexed enough. Withdraw the needle into the introducer a little, withdraw the introducer itself a little, change its direction slightly, and push it in again. Then push the needle through it.

CAUTION ! Always withdraw the needle into the introducer, before changing its direction, even a little.

If pure blood comes out of the needle, it is in a vein. Withdraw the needle and introducer and try another space.

If the CSF that comes out is mixed with blood, this is not important. It will probably become clear after a few millilitres have flowed.

If you fail 2 or 3 times, try another space. If you fail there also, try a general anaesthetic.

DOSE FOR ISOBARIC SUBARACHNOID ANAESTHESIA

For routine purposes use 0.5% bupivacaine without adrenaline. Take it from a single-dose ampoule without a preservative, which might harm the cord. Use 3 ml if you want the block to go to T10, and 4 ml if you want it to go to T6. For most purposes don't use smaller volumes, or you will get a patchy block. 4 ml is the maximum dose. In pregnancy, in very old patients, or in very short ones, and for perineal operations, use only 2 ml of bupivacaine.

If you are using lignocaine, inject 1.5 or 2 ml of 2% solution without added dextrose or adrenaline, and without barbotage, between L1 and L2. After 10 minutes the patient will be anaesthetic 2 finger's breadth above his umbilicus.

BARBOTAGE is optional. Instead of injecting the bupivacaine as above, attach a 5 ml syringe containing 2 to 2.5 ml of 0.5 bupivacaine to the spinal needle. Aspirate 0.4 ml of CSF into the syringe. This will confirm that your needle is in the right place. The patient's CSF will mix with the drug.

Slowly inject the mixture of bupivacaine and CSF. Then aspirate another 0.5 ml of CSF, and reinject it.

AFTER INJECTING BUPIVACAINE (or lignocaine) you can put the patient into any position which is convenient for the operation. If necessary, you can safely give the table a slight head down tilt. The isobaric bupivacaine solution will not flow to higher segments in his cord, and raising his legs a little will compensate for the venous pooling that will take place in them.

The latent period lasts 7 minutes, and the block is maximal at 15 minutes. Test the height of the block with a pin; if it is high (above T8) watch his blood pressure with particular care.

CARE DURING THE OPERATION WITH SUBARACHNOID ANAESTHESIA

Ask a nurse to sit by the patient, to watch his respiration, and to take his pulse and blood pressure every 5 minutes. Bradycardia is not pronounced with bupivacaine, but it may be with hyperbaric agents. The fluid you have already given him should prevent his blood pressure falling. Give him more as necessary.

POST OPERATIVE CARE WITH SUBARACHNOID ANAESTHESIA

Keep the patient lying flat for 6 hours with only a single pillow, to prevent the "post spinal headache" that can be so distressing. Explain carefully that he must not sit up or strain at any time during this period.

DIFFICULTIES WITH SUBARACHNOID ANAESTHESIA

These difficulties apply to isobaric and hyperbaric subarachnoid anaesthesia.

If the patient's blood pressure falls, give him more fluid. This will usually restore his blood pressure to normal. If it does not, give a vasopressor, such as methoxamine or ephedrine in the dose advised in Fig. 2-4, either intramuscularly or intravenously as required (2.10). If you give methoxamine, give him atropine 0.5 mg intravenously first. Lay the patient flat, give him oxygen, raise his legs.

CAUTION ! If you have used a hyperbaric solution, don't tip the patient head downwards! If some of the anaesthetic is still free in his CSF, a head–down tilt will certainly raise the level of the block and may give him a "total spinal", if he has not already got one. You can however raise his legs while keeping his spine horizontal.

Next time, take these measures to prevent a patient's blood pressure falling: (1) Don't give him a subarachnoid anaesthesia if he is hypovolaemic. (2) Don't exceed the recommended dose. (3) Preload him with saline. (4) Don't raise the upper part of his body. A patient under spinal anaesthesia is very sensitive to position. Raising the upper part of his body causes gravitational pooling, and sudden hypotension.

If the block extends above the patient's umbilicus, his lower intercostal muscles will be paralysed and his respiration weakened, so be prepared to assist his ventilation and give him oxygen. This is especially important if he has a large abdominal tumour which may splint his diaphragm.

If the patient becomes nauseated, or cyanosed, he may not be breathing well enough to keep himself oxygenated, so give him oxygen.

If he cannot speak, he probably has a "high spinal", or even a total one, or severe hypotension. The drug may have spread far up his spinal canal and paralysed his intercostal muscles and even his diaphragm. If this is likely, assist his respiration, first with a face mask and a self–inflating bag.

If necessary, intubate him, pass a tracheal tube, and connect that to the bag. You may have to keep respiring him for two hours or more, but eventually he will breathe spontaneously again. His blood pressure is low, so treat this as above.

If he is awake and worried and you have intubated him, be kind and give him 0.25 mg/kg of ketamine every 15 minutes. This is much less important than keeping him alive with adequate ventilation.

DON'T DO "SUBARACHNOIDS" OR "EPIDURALS" ON SHOCKED PATIENTS

7.6 Hyperbaric subarachnoid (spinal) anaesthesia

Hyperbaric spinal anaesthesia has been the standard method for many years. It is not quite so straightforward as isobaric anaesthesia, but it is more consistently successful. One of its advantages is that you can choose the nerve roots you wish to anaesthetize. *If you are attempting subarachnoid anaesthesia for the first time, this is the method to start with.*

The first step is a lumbar puncture to inject the anaesthetic solution. For this the patient can be sitting, or lying on his side, whichever is most convenient. As soon as the anaesthetic solution is safely inside his subarachnoid space, you must quickly turn him into the position that will let the anaesthetic solution fall through the CSF to reach the nerve roots you want to anaesthetize. He must stay in this position for about 10 minutes, while his nerve roots fix the drug and are blocked by it. After this has happened, you can turn him into any position that is convenient for surgery.

If a patient is lying on his side, on a horizontal table, the curves of his spine have no effect, and a heavy solution will tend to anaesthetize the roots of the side that is lowest. If you tilt the table at this stage you can further influence the roots that will be anaesthetized. For all methods except anaesthetizing a patient's perineum, give the table a 5° head–down tilt while you are injecting. If you are anaesthetizing his perineum give it a feet–down tilt, or do a lumbar puncture while he is in the sitting position.

When you turn the patient onto his back, the way a heavy solution flows is determined by the fact that his spine is concave in his thoracic region and convex in his lumbar region. If you inject it at the top of the lumbar curve and put the patient on his back, some of the anaesthetic solution will roll down towards his sacrum, and some towards his thorax. You can determine how much solution flows in each direction by carefully adjusting the tilt of the table.

How high a block goes depends on: (1) The level at which you do the lumbar puncture. (2) The dose of the drug you inject. (3) The volume of the solution. (4) Its specific gravity. (5) The slope of the table (and the patient's spine): (a) while you are injecting the anaesthetic solution and (b) while it is being fixed. *The details of positioning, tilting and timing are critical.* Although they may seem similar, the small differences between these details are all important. By combining position, tilt and timing in various ways, you can do three kinds of low subarachnoid (called A, B, and C in the account below). You can do a mid subarachnoid, or a unilateral subarachnoid on one leg only. A high subarachnoid is not for beginners, because of the danger of it spreading too high and affecting a patient's vital centres. The segments you can expect to be blocked are given with each method. To see exactly which dermatones are anaesthetized by each block, consult Fig. 6-8. If you want an accurately determined block, follow the details carefully.

A method for Caesarean section is described in the next section. Should you be so unwise as to give a mother an ordinary subarachnoid anaesthetic, don't inject the drug during a labour pain, or the block will go much higher.

The position of a patient's upper spine during the 10 minutes following the injection of a heavy anaesthetic solution is critical. If, by mistake, during this time, you allow the his head and neck to fall backwards, the anaesthetic will flow down his thoracic spine, and may even reach his neck, so causing a "total spinal". This may paralyse both his intercostal muscles and his diaphragm. *So when the patient lies on his back after the injection, always place a pillow under his neck and shoulders to prevent the anaesthetic solution flowing down his thoracic spine.* At no time should any part of his spine above T6 ever become lowermost on the table or his intercostal muscles will be paralysed.

ESTON (29) was being given a hyperbaric subarachnoid anaesthetic by a doctor who had never given one before. The doctor was suprised to find that Eston's blood pressure dropped alarmingly, so he gave the table a steep head—down tilt—"to counteract hypotension while he put up a drip". Eston's respiration failed, he was not ventilated, and he rapidly died.

WESTON (39) was given a subarachnoid anaesthetic for an ENT operation. He died, and when last heard of, the case was still going through the high court.

PATSON (54) was having his varicose veins tied under epidural anaesthesia. His breathing became shallow, he became cyanosed, he started twitching, and his blood pressure fell. He was immediately suspected of having a "total spinal" so he was intubated and ventilated; the drip he was already receiving was speeded up, whereupon he rapidly improved. He was given a little ether to keep him asleep and to abolish the discomfort of the tube, and the operation was completed. LESSONS FROM ALL THREE CASES: (1) Subarachnoid anaesthetics should always be given with a drip running so that you can give fluid or a vasopressor quickly. (2) If you tip a patient having a hyperbaric subarachnoid anaesthetic head down, the solution will flow towards his upper thoracic and cervical segments and depress his respiration, so don't! However, provided you can support his respiration, this should not be fatal, as PATSON shows. (3) You must have the equipment for cardiopulmonary resuscitation available before you anaesthetize any patient. (4) As the example of WESTON shows, there are cases for which subarachnoid anaesthesia is NOT suitable. You would be wise not to use it on the upper abdomen (unless you are expert), and certainly not on the chest, neck or head!

HYPERBARIC SUBARACHNOID (SPINAL) ANAESTHESIA

The indications and contraindications, equipment, preloading, premedication, explanation, preparation, lumbar puncture, the care during the operation, and the difficulties, are the same as for hypobaric anaesthesia (7.4). Here we give only those parts of the procedure that differ from the hypobaric technique—the drugs and their doses, and the method of positioning the patient for particular blocks.

DRUGS All these drugs are "heavy" in that they are mixed with 5 to 10% dextrose. They must be in single dose ampoules, without preservative. Dextrose chars and goes slightly brown if you autoclave it. Although it is not advisable, you can if necessary use it in this state. Don't add adrenaline.

All the doses in the methods below are for heavy cinchocaine. Note that the dose gets slightly larger (from 0.6 to 2 ml) the higher the block goes. The doses given are for average adults, so adjust them for large or small ones. If you don't have heavy cinchocaine and have to use any of the other drugs listed below, you will probably get satisfactory results if you use the same dose as indicated for cinchocaine.

Cinchocaine, 0.5% in 6% dextrose. Before use, mix it with an equal or greater volume of CSF in the syringe. Analgesia lasts 2 to 3 hours.

Prilocaine, 5% solution in 5% dextrose. Don't use it for operations lasting more than an hour.

Amethocaine ('Tetracaine'), Use a 1% solution in 5 or 6% dextrose.

Bupivacaine, 0.5% solution in 5% dextrose.

Mepivacaine hydrochloride, 4% in 10% dextrose.

Lignocaine, 4% or 5% solution in 5% dextrose. Alternatively, mix 2.5 ml of 2% lignocaine with 2.5 ml of 10% dextrose.

PILLOWS When you do the lumbar puncture, put a pillow under the patient's head to keep his spine straight. When you have given him the anaesthetic, put a pillow under his head and neck for comfort.

PARTICULAR BLOCKS FOR SUBARACHNOID ANAESTHESIA

Do a lumbar puncture as in Section 7.5.

CAUTION ! (1) These methods make a distinction between the table and the patient's spine having a tilt. If the patient has a broad pelvis and narrow shoulders, the tilt of the table and his spine may not be the same. (2) When you need to change the patient's position after injection, ask an assistant to help you move the patient, don't allow the patient to change his position himself. If he moves about actively, the solution may move unpredictably in his spinal canal.

LOW SUBARACHNOID–A (S2 to S5)

INDICATIONS Haemorrhoids, anal fissure etc.

METHOD Puncture the patient's subarachnoid space between L4 and L5 while he is sitting, or lying with the table in a definite (at least 10°) *feet–down* tilt.

Slowly inject heavy cinchocaine 0.6 ml, mixed with an equal volume of his CSF. It will sink to the bottom of his subarachnoid space.

After 1 minute, he can lie flat with a pillow under his neck and shoulders. The curve of his lumbar spine will prevent the drug spreading upwards.

LOW SUBARACHNOID–B (S1 to S5)

INDICATIONS Operations on the urethra, bladder neck or prostate etc.

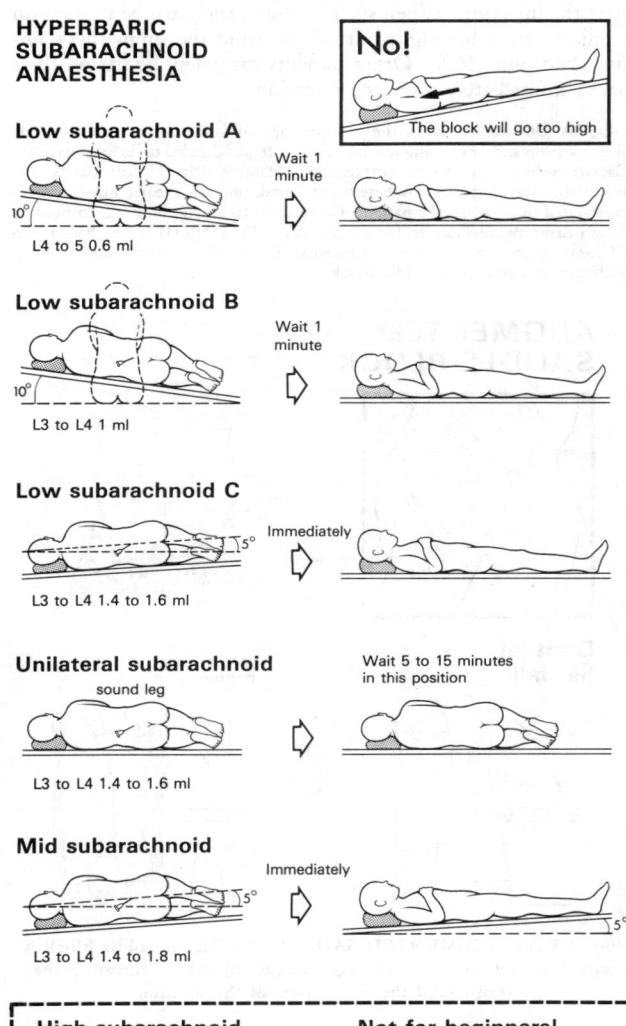

Fig. 7-7 HYPERBARIC SUBARACHNOID ANAESTHESIA. The site at which you do the lumbar puncture, the volume of heavy cinchocaine you inject and how you tilt the table before and after the injection all determine how high the block goes. All these doses are for heavy cinchocaine. Mix the cinchocaine with an equal volume of CSF. The figures on the left show the positions for injection, the column in the middle tells you how long to wait before turning the patient. The figures on the right show the position in which he should wait while the drug is fixed.

METHOD Puncture the patient's space between L3 and L4, while he is sitting, or lying on his side with the table in a 10° *feet–down* tilt.

Slowly inject 1 ml of cinchocaine, mixed with an equal volume of CSF.

Lay him level after one minute with a pillow under his neck and shoulders.

LOW SUBARACHNOID–C (L1 to S5)

INDICATIONS Operations on both legs.

METHOD Lay the patient on his side, *with his spine* tilted 5° head down to prevent the solution running towards his sacrum, and puncture his subarachnoid space between L3 and L4.

Slowly inject 1.4 to 1.6 ml of cinchocaine mixed with an equal volume of CSF.

Immediately after the injection turn him onto his back with a pillow under his neck and shoulders, and level the table.

UNILATERAL SUBARACHNOID (L1 to L5)

INDICATIONS Operations on one leg.

METHOD Lay the patient on his side, with the table level and his sound leg upwards, and puncture his subarachnoid space between L3 and L4.

Slowly inject 1.4 to 1.6 ml of cinchocaine mixed with an equal volume of CSF.

Keep him in this position from 5 to 15 minutes. His lower leg will slowly become anaesthetic. Unless he stays in this position, his other leg will also become anaesthetic during the operation.

MID SUBARACHNOID (T7–T8 to L4)

INDICATIONS Hernia, hydrocoele, cystoscopy, suprapubic prostatectomy, appendectomy.

METHOD Lay the patient on his side with *his spine* tilting 5° head down. Puncture his subarachnoid space between L3 and L4. Inject heavy cinchocaine 1.4 to 1.8 ml mixed with an equal volume of CSF.

Immediately turn him on his back for 5 minutes with a pillow under his neck and shoulders, maintaining the 5° head–down tilt.

HIGH SUBARACHNOID (T2-T5 to L4)

INDICATIONS Upper abdominal anaesthesia.

CAUTION ! This is not for the inexperienced operator. There is a danger of a total spinal if you are not careful.

METHOD Lay the patient on his side with the table tilting 5° head down. Puncture his subarachnoid space between L2 and L3.

Inject 2 ml of heavy cinchocaine mixed with an equal volume of CSF, using a little barbotage.

Immediately after injection turn the patient passively onto on his back, maintain the 5° head–down tilt, and put a pillow under his neck and shoulders. Any excess solution will pool at the bottom of his thoracic curve opposite T5.

CAUTION ! With all methods make quite sure there is no *steep* head–down tilt for 15 minutes after the injection.

IS THE ANAESTHETIC SUCCESSFUL?

As soon as the patient has been in the required position for 10 minutes, you can turn him into any position. Run a needle up his abdomen and chest to see how high the block has risen. If the block is not completely successful during a further period of waiting, give him a general anaesthetic. This requires special precautions, so see Section 6.2.

For care during and after the operation, go to Section 7.5.

7.7 Augmented saddle block

In this block the patient sits up so that a heavy anaesthetic solution falls through his subarachnoid space, blocks his sacral nerve roots, and anaesthetizes the part of his body on which he sits (his saddle area), so that you can do anal and perineal operations.

A saddle block will also anaesthetize a mother's pelvic organs, including her uterus, and her abdominal wall, but only for about three fingers' breadth above her pubis. This is not high enough to anaesthetize the whole incision site for Caesarean section, but you can easily anaesthetize the rest of it by local infiltration. Only a limited area is anaesthetized, so she is in no danger from hypotension, as she would be if the block went higher. This method combines the advantages of subarachnoid anaesthesia and those of local infiltration without their disadvantages. It also provides better anaesthesia if her lower segment tears behind her bladder. Augmented saddle block is probably the ideal method of anaesthesia for Caesarean section if you are single–handed and are working under difficult conditions. Anaesthesia lasts 60 to 90 minutes. To be safe, you should be able to intubate her and control her ventilation, if necessary.

Keep a pregnant mother sitting up for 5 minutes immediately after the injection. When she lies down, she must be tilted with a pillow under her right buttock to avoid the supine hypotensive syndrome (16.6). Other patients can safely lie flat on their backs immediately after the injection.

PRISCA (36) had delay in the second stage of labour, with cephalopelvic disproportion and impending uterine rupture. It was decided to do an emergency Caesarean section under an intravenous ketamine drip. Unfortunately, the anaesthetic assistant was nowhere to be found, and the theatre nurse was incapacitated in a bar, so the patient was referred to a neighbouring hospital an hour's drive away. She died before arriving. LESSONS (1) If you have to do a Caesarean section, more or less unassisted, the most suitable anaesthetic is probably an augmented saddle block.

AUGMENTED SADDLE BLOCK

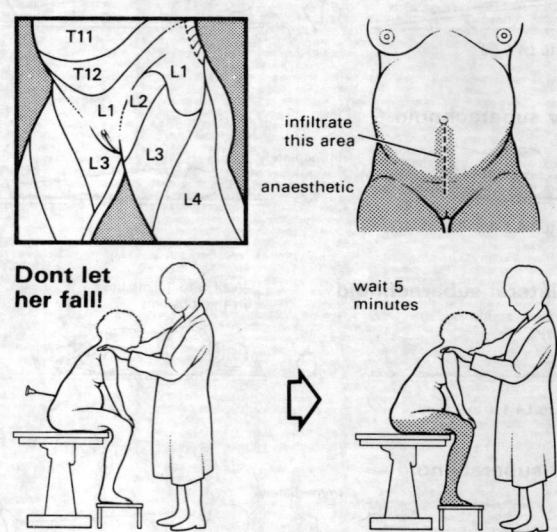

Fig. 7-8 AN AUGMENTED SADDLE BLOCK. A saddle block is safe, but you will have to augment (assist) it by infiltrating the skin round the upper part of the incision.

COMBINED SADDLE BLOCK AND LOCAL INFILTRATION

This method is described as if the patient was for Caesarean section. It is equally suitable for anal and perineal operations in men.

PRELOADING Preload the patient with 500 or 1000 ml of saline or Ringer's lactate.

PREMEDICATION Give the mother atropine (2.7). If she is conscious you may have to sedate her with diazepam or pethidine or both, even though this is not ideal for the baby, but avoid it if you can.

OTHER MEASURES FOR CAESAREAN SECTION **Give her oral antacids (16.3), tilt her with a pillow under her right buttock, (16.6), and avoid ergometrine (6.9).**

METHOD **Sit the mother up on the table; prepare and drape her lumbar region. Introduce a 0.6 mm needle (ideally use a 0.6 mm needle with an introducer) between the spines of L3 and L4. When CSF appears inject one of the following drugs and withdraw the needle.** *Don't add adrenaline to any of them.*

5.0% heavy (hyperbaric) lignocaine 0.8 to 1.0 ml (40 to 50 mg).

0.5% heavy chinchocaine (nupercaine) 0.8 to 1.0 ml.

1% heavy tetracaine (pontocaine, amethocaine) 1 ml (10 mg).

0.5% isobaric bupivacaine 1 to 1.5 ml (5 to 7.5 mg).

Keep her sitting up for exactly 5 minutes, while you scrub up.

CAUTION ! Make sure someone stays with her and supports her during this period. She may faint and fall off the table. (One patient sustained a cervical fracture and quadriplegia by doing this!)

After 5 minutes allow her to lie down; clean and drape her abdomen for a midline incision in the usual way. Tilt the table 15° to the left to avoid the supine hypotensive syndrome (16.6).

ALTERNATIVELY **Do a low subarachnoid in the lateral position with the table tilted foot down.**

LOCAL INFILTRATION **Use 20 ml of solution to infiltrate a path 5 cm wide along the site of the incision from her umbilicus to the zone that is already anaesthetic.**

8 Dissociative anaesthesia and intravenous analgesia

8.1 Dissociative anaesthesia with ketamine

Ketamine produces a most useful state of dissociative anaesthesia. The patient rapidly goes into a trance–like state, with widely open eyes and nystagmus. He is unconscious, amnesic and deeply analgesic. His airway is remarkably preserved, with his head in almost any position, far more so than with any other anaesthetic. Not suprisingly, this remarkable drug has made many operations possible that would otherwise have been impossible for lack of a trained anaesthetist. Ketamine is especially useful if you have no recovery ward and patients have to recover in their own beds. Ketamine is remarkably safe and is certainly the safest anaesthetic if you are inexperienced. Nevertheless, it is not absolutely safe, so be vigilant. In some hospitals without a trained anaesthetist, 90% of the operations are done with ketamine. Intramuscular ketamine acts rapidly. You can also give it intravenously as a bolus injection or as a drip, either alone or with relaxants.

Although ketamine anaesthesia has many advantages, it should not replace conventional anaesthesia, especially ether and air, or local anaesthesia where these are more appropriate.

Ketamine also has a few disadvantages: (1) Used alone it causes unpleasant emergence reactions in the form of frightening hallucinations. You can reduce their incidence, but not entirely eliminate them, by giving a patient suitable drugs. (2) By itself, ketamine provides no muscular relaxation. (3) From its original manufacturers Ketamine is expensive, but from other suppliers it is now much cheaper. (4) Ketamine is not ideal for outpatient anaesthesia, because its effects take some hours to pass off, so you have usually to admit a patient to recover from them overnight.

Although a patient's pharyngeal and laryngeal reflexes may seem to be normally active after ketamine, *they are not completely normal,* so he can regurgitate and aspirate his vomit, especially if he has been heavily premedicated. Fortunately, this is rare. Even so, preserve his airway carefully and take the necessary precautions: (1) Starve him. (2) Anaesthetize him on a table that can tip. (3) Keep a sucker instantly ready. (4) Remember that aspiration can still occur with ketamine, unless he has been intubated. This is ketamine's most serious risk, but it is fortunately not common.

Because the patient's laryngeal reflexes are largely preserved, you need not, and cannot, laryngoscope or intubate him under ketamine alone. But you can and must do both these things when you use ketamine with relaxants. Don't insert an oral airway routinely, except in babies. In adults, only insert one when necessary.

A patient receiving ketamine tends to breathe faster and more deeply than normal. His pulse also becomes faster and his blood pressure rises about 25 mm. This makes ketamine a useful induction agent for shocked patients (16.7).

Ketamine also increases a patient's intracranial and intraocular pressure, so it is unsuitable for operations inside his eye or his skull.

Emergence reactions are common in young adults recovering from ketamine alone, but are much less common in young children and in the very old. The patient has vivid dreams, which may be pleasant or unpleasant. He may also have visual or auditory hallucinations and become restless, or shout, or cry. He may talk in his sleep or move about. The incidence of all these reactions is markedly increased if he is disturbed during recovery. Fortunately, they do not threaten his life and he soon recovers.

Several drugs, including haloperidol, will usually prevent these emergence reactions, but promethazine or diazepam are the best. Although these drugs are often referred to as "premedication", with ketamine they are not given for their sedative effect, but specifically to counter one of ketamine's less desirable properties. They are mainly required during recovery, which is useful because you can give ketamine alone at the start of a Caesarean section, and then give intravenous diazepam after delivery, when it can no longer affect the baby (6.9).

The incidence of emergence reactions seems to vary from one country to another. This may be one reason why ketamine is much used in some parts of Africa and little used in Europe, America, or India. Some hospitals in Africa routinely give ketamine without premedication, and only give it if a patient is obviously restless.

Muscular relaxation is not produced by ketamine, so it is not ideal for abdominal surgery, unless you combine it with relaxants (8.4), or intercostal blocks (6.7). Operations, such as hysterectomy, which need abdominal relaxation, have been done under ketamine alone, but they are not easy.

An increased flow of saliva is another disadvantage of ketamine. You can minimise this by giving the patient atropine (2.7). Unfortunately, this makes his secretions thick and sticky and less easy to suck out. But, if you don't give atropine, his secretions may accumulate dangerously; so, if you decide not to use it, you must have tracheal suction available. Increased secretions are a greater problem in children, so always give them atropine. Atropine with ketamine makes the heart beat faster, but this is not important. Hyoscine, if you have it, is better than atropine, because it 'dries' more, and is sedative and anti–emetic.

Respiratory arrest is very rare indeed with intramuscular ketamine, except in babies, and if you give too much. It is also rare with intravenous ketamine, *but only if you inject it slowly taking at least a minute, and don't give too much.* If you inject Ketamine fast, or give too large a doses, the patient is sure to stop breathing. If he does so, ventilate him.

GIVE KETAMINE SLOWLY

Laryngeal spasm is a rare, and alarming complication of ketamine anaesthesia. It should not be disastrous if you treat it properly. Secretions or blood falling onto the patient's vocal cords may cause it.

The dose range of ketamine is wide, and an overdose is rare. Patients have recovered uneventfully after 10 times the normal dose. This seems to vary from one country to another. Fig. 2-4 calculates the *intravenous dose* at 2 mg/kg, but you may need to give more than this. In Kenya 6 to 10 mg/kg is the standard intramuscular dose but in Nepal 4 mg/kg is said to be enough.

This variation in dosage may be related to the extent to which alcohol is drunk by a community. Alcoholic patients usually need more ketamine. Occasionally, a patient shows no sign of surgical anaesthesia after three times the normal dose. Patients like this usually need to be anaesthetized in some other way.

One difficulty in estimating the dose is not knowing when a patient is adequately anaesthetized. His eyes may be wide open and he may make occasional spontaneous movements, and yet anaesthesia may be adequate for surgery. The best test is to prick him with a needle.

Caesarean section can be done under ketamine anaesthesia, but ketamine is not the ideal agent for it. Ketamine does however rival a saddle block (7.7) as one of the methods of choice if you are very inexperienced and are working under difficult conditions. It crosses the placental barrier rapidly. A dose of 1 mg/kg causes little respiratory depression in the baby, but in doses above 2 mg/kg it may cause both respiratory depression and cause chest wall rigidity and make resuscitation difficult. In analgesic doses of 0.25 mg/kg ketamine is a useful addition to local or regional anaesthesia for Caesarean section.

The main purpose of promethazine or diazepam is to prevent emergence reactions, so wait to give it during Caesarean section until after she has been delivered when it can no longer reach her baby.

A possible disadvantage of ketamine anaesthesia is the adverse effect that it may have on the establishment of bonding between a mother and her baby. Ketamine also makes the uterus contract, so avoid it if you are doing a Caesarean section for fetal distress.

Safety is one of ketamine's great advantages. As Fig. 8-1 shows, there are fewer opportunities to make mistakes with it. You are much more likely to make a mistake with a complex anaesthetic machine like that in Fig. 8-2. Although ketamine is about as safe as any anaesthetic could be, it is not completely safe. If a patient with intestinal obstruction, for example, is going to vomit, and inhale his vomit, ketamine will not stop him doing so. Disaster can still happen, so don't give ketamine unless you have all the equipment ready to resuscitate the patient.

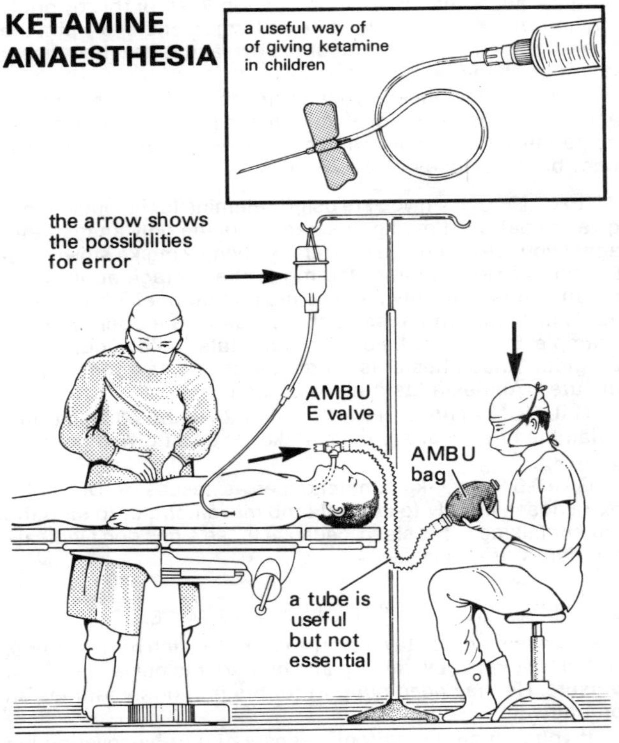

TAKE ALL THE USUAL ANAESTHETIC PRECAUTIONS STARVE PATIENTS RECEIVING KETAMINE

GAIA (40 years) was referred because of a delay in the second stage of labour. One of the baby's arms had prolapsed two days previously, and traditional midwives had been unable to help the mother. The infant was macerated, and a destructive operation was indicated. The anaesthetic assistant was taking his annual leave, so it was decided to operate under an intravenous ketamine drip. A gram of ketamine (about 10 times the standard dose) only made her slightly drowsy, without in any way anaesthetizing her. It appeared she was a well-known alcoholic. There being no staff who could be trusted with a difficult anaesthetic, she was transferred to another hospital, where she recovered. LESSONS (1) Ketamine is unsuitable for alcoholics. (2) If you can avoid operating under very difficult conditions, do so. (3) If you had been unable to refer her, a saddle block would probably have been the most suitable anaesthetic.

White PF, Way WL. Trevor AJ, Ketamine—its pharmacology and therapeutic uses. Anaesthesiology 1982, 56:119-136.
Ellingson A, et al, Transplacental passage of ketamine after intravenous administration. Acta. anaesth. Scand. 1977, 21:41-44.

WHEN IS KETAMINE ANAESTHESIA APPROPRIATE?
KETAMINE WITHOUT RELAXANTS

INDICATIONS Any operation not requiring deep muscular relaxation, or the absence of pharyngeal reflexes.

(1) Short operations, such as reducing fractures and dressing burnt children. A low dose of 1 mg/kg is excellent for changing painful dressings when analgesia is wanted without anaesthesia. (2) Operations on the head and neck that are not suitable for local anaesthesia and where access to the airway is difficult. Ordinary ketamine is not suitable for operations inside the mouth. You can however wire teeth under ketamine. (3) Operations on several parts of the body that would require too many local anaesthetics at once (desloughing the chest, or skin grafting the chest from the thigh). (4) Operations where the patient lies face downwards, and which would be difficult for a non-specialist anaesthetist, for example, disarticulating the knee, or amputating through the lower leg may require this position. (5) Emergency operations when the equipment for general or subarachnoid anaesthesia is not available. (6) Limb operations, biopsies. (7) Patients who are difficult to intubate for any reason. (8) Extracting injured patients trapped in buildings or vehicles.

For the induction of anaesthesia, especially before ether in children, and in patients with incompletely corrected hypovolaemic shock, when an operation is urgent, for example, rupture of the spleen or ectopic pregnancy. Ketamine is particularly useful for raising the blood pressure of these patients. Give it intramuscularly or better intravenously.

CONTRAINDICATIONS Some of these are only relative contraindications. (1) Because ketamine does not relax the muscles, relaxants should in theory be required for all operations in which a patient's abdominal muscles should be relaxed. Nevertheless, in an emergency, and depending on how much relaxation you need, you can use ketamine without relaxants for such indications as ruptured ectopic pregnancy, Caesarean section, and even for some intestinal operations in children. It is however far from ideal. (2) Ketamine is also not ideal for reducing dislocations and fractures, when these need relaxation of the limb muscles. (3) Patients in whom a rise in blood pressure would be undesirable, such as those with PIH (pregnancy induced hypertension or pre—eclamptic toxaemia), eclampsia, severe hypertension, or heart failure. (4) Internal version, and Caesarean section for fetal distress, because ketamine increases uterine tone. (5) Intracranial operations, particularly head injuries, because it raises the intracranial pressure. (6) Eye operations, because ketamine raises the intraocular pressure and does not abolish eye movements, unless you

Fig. 8-1 THERE ARE FEW OPPORTUNITIES FOR ERROR WITH KETAMINE ANAESTHESIA. *Kindly contributed by Peter Bewes and Georg Kamm*

give larger doses—see Section 16.9. (7) Glaucoma is an absolute contraindication. (8) Bronchoscopy, unless relaxants are used, and most throat and dental operations, or any operation in which blood, tissues, or instruments may cause "gagging" or spasm of the larynx. Ketamine has however been used successfully for severe maxillofacial injuries, where intubation would be impossible. (9) Psychiatric patients, because of the hallucinations that ketamine may cause. (10) Any case that could be anaesthetized more simply in some other way, such as by local anaesthesia. (11) Alcoholics and drunk outpatients.

If you don't have equipment for intubation and ventilation, and yet you have to anaesthetize a patient, ketamine is likely to be the safest anaesthetic for him. Even so, equipment for it should always be available.

KETAMINE DRIP WITH RELAXANTS

INDICATIONS Any of the above indications, and any patient requiring muscle relaxation. Almost any operation could be done this way.

NEVER GIVE KETAMINE WITHOUT EQUIPMENT FOR CONTROLLING THE RESPIRATION

THERE ARE MANY POSSIBILITIES FOR ERROR WITH A COMPLEX ANAESTHETIC

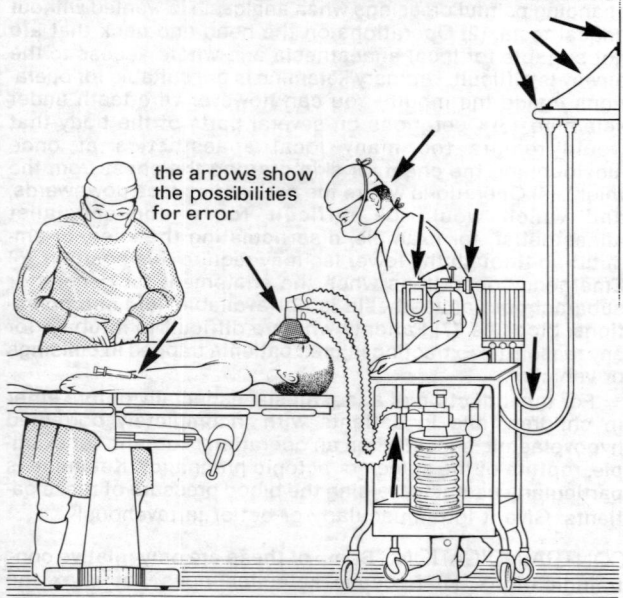

Fig. 8-2 THERE ARE MANY MORE OPPORTUNITIES FOR ERROR WITH COMPLEX ANAESTHETIC APPARATUS THAN WITH KETAMINE. *Kindly contributed by Peter Bewes and Georg Kamm*

8.2 Intramuscular and bolus intravenous ketamine

These are two very useful methods, with few serious side effects. Intravenous ketamine acts more quickly than ketamine by the intramuscular route, and it is cheaper because the dose is smaller. In some district hospitals it is the standard method for most patients. Intramuscular ketamine, on the other hand, is particularly useful for small children with difficult veins.

INTRMUSCULAR AND BOLUS INTRAVENOUS KETAMINE

INDICATIONS AND CONTRAINDICATIONS See also Section 8.1. Short procedures such as reducing fractures. Intramuscular ketamine takes 5 to 10 minutes to act. If you want immediate anaesthesia, give ketamine intravenously.

Starve the patient preoperatively. Have resuscitation equipment available.

PREMEDICATION Always premedicate an adult; premedication is less important in children, especially small ones. Two hours before the operation give an adult promethazine 50 mg. Give children 1 mg/kg. Or, give them diazepam (2-4).

CAUTION ! Don't mix ketamine and diazepam or barbiturates, like thiopentone, in the same syringe, because they react to form a white precipitate. Give the diazepam first, then the ketamine. Or, less satisfactorily, give the promethazine or diazepam as the patient is recovering.

If a mother is having a Caesarean section, give promethazine, or diazepam (or pethidine) after her baby is delivered, so that the drug will not affect him.

ATROPINE For adults this is optional, for children it is essential. Give adults 0.75 mg, and children the doses in Fig. 2-4.

If necessary, give atropine and promethazine (or diazepam) intravenously.

AIRWAYS When you have given ketamine, don't try to put in an airway routinely in an adult, because he will probably reject it. Some adults will tolerate an airway, others will not. One of the dangers of inserting an airway in a patient under ketamine is that it can precipitate severe laryngospasm. Insert an airway routinely in small babies.

GIVING THE KETAMINE

INTRAMUSCULARLY Give 6 to 10 mg/kg of ketamine. It is supppplied in 3 strengths 10 mg/ml, 50 mg/ml, and 100 mg/ml, so check the strength.

The patient will start to look sleepy. He will stop following things with his eyes, and then become "glassy-eyed". Surgical anaesthesia will then develop. Test for this by pricking him with a needle. When he no longer reacts to a pin, the operation can start. Don't test his eyelash reflex, because it is not abolished.

Surgical anaesthesia is usually reached in about 5 minutes, and occasionally not for 10 minutes. It lasts 25 minutes, and sometimes up to an hour and more. If necessary, give the patient booster doses of 2 to 5 mg/kg.

INTRAVENOUSLY If you are using ketamine for induction only, give the patient 1 mg/kg. If ketamine is the only anaesthetic agent you are going to use, start by giving 2 mg/kg slowly during one or two minutes. 100 mg is the average adult dose. Small adults may only need 50 mg and fat or alcoholic ones 200 mg. Adjust the dose to the needs of the operation, for example, 50 mg may be enough for dilatation and curettage. Surgical anaesthesia is immediate and lasts about 20 minutes. Amnesia lasts up to an hour.

CAUTION ! (1)*Inject slowly—over 1 or 2 minutes.* (2) Don't give ketamine into an artery by mistake. (3) Don't give more than 3 mg/kg.

Give 0.5 to 1 mg/kg booster doses as necessary. Don't give extra doses merely to control limb movement, or to stop the patient talking in his sleep, because those signs don't indicate the depth of anaesthesia.

DURING THE OPERATION WITH KETAMINE

Ask an assistant to stay near the patient, watch his breathing, watch for signs of vomiting, and monitor his pulse and blood presure. He may need support for his jaw, or sometimes an oral airway.

If you reduce the patient's sensory input by covering his eyes and ears, this will reduce postoperative excitement. If you do cover the eyes, make quite sure you close them first, or you may injure his cornea.

POSTOPERATIVE CARE WITH KETAMINE
The patient will be sleepy for about 2 hours, so take him to a quiet place to recover. Noises will wake him while he is still in a dreamy stage, and may make him noisy and restless. Let him wake naturally, and don't try to wake him forcibly, or he may have emergence reactions. His airway is comparatively safe, so he is in much less danger than he would be if he was recovering from a conventional general anaesthetic, but he may fall out of bed.

Keep the patient in the hospital grounds for at least 4 hours after he has apparently recovered completely. Tell him, in the presence of his guardian, not to climb trees or ladders, or to ride a bicycle, or to operate a car or machinery, or drink alcohol for 24 hours. He should not go by plane for 3 days, because violent behaviour in a light plane can be dangerous.

DIFFICULTIES WITH KETAMINE

If the patient stops breathing, control his ventilation. Respiratory arrest is rare, and is more common after intravenous ketamine. It is said never to last more than a minute or two, and it should not happen if you give ketamine slowly. If you don't have a self-inflating bag, ventilate him mouth to mouth.

If he appears to feel pain, and keeps moving about: (1) He may need more ketamine. (2) Premedication may have been inadequate. (3) Muscular relaxation may be needed. (4) He may be an alcoholic, and need larger doses.

If you know he is an alcoholic, give him a second dose of ketamine immediately.

If he is not an alcoholic, don't give more ketamine. Don't try to control him with pethidine and morphine. Either abandon the operation, and try ketamine again later after adequate premedication, or give the patient a relaxant and intubate him.

If he shows purposeless tonic–clonic movements of his limbs, they do not indicate that anaesthesia is light and do not indicate the need for more ketamine.

If he becomes catatonic with stiff muscles, give him suxamethonium, and intubate him. This is rare.

If ketamine is in short supply, you can reduce the amount you need by premedicating him with morphine.

If he shouts, swears, and struggles as he emerges from the anesthetic, give him diazepam, 5 to 10 mg intravenously. These emergence reactions last a variable time, they are shorter after intravenous ketamine, and always pass off rapidly. If many patients behave like this, your routine premedication is probably unsatisfactory, or you are giving it at the wrong time.

8.3 Plain ketamine drip

A ketamine drip: (1) Allows you to control the depth of anaesthesia more easily than ketamine by the intramuscular or the bolus intravenous route. (2) Is simple and fast. (3) Needs little equipment. (4) Is safe, if you use it with care. (5) Makes induction and recovery quick. (6) Is cheap (provided intravenous fluid is cheap), because you need a smaller dose (about 4 mg/kg/hour) than by the intramuscular route. (7) Is even less likely to cause respiratory arrest than ketamine by the other routes. A ketamine drip is slightly more demanding than giving an intramuscular injection, and it does require a bottle of intravenous fluid.

A simple ketamine drip has two other disadvantages: (1) It does not relax a patient's abdominal muscles. (2) His pharyngeal reflexes, which are so useful in protecting his respiratory tract, are still present, so they make operations on his mouth difficult. If necessary, you can overcome both these disadvantages by giving him a relaxant (8.4) and intubating him. To begin with his pulse and blood pressure will rise slightly and then fall again. Although this method has a wide margin of safety with few opportunities for human or technical error, you can still make mistakes with the drip. If you use relaxants, there is also room for error when you intubate the patient and control his ventilation.

PLAIN KETAMINE DRIP

INDICATIONS AND CONTRAINDICATIONS See Section 8.1. Larger procedures, such as prostatecomy, not requiring abdominal relaxation.

Starve the patient preoperatively. Have resuscitation equipment available.

EQUIPMENT An intravenous infusion set and a cannula or large bore needle, 500 ml of 5% dextrose or 0.9% saline, ketamine. A sphygmomanometer, a self-inflating bag or bellows, equipment for tracheal intubation (13.2), and a sucker.

PREMEDICATION Sedate the patient with promethazine or diazepam (2-4), as for intramuscular or intravenous ketamine. Give him atropine (2-4).

KETAMINE SOLUTION Make a solution of 1 mg/ml. Dissolve a 10 ml bottle of ketamine containing 50 mg/ml in 500 ml of 5% dextrose, or 0.9% saline. For short procedures mix smaller volumes.

Before the operation, set up a free-flowing drip using plain 5% dextrose and a cannula or large needle in an adequate vein. Don't try to give ketamine through a poorly flowing drip into a small vein. If you are using a ketamine drip routinely, arrange for each case to come to the theatre early enough for you to set up a saline drip. When you want to anaesthetise them, exchange the bottle of saline for the bottle containing ketamine. This will enable you to work faster.

If a patient needs a blood transfusion, or a drip for some other purpose, don't combine it with the ketamine. Put the blood through another needle into another vein.

INDUCTION Before you scrub up, change the 5% dextrose for the ketamine solution.

For an average sized adult, start the drip at 140 drops a minute. This is about 2 drops a minute per kilogram body weight.

Continue the drip beyond the point at which the patient becomes unconscious, until surgical anaesthesia is reached. This is easy to recognise, but difficult to describe. He develops a vacant stare, he does not respond to pain, but he still has his eyelash, corneal, and pharyngeal reflexes. Test his sensation of pain by pricking him with a pin.

MAINTENANCE When surgical anaesthesia has been reached slow the drip to 60 to 80 drops a minute. This is about one drop per minute per kilogram body weight (4 mg/kg/hour). If the patient is shocked, give him the smallest dose of ketamine that will keep him quiet.

Monitor his respiration, his pulse rate and his blood pressure.

If he seems to react to the pain of the operation, increase the speed of the drip, say to 120 drops a minute. Stop operating until conditions are again satisfactory. Later, you may be able to slow the drip.

Stop the drip about 10 minutes before the operation ends.

POSTOPERATIVE CARE This is the same as for intramuscular and intravenous ketamine.

8.4 Ketamine drip with relaxants

This is the cheapest way of giving a patient ketamine, because it uses only 2 mg/kg/hour, which is half as much as a simple drip. It provides good analgesia and relaxation; induction and recovery are smooth; he does not normally need oxygen; there are no infammable vapours, and he does not usually complain of unpleasant hallucinations or dreams. You need the absolute minimum of equipment. The most convenient way of controlling his ventilation is to use a self-inflating bag. Provided that you maintain his depth of anaesthesia, and his ventilation correctly, his blood pressure will not change. Occasionally, he will salivate so severely that you will have to suck out his pharynx.

KETAMINE DRIP WITH RELAXANTS AND CONTROLLED RESPIRATION

EQUIPMENT A freely flowing drip of 5% dextrose or 0.9% saline, a self-inflating bag or bellows, a non-rebreathing valve, a laryngoscope and suitable blades, a range of tracheal tubes, suitable adaptors from the non-rebreathing valve to the tracheal tubes, a syringe and artery forceps for the cuff of the tracheal tube, pharyngeal and endotracheal suction catheters, a foot sucker, oxygen (for patients who are anaemic or shocked or undergoing lung surgery), ketamine, promethazine, suxamethonium, and alcuronium or d-tubocurarine or any other long acting muscle relaxant. Gallamine is better avoided.

PREMEDICATION This is the same as for intramuscular or intravenous ketamine. Give the patient atropine. Starve him.

DRIP Set this up in the same way as for a simple ketamine drip.

INDUCTION AND MAINTENANCE OF A KETAMINE DRIP WITH RELAXANTS

Start the drip at 140 drops a minute, or about 2 drops per minute per kilogram body weight. Continue the drip at this rate only until the patient is asleep. As soon as he is asleep, give him suxamethonium 1mg/kg and intubate him. After intubation, control his ventilation with bellows or a self-inflating bag and air.

When his muscles recover from the suxamethonium, give him a non-depolarising relaxant, such as alcuronium, d-tubocurarine or gallamine. Continue to control his respiration. A comfortable squeeze of the bag yields about 500 ml. Aim for a minute volume of 1 litre per 10 kg per minute. This is about 12 squeezes a minute for a 60 kg adult.

Reduce the speed of the ketamine drip to 30 to 40 drops a minute. This is about half a drop per minute, per kilogram body weight.

If saliva accumulates in his pharynx, suck it out.

If there are sounds that fluid is accumulating in his trachea, suck this out too.

If he needs fluid or blood during the operation, either give these with separate drips, or put the needle of one drip into the tube of the other.

If he needs oxygen, add this to the inlet port of the self-inflating bag at 1 litre per minute.

REVERSAL Stop the ketamine drip about 10 minutes before the end of the operation. Keep ventilating.

Ten to 15 minutes before the end of the operation prepare to reverse the patient's residual muscle paralysis. Give him intravenous atropine, 0.02 or 0.04 mg/kg.

Then give him intravenous neostigmine 0.04 mg/kg.

Ventilate him until adequate neuromuscular function returns. If necessary, underventilate him a little so that his carbon dioxide tension rises a little and provides a stimulus to spontaneous respiration.

Suck out his pharynx, turn him onto this side and then remove the tracheal tube in the usual way.

POSTOPERATIVE CARE This is the same as for intramuscular and intravenous ketamine.

8.5 Ketamine in children

The anaesthetic problems of children are discussed in Chapter 18. Here we only discuss ketamine, which is an excellent anaesthetic for children. In hospitals where they are operated on only occasionally, ketamine is certainly the safest anaesthetic for them. It does not give a child serious nightmares or hallucinations, so you need not premedicate him. Because he only needs a small dose, it is cheap. You can give it intramuscularly, so you don't have to find a vein.

Usually, all you need do is to support the child's chin, and there is seldom any need to intubate him. But respiratory obstruction and apnoea can occur, so be ready to intubate him and control his ventilation if necessary.

Neonates and newborn babies may stop breathing at any time as the result of quite minor changes in the oxygenation, pH, and volume of their circulating blood, or of the depth of anaesthesia. So they are best intubated, allowed to breathe an inhalation anaesthetic spontaneously, and ventilated when necessary. This needs skill and equipment; if you don't have these, use ketamine—it may even be the method of choice for short procedures. You can combine it with chloral hydrate, and if necessary with awake intubation, or with local infiltration with 0.25% bupivacaine or 0.5% lignocaine. Avoid relaxants.

Hypoglycaemia can occur, as after any operation, so see Section 18.1.

Cardiac arrest has been reported after ketamine in dehydrated and malnourished children. If you have to give them ketamine, give them the smallest possible dose.

KETAMINE IN THE VERY YOUNG

Have an adequate supply of oxygen, and a use a well fitting paediatric mask. Be sure to insert an airway. Have tracheal tubes and a infant laryngoscope ready. Suction is essential. All but the smallest operations in young children require a drip so that you can replace any blood that is lost ml for ml. This is usually best put up when the child is asleep. Weigh the swabs and inject blood of equal volume into the rubber section of the drip—don't wait until 5 or 10% of a child's blood volume is lost.

Strap a precordial stethoscope to his chest, and monitor him with this. Monitor his circulation by observing his fingers.

Give him intramuscular atropine 15 to 30 minutes before the operation. If you don't do this, crying may have made him very "wet", when the time comes to give him ketamine. In very hot climates, where hyperthermia is a real danger (2.7), don't give atropine.

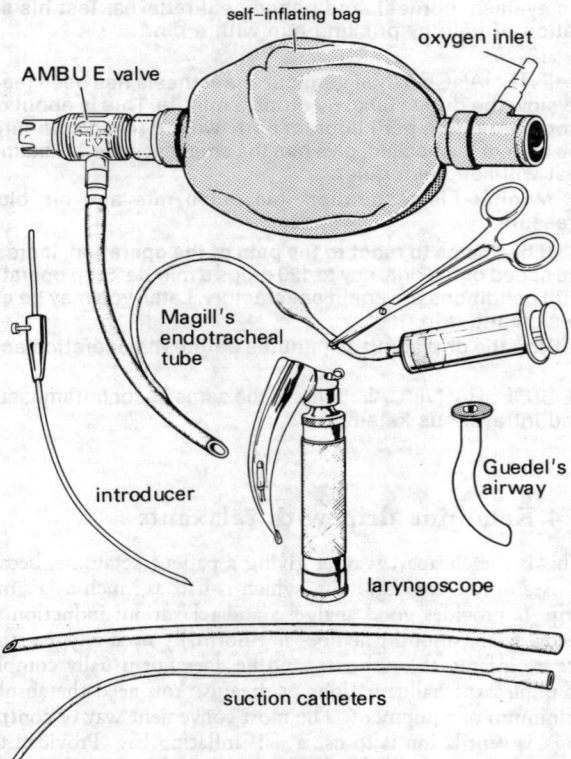

Fig. 8-3 THE EQUIPMENT FOR KETAMINE DRIP WITH RELAXANTS. *Kindly contributed by Peter Bewes and Georg Kamm*

Give him his first dose of ketamine 10 mg/kg intramuscularly. One intramuscular dose is usually enough. If necessary, supplement this with 2 mg/kg intravenously, or, less satisfactorily 10 mg/kg intramuscularly.

CAUTION ! See also Chapter 18.

8.6 Intravenous analgesia

For changing plasters or burns dressings, try giving a patient a low dose of ketamine (1 mg/kg) intravenously. He won't be deeply anaesthetized and there is little chance of delirium.

For short procedures such as reducing fractures, it is useful to be able to abolish pain and produce amnesia without having to make special provision for the patient's airway, although you should always watch it. You can conveniently do this by giving a bolus intravenous injection of: (1) Ketamine with diazepam, as in Section 2.8, either intramuscularly or intravenously—*this is much the safest method, especially in children.* (2) Morphine alone. (3) Pethidine with diazepam, or chlorpromazine, or promethazine. (4) Thiopentone with pethidine. None of these agents relax the patient's muscles satisfactorily, so they are far from ideal for reducing fractures and dislocations, which is one of the commonest occasions on which you need a short anaesthetic. Intravenous ketamine with diazepam is the safest of these methods, and is discussed in Section 8.2. It is more expensive than thiopentone, and lasts longer, so it is less satisfactory for outpatients.

Provided you only use *moderate* doses of these drugs—pethidine, promethazine, chlorpromazine or promethazine—a patient's pharyngeal and laryngeal reflexes are sufficiently preserved for them to be *comparatively* safe. Larger doses act as general anaesthetics, and so does thiopentone. They may nauseate the patient, and depress his reflexes sufficiently for the inhalation of vomit to be a real danger. In general, a patient who is not fit for a general anaesthetic is not fit for one of these intravenous analgesics either. So you had better anaesthetize him in some other way.

If you use intravenous analgesics carelessly, they can be and often are, disastrous. So take all the standard precautions for a general anaesthetic: (1) Starve the patient, (2) Put him on a table that tips. (3) Give him atropine, because this will reduce the incidence of laryngeal spasm due to secretions. (4) Have the equipment for suction, intubation and controlled ventilation instantly available, because respiratory arrest, laryngeal spasm and vomiting can all occur.

8.7 Intravenous morphine

This is useful in an emergency for reducing fractures and dislocations, for dressing wounds, for relieving pain, for evacuating disaster casualties, and for extracting patients trapped in machinery or collapsed buildings. *The secret of giving it is to give it slowly, until pain is sufficiently relieved.* This needs a larger dose than that used for premedication. Thus you may occasionally need to give up to 0.5 mg/kg, or more (30 mg for an adult), compared with the premedication dose of only 0.2 mg/kg (10 to 15 mg for an adult). If you give it too fast, or give an unnecessarily large dose, the patient's respiration will be depressed and he may stop breathing completely. But, if you judge the dose correctly, he will be in a state of analgesia short of full anaesthesia and will have considerable amnesia, even for cutting surgery. His pharyngeal and laryngeal reflexes will be largely preserved, and respiratory depression will not be marked.

THERE IS NO STANDARD DOSE OF INTRAVENOUS MORPHINE

8.8 Anaesthetic mixtures based on intravenous pethidine

Pethidine is a powerful analgesic, but it has little anaesthetic or sedative action, so you cannot operate under it alone. But, if you combine it with diazepam, or chlorpromazine, or promethazine, or thiopentone, the pair of drugs will provide enough anaesthetic and sedative action to enable you to operate. Two drugs are enough and there is no need to add more.

Pethidine with one or more of these drugs is often mixed together in the same syringe to make a "cocktail" for short procedures. This is bad practice because: (1) You cannot titrate the effect of the two drugs separately. (2) Pethidine and diazepam form a precipitate when they are mixed in a syringe. Instead, give the required dose of intravenous pethidine in mg/kg and then 'titrate' the dose of the other drug until you get just the effect you want.

For very short procedures pethidine with thiopentone is best, because the patient recovers more quickly and can go home sooner than after pethidine with diazepam or ketamine. *But thiopentone is only suitable for procedures that you are sure are going to last less than 3 minutes.* It is a poor analgesic, so don't give it without pethidine. If you don't have pethidine, you would be wise not to give him thiopentone alone.

For procedures lasting between 3 and 20 minutes, use pethidine and diazepam. The patient sleeps, but you can rouse him if necessary. Unfortunately he is likely to sleep for many hours afterwards, which is undesirable if nursing skills are scarce.

When you give these intravenous pethidine combinations, remember that that they are full anaesthetics, with all the anaesthetic risks and complications. So, follow the "ten golden rules" in Section 3.1, starve the patient, put him on a table that tips, and have suction ready.

Evacuating an incomplete abortion is the most frequent indication for a intravenous pethidine cocktail. Because so many women have abortions, this is one of the most frequently used forms of anaesthesia in many hospitals. Even so, use pethidine cocktails with caution. They are not as safe as ketamine, especially in children, so use ketamine where you can. It produces better and safer analgesia than pethidine, and less respiratory depression than diazepam. The patient's laryngeal and pharyngeal reflexes are better preserved, and his slow recovery from it not a threat to his life and is seldom important.

DAISY (3 years) was in the children's ward with an abscess in her thigh that needed draining. The ethyl chloride was finished and the hospital had a rule that ketamine was an anaesthetic and so had to be given by an anaesthetic assistant. None was available, so she was taken to the side room and 25 mg of pethidine and 20 mg of diazepam were mixed in a syringe. While this was being given she collapsed; oxygen and a self inflating bag were fetched from another part of the hospital, but by the time they arrived they were too late to revive her. LESSONS (1) 20 mg of diazepam was about 10 times and 25 mg of pethidine about 5 times the correct dose. Stick the spare copy of Figure 2-4 up on the wall and use it. (2) They should not have been mixed in the same syringe. She should have been given 5 mg of intravenous pethidine, and then given just enough diazepam (about 2 mg), diluted in a larger volume of saline, to send her to sleep. (3) Ketamine is safer than "cocktails", especially in childen. (4) The large dose she was given probably produced death by respiratory arrest. Had she been ventilated immediately, even mouth to mouth, she would probably have survived—the equipment for controlled ventilation must be instantly available when these drugs are given. (5) Ethyl chloride may be an ineffective local anaesthetic, but at least it would not have killed her.

WHEN YOU USE THIOPENTONE FOR SHORT PROCEDURES, GIVE PETHIDINE

INTRAVENOUS PETHIDINE

Before you start *any* of the following methods: (1) The patient must be on a table that can tip. (2) Airways and equipment for intubation and controlled ventilation must be available. (3) Starve him. (4) Give him atropine. (5) Insert a diaphragm needle. (6) Be prepared to continue with an inhalational anaesthetic if necessary. (7) Maintain a clear airway and monitor his pulse and respiration.

CAUTION ! Don't use intravenous pethidine cocktails in children if you can possibly avoid doing so.

PETHIDINE AND THIOPENTONE

INDICATIONS (1) Ultra-short procedures not requiring relaxation and lasting less that 3 minutes, such as opening an abscess. (2) Extraction of a single tooth if the dentist is skilled.

PREPARATION The surgeon must be scrubbed up and completely ready to cut, with his instruments ready. The patient must be towelled up with his skin prepared. Have an assistant standing by to restrain the patient if he moves.

METHOD Slowly give pethidine intravenously in the dose in Fig.2-4. When the surgeon is completely ready, give intravenous thiopentone, until the patient just sleeps. You will probably need about the dose shown in Fig. 2-4 for a patient who has been premedicated. The usual adult dose is about 250 mg.

Perform the procedure as soon as the patient is unconscious. Care for his airway as usual. Put him in the recovery position as soon as the procedure is complete and, if possible, while the dressings are being applied. After 10 minutes he will respond to questions, and after an hour he can go home *under supervision*.

CAUTION ! (1) Don't try to prolong anaesthesia with more thiopentone. (2) The main danger with this method is laryngeal spasm, so be prepared for it (3.2).

If you have no pethidine, so that you have to give thiopentone alone, don't give more than 500 mg in all.

PETHIDINE WITH EITHER DIAZEPAM, OR CHLORPROMAZINE, OR PROMETHAZINE

INDICATIONS Procedures lasting more than three but less than 20 minutes, such as wound dressings, or dilation and curettage. You can use pethidine/diazepam for almost any obstetric procedure, except Caesarean section.

METHOD Give the intravenous pethidine first in the dose in Fig. 2-4. 25 or 50 mg is the usual adult dose. Follow this by intravenous diazepam until the patient just sleeps. He usually needs 5 to 10 mg. Or, give intravenous promethazine, the usual adult intravenous dose is 50 mg. Or, give intravenous chlorpromazine the usual adult intravenous dose is 25 mg. With all three of these drugs, give only enough to send him to sleep.

CAUTION ! (1) The pethidine should be labelled as suitable for intravenous use. (2) Don't give pethidine and diazepam in the same syringe, because a precipitate forms. (3) Don't exceed 1 mg/kg of pethidine, or the patient may stop breathing. If he does, control his ventilation. (4) Avoid this method in young children.

DON'T GIVE COCKTAILS WITHOUT RESUSCITATION EQUIPMENT

8.9 Ketamine and morphine drips

If you give low doses of these drugs, you can keep a patient alert, and free from pain for days or weeks if necessary. When used like this, morphine causes little respiratory depression, and ketamine none.

ANALGESIC DRIPS

INDICATIONS Intractable pain, as from multiple fractured ribs.

CONTRAINDICATIONS Nurses who cannot manage drips reliably.

MORPHINE

LOADING DOSE Give the patient just enough morphine by slow bolus intravenous injection to abolish pain.

MAINTENANCE DOSE Dissolve 25 mg of morphine in 500 ml of 5% dextrose (or 15 mg in 300 ml). The adult dose is 12 to 25 drops per minute (0.5 to 1.0 mg/kg/hour, or 1 to 2 ml/kg/hour).

KETAMINE

LOADING DOSE Give just enough ketamine by slow bolus intravenous injection to abolish pain.

MAINTENANCE DOSE Make a solution of 0.5 mg/ml by dissolving 250 mg of ketamine (5 ml of a 50 mg/ml) in 500 ml of saline. Adjust the rate of the drip to keep him just free from pain. The drip rate will probably vary between 15 and 30 drops a minute (0.5 to 1 mg/kg/hour). This is between a quarter and eighth of the maintenance dose needed for a simple ketamine drip (8.3). 15 drops a minute will give him about a litre and a half of fluid in 24 hours.

CAUTION ! Make sure that the fluid you give him in his analgesic drip is reckoned as part of his total fluid needs and does not exceed them.

9 Nitrous oxide, air, and oxygen

9.1 An introduction to inhalational anaesthesia

A general anaesthetic has many advantages. You can give it quickly, it makes the patient's whole body insensitive to pain, and it makes him unconscious. But: (1) A general anaesthetic may cause both respiratory and cardiovascular complications. (2) You must keep one of his veins open, so that you can give him any drugs he needs quickly. (3) He must have a clear airway. (4) You must be able to assist or control his ventilation, if this becomes depressed.

A general anaesthetic follows the stages of premedication, induction, maintenance and recovery as shown in Fig. 9-1.

Premedication. During this phase (1), sedate the patient with oral or intramuscular diazepam and/or pethidine (2) to relieve his anxiety. Give him atropine (3).

Induction. Induce the patient (4) with one of the inhalation agents: ether, halothane, or trichloroethylene (5). Alternatively, you can induce him with one of the intravenous agents: thiopentone, ketamine, or diazepam (6).

The patient loses consciousness (7) and passes into the stage of pre-surgical anaesthesia (8). During this stage he "settles" and you can prepare him for surgery. You can now continue with an inhalation agent only (9), or you can intubate him, either under the inhalation agent alone or with a short-acting relaxant, such as suxamethonium to paralyse him; and then intubate him. (10). Alternatively, you can continue to give him ketamine alone (11).

Maintenance. This is the phase when the operation is done. You can maintain the patient on one of the inhalation agents (12), usually ether or trichloroethylene. Or, if good muscular relaxation is needed, you can give him a long-acting relaxant such as alcuronium and control his ventilation (13). Or, you can continue with ketamine (14) alone, or combine this with a long-acting relaxant.

Recovery. During this phase the patient exhales and, or, metabolises his inhalation agent (15). He also excretes or metabolises his relaxant, or has its activity reversed with neostigmine (16). If you have given him ketamine, he excretes and metabolises it (17).

The thicker arrows show some of the more usual ways in which you can combine the various forms of anaesthesia. A commom sequence is intravenous induction (a), followed by inhalation anaesthesia, usually with ether. You can vary this by (b)

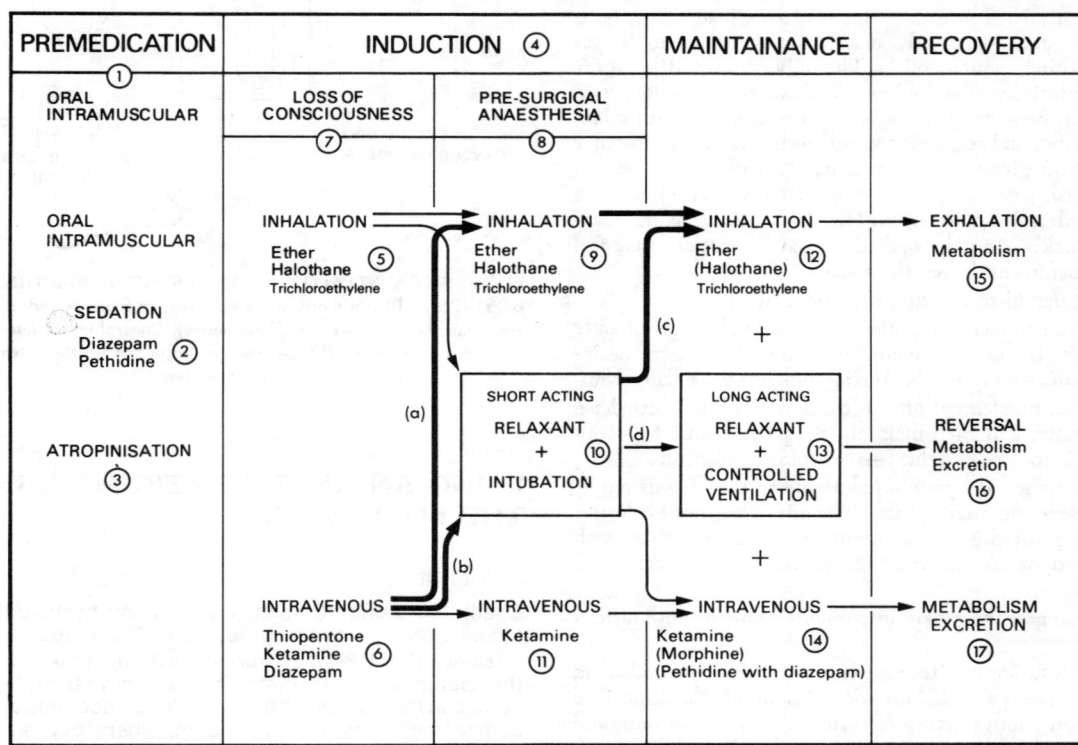

Fig. 9-1 THE MAIN PHASES OF GENERAL ANAESTHESIA and some of the alternatives. *Kindly contributed by John Farman.*

intubating him under suxamethonium and maintaining him with an inhalation agent (c). Alternatively, you can use inhalation agents without a relaxant. If you do decide to use a relaxant, you can either use a short—acting one (suxamethonium) alone, or (d) you can use suxamethonium followed by a long—acting relaxant such as alcuronium. You would be wise not to use a long—acting relaxant alone for both intubation and maintenance, although some expert anaesthetists do.

One of the most practical ways to produce general anaesthesia is to let a patient inhale ether, trichloroethylene, or, if necessary, chloroform, vapourised in a carrier gas. This can be air, or nitrous oxide and oxygen.

Atmospheric air has many advantages. It costs nothing, and in routine use you do not have to add oxygen to it. Most important, air cannot run out, and when mixed with ether alone, it cannot explode. When air is trapped in the alveoli of a patient's lungs, the nitrogen it contains is only slowly absorbed, so his alveoli have little tendency to collapse.

Nitrous oxide has many disadvantages. It is expensive (2-1), and supplies are likely to be unreliable in remote hospitals. You must give it with oxygen, and if the oxygen runs out without you noticing, the patient is at risk of grave anoxia and may die. When oxygen is mixed with ether, it may explode. When it is trapped in the alveoli oxygen is rapidly absorbed, so that the alveoli easily collapse.

For all these reasons, air is much the most appropriate carrier gas for the hospitals for which we write, and nitrous, oxide has little place in Primary Anaesthesia. You may however find yourself in a hospital where you have to use it on a machine of the Boyle's type, so the next section tells you what to do.

9.2 Using nitrous oxide

Nitrous oxide is a strong analgesic, but a weak anaesthetic. It is relatively non—toxic, and the patient recovers quickly. Mixing nitrous oxide with even the minimum amount of air to keep the patient alive (not less than 30% to allow for possible errors in measurement) makes it even weaker. The resulting mixture, containing only 70% nitrous oxide, is usually inadequate, both for induction and as the only anaesthetic agent when the patient is breathing spontaneously. The only exceptions are short minor procedures, which don't need relaxation, such as extracting teeth. If, however, you combine nitrous oxide with relaxants, intubation, and controlled ventilation, it is useful for major surgery. If you give it this way it has two disadvantages: (1) There is a risk that the patient may be conscious while he is still paralysed and unable to protest. (2) Nitrous oxide is excreted so quickly after the operation that the patient may feel pain, even before he leaves the theatre.

You can use nitrous oxide in various ways—

(1) You can induce the patient with a *few* breaths of pure nitrous oxide. Because he is not breathing any oxygen, he inevitably becomes temporarily anoxic, which may be dangerous.

(2) You can supplement nitrous oxide with trichloroethylene, change to ether, and then maintain the patient on a low concentration (2 to 4% of ether)—an explosive mixture!

(3) You can add 0.5 to 1% halothane to the nitrous oxide. You must use a calibrated inhaler. The mixture is not explosive. The advantage of this is that induction is quicker than with halothane and air, so that you can operate on more patients in a given time.

(4) You can give the patient intravenous pethidine with nitrous oxide.

(5) You can induce the patient with nitrous oxide and trichloroethylene, paralyse him with suxamethonium, intubate him, give him a long—acting relaxant such as alcuronium, and then maintain him on nitrous oxide with a little ether.

Modern anaesthetic machines have calibrated vapourisers for inhalation agents which allow you to measure the concentration of the vapour they deliver. Older machines have glass bottles for ether and trichloroethylene (never give halothane from a bottle—it is much too powerful) each with a control lever to divert the mixture of nitrous oxide and oxygen over the surface of the agent, or to by-pass it, as required. Each bottle also has a rod that can be used to push a hood into the bottle. The further into the bottle this hood goes, the higher the concentration of the vapour delivered. When the rod is fully inserted into the ether bottle, the mixture of nitrous oxide and oxygen bubbles under the surface of the liquid ether. With these bottles you have no way of measuring how much vapour the patient is breathing. Unlike a vapouriser, an ether bottle does not compensate for changes in temperature, so that with a given setting of the control lever and the hood, the vapour concentration falls steadily as the ether cools.

Nitrous oxide is more economical if it is used on a closed circuit and the carbon dioxide that the patient exhales is absorbed with soda lime. Don't use a closed circuit if you don't understand it (we don't describe it here), and never use soda lime with trichloroethylene, because the poisonous gas, phosgene, is produced! If you use an anaesthetic machine of the Boyle's type, use an open circuit. Don't use carbon dioxide, cyclopropane, or any anaesthetic you don't understand. The simplest method is to induce the patient with trichloroethylene and nitrous oxide with oxygen, and then change to ether, as described below.

THE SYSTEM ON A BOYLE'S MACHINE

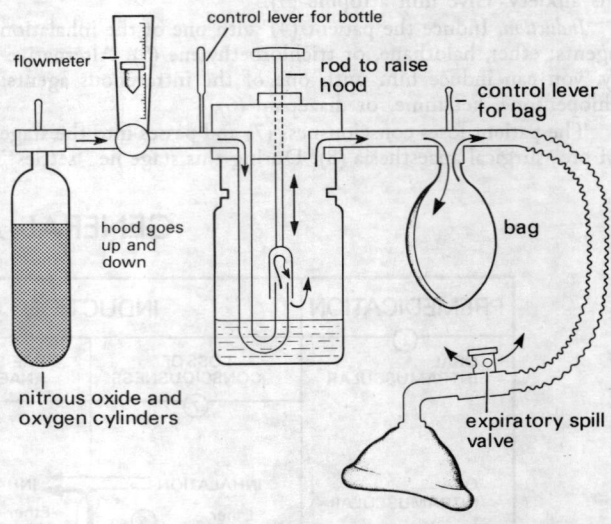

Fig. 9-2 THE SYSTEM ON AN ANAESTHETIC MACHINE OF THE BOYLE'S TYPE. Nitrous oxide and oxygen from cylinders on the left are measured by rotameters (flowmeters). Control levers determine what proportion of the total flow goes through the bottle. A rod raises or lowers the hood.

USING AN ANAESTHETIC MACHINE OF THE BOYLES TYPE

CHECKING

Check that none of the cylinders is empty, including those labelled "full". When you open a cylinder, open it slowly.

Check that the leads from the cylinders are connected to the appropriate flowmeters. Cylinders have the following colours: Oxygen-black with a white shoulder, unless you happen to have American cylinders, where oxygen is green. Nitrous oxide-blue. Carbon dioxide-grey.

In a cylinder, oxygen is a compressed gas (full 136 kPa, 135 atmospheres), so that its pressure is a good indication of how much it contains. Most of the nitrous oxide in a cylinder in is in liquid form, so that just before it is empty, the pressure quickly falls to zero. The pressure in the nitrous oxide cylinder is thus not a reliable indication of how much the cylinder contains.

Rotameters (flowmeters) consist of a bobbin in a glass tube. Make sure that each bobbin rotates when the appropriate gas is flowing, and has not stuck to the side of the tube.

Are the right liquid inhalation agents in the right bottles? If you are not sure, smell the contents of each bottle or replace them.

Turn off the gases and lower the sleeve. Gently turn on the control lever and note the point at which bubbles start. This shows the point at which the control lever starts to be "on", and varies from one machine to another.

TRICHLOROETHYLENE INDUCTION FOR ETHER
Premedicate the patient with pethidine and diazepam (8.8).

Use an expiratory spill valve of the Heidbrinck type, and the smallest mask that will comfortably fit the patient's face.

Adjust the flow of nitrous oxide to 8 to 10 litres a minute. Hold the mask 6 cm from his face and gradually lower it until he loses consciousness.

As soon as the mask touches his face, reduce the nitrous oxide to 6 litres a minute, and turn up the oxygen to 3 litres a minute.

Steadily turn the trichloroethylene lever to fully "on" as fast as he will tolerate it. Don't lower the hood.

As soon as he is breathing trichloroethylene satisfactorily, turn the ether lever to the first mark, move it 1 mm forward every fourth breath, in the same way that you would with an ether vapouriser (11.3).

If he coughs or holds his breath, turn the ether off, then turn it on again, a little less than before.

The maximum increase in vapour occurs at about the third mark on the scale of the control lever, so be extra careful there. Once this has passed, you can usually advance the lever more rapidly.

When the ether control lever is fully "on", turn off the trichoroethylene. Now gradually depress the ether hood until the right level of anaesthesia has been reached.

CAUTION ! (1) Machines vary, and there may be a point on the scale where moving the lever one division doubles the concentration of ether the patient breathes. (2) Watch the oxygen gauge carefully, because 100% nitrous oxide without any oxygen is very quickly fatal. (3) Use trichoroethylene cautiously in an anaesthetic machine of the Boyle's type. This is where it got its reputation for causing cardiac arrest!

If you want to intubate the patient under suxamethonium, do so as soon as he is unconscious. Give him suxamethonium, wait for relaxation or fasciculation, preoxygenate him and then pass the tube quickly.

THIOPENTONE INDUCTION Give the patient a suitable dose of thiopentone (2-4), then follow the sequence of trichloroethylene and ether, as above. This is much the most pleasant way of inducing him.

SUPPLMENTATION WITH INTRAVENOUS PETHIDINE For most adults give an initial dose of 20 to 30 mg after induction, then repeat it as necessary in half hourly increments to a maximum of 100 mg. You can give a patient suxamethonium and intubate him under this mixture.

DIFFICULTIES WITH AN ANAESTHETIC MACHINE

If the patient is very sick, induce him with nitrous oxide and 30 to 50% oxygen until he loses consciousness. This takes time. Then continue as above. You will need less ether. Better still is intravenous induction with a small dose of ketamine or diazepam.

If the oxygen or nitrous oxide cylinders are running low, and you are unable to replace them, pull out the cork of the ether bottle, and loosen the spring of the expiratory spill valve. Use the ether bottle as a draw-over vapouriser. Each time the patient breathes out, block the ether inlet with your thumb.

If you don't have oxygen, "preoxygenate "him with air.

If he is cyanosed with a fast pulse and a low blood pressure, you are probably giving him a hypoxic mixture, so check his airway and increase the percentage of oxygen.

THE ETHER BOTTLE ON A BOYLE'S MACHINE

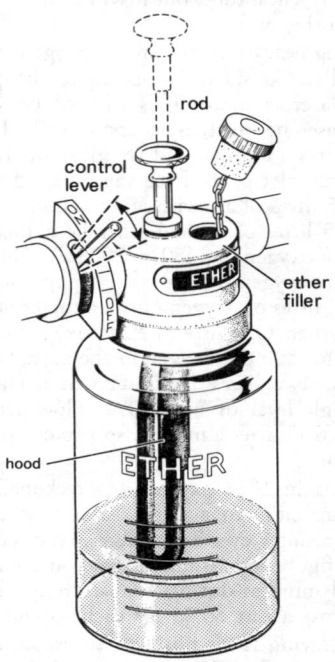

Fig. 9-3 THE BOTTLE ON AN ANAESTHETIC MACHINE OF THE BOYLE'S TYPE. A hood on the end of a rod can be raised and lowered. A control lever directs gases through the bottle or byepasses it.

9.3 Using oxygen economically

If you are using air as the carrier gas for ether, when do you need to add more oxygen to the 21% that is already in the air?

Consider the case of the fit patient whose haemoglobin is 10 g/dl or more and who is breathing 6% ether in air, at a medium depth of surgical anaesthesia. He has enough oxygen in his blood without the need to breathe any more. His arterial oxygen saturation is reduced, but no more than it would be if he were climbing a moderately high mountain. His favourable arterial oxygen saturation is caused by ether's stimulating effect on his respiration and cardiac output, during light and medium anaesthesia. Only when he is deeply anaesthetized does ether depress his respiration so much that he becomes significantly hypoxic.

There are however some occasions when a patient's arterial oxygen saturation may fall, and when extra oxygen is useful. The fall may be dangerous in itself, or it may only be dangerous if he has some special need for extra oxygen. You can give him extra oxygen in three ways:

(1) You can give him a high concentration of oxygen for about 2 minutes before you do some procedure that is likely to cause anoxia. This is *preoxygenation*. With air alone in his lungs, the safe period of apnoea is only one minute, but after preoxygenation it is 2 minutes. Preoxygenation is especially important in old, anaemic, or shocked patients, in patients with cardiac and respiratory problems and in small children.

(2) You can give him a high concentration of oxygen in an emergency, such as laryngeal spasm.

(3) You can give him a lesser concentration of oxygen throughout the operation. This is *continous oxygenation*.

If you find that the indications for preoxygenation that we give below are difficult to remember, give extra oxygen *whenever something unusual happens during anaesthesia*. Giving extra oxygen is never wrong, but it may be unncessary. When you give it, don't give it under such high pressure that you blow up a patient's stomach, because he may regurgitate fluid with it, and perhaps aspirate the fluid. This may not be a danger if you are using a cuffed tracheal tube, but it will be if you are anaethetizing him any other way.

Transporting heavy cylinders makes oxygen expensive. So use it economically. Consider, for example, the patient who is breathing 15% ether in air. This will reduce the oxygen content of the gases he breathes to about 18%. Let us say he is breathing 6 litres a minute, and we give him 1 litre of oxygen a minute at the inlet port of the vapouriser. He will therefore be breathing 5 litres of air with ether and one litre of pure oxygen. In the 5 litres of air and ether he is breathing, there is nearly a litre of oxygen ($5 \times 180 = 900$ ml). This together with the litre of pure oxygen that he is breathing, means that he will be breathing 2 litres of oxygen out of a total of 6 litres, or 33% oxygen altogether. One litre of extra oxygen each minute has been enough to raise the oxygen in the gases he breathes from 18% to 33%. Two litres a minute would raise it to be unnecessarily high level of over 40%. Flowmeters are usually calibrated up to 15 litres a minute, so you can give oxygen very wastefully indeed.

In Tanzania in 1978 oxygen was reckoned to cost about $0.0025 a litre close to a depot. Transport several hundred kilometres upcountry over bad roads raised its cost 4 times. Taking the latter figure and assuming that you use 2 litres a minute for 10 critical minutes during a laparotomy, the oxygen used would only cost about $0.25 for each patient.

A further saving is for hospitals to use an oxygen concentrator, like that in Fig. 9-4 to prepare 90% oxygen from ordinary air. Unfortunately, an oxygen concentrator needs maintenance, whereas a cylinder of oxygen does not.

• OXYGEN, *in cylinders.* Use the largest cylinders that are practical.

• VALVE, *reducing, for oxygen cylinder, with screw handwheel and flowmeter, two only of each.* Remember to close the cylinder with a spanner when it is not being used, or it may slowly leak. The valve must fit the cylinder.

• OXYGEN CONCENTRATOR, *air or water cooled, closed system with oxygen boost, and alarms for low pressure, low vacuum, or low oxygen concentration, (DRA), (RIM), one only.* It is now possible to have a machine which concentrates oxygen from atmospheric air, as in Fig. 9-4. The difficulty is maintaining them. If you decide to get one, get a bigger machine than you think you will need. If the district is hot, get one that is cooled with water, rather than with air.

• OXYGEN ANALYSLER, *simple type, powered by a fuel cell, one only.* This is not included as part of an oxygen concentrator, but is essential. Small oxygen analysers are available, powered by renewable fuel cells, and last about a year. The paramagnetic type are much better but much more expensive.

WHEN SHOULD I GIVE EXTRA OXYGEN?

CONTRAINDICATIONS Don't give oxygen during surgery if you are giving ether and are using diathermy.

PREOXYGENATION

Give the patient enough oxygen and don't mix it with air. The minimum flow is 6 litres a minute. Preoxygenate him:—
Before you do anything, such as using a laryngoscope or

WAYS OF GIVING OXYGEN WITH THE EMO

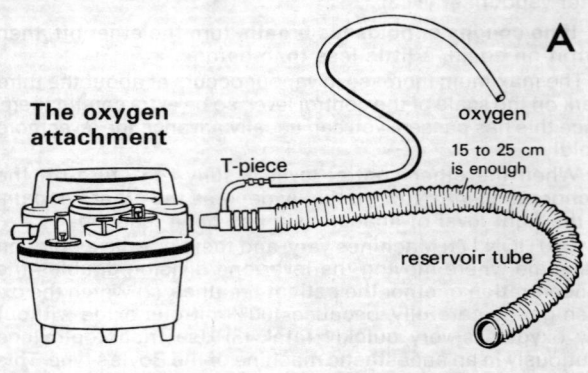

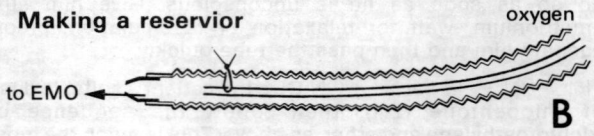

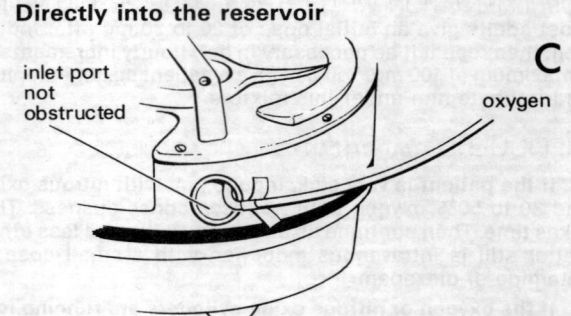

AN OXYGEN CONCENTRATOR

Fig. 9-4 AN OXYGEN CONCENTRATOR. Air is compressed and filtered and passed to one of two chambers filled with crystalised zeolites. The nitrogen is absorbed, after which the oxygen is passed to a storage tank. The nitrogen absorbed on the zeolite is then discharged and the first chamber of zeolite is regenerated, while air is being compressed into the second chamber. *As supplied by Drägerwerke AG.*

Fig. 9-5 WAYS OF GIVING OXYGEN WITH THE EMO. When you use oxygen with a vapouriser, add it to the air upstream of the point at which the agent is vapourised. *Kindly contributed by Michael Wood.*

passing an a tracheal tube or removing one, that may result in a brief period of anoxia if it is quickly successful, or a longer one, if you have difficulty.

For 2 or 3 minutes after you have given him thiopentone.

Before you intubate him with suxamethonium. The fasciculation suxamethonium causes will increase the patient's oxygen demand, and at the same time there will be a period of apnoea.

OXYGEN FOR EMERGENCIES

Give oxygen from a mask when a patient's airway is obstructed, for example, by laryngeal spasm, or a foreign body.

CONTINOUS EXTRA OXYGEN

When the patient's oxygen demand is increased over longer periods, give him 2 litres a minute. Give it—:

When you are inducing him with ether and air. He may be breathing irregularly, or coughing, or holding his breath.

Whenever you give more that 8% ether. For example, the oxygen content of a mixture of 15% ether in air is only 18%.

When you are giving halothane or chloroform, which will depress the patient's respiration. Oxygen lack with these agents increases the risk of cardiac arrest.

During Caesarean section from the period of preoxygenation until you deliver the baby.

When the patient's haemoglobin is 9 g/dl or less, or he has sickle cell disease, or when he has any respiratory abnormality or has troublesome secretions in his airway.

When his preoperative blood pressure has fallen by more than 30%.

When he is breathing spontaneously in a steep Trendelenburg or prone position. Both these positions make breathing more difficult (16.12).

Give oxygen routinely to patients with: (1) Anaemia. (2) Shock. (3) Heart or lung disease. (4) To all patients at altitudes over 3,000 metres.

WAYS OF GIVING EXTRA OXYGEN

When you use oxygen with a vapouriser, add it to the air upstream of the point at which the agent is vapourised. If you add it downstream, it will dilute the air–agent mixture, and the advantage of an accurate vapouriser will be lost. For example, don't use the oxygen nipple on the Oxford bellows. Instead, give oxygen in one of these three ways.

(1) Fix the special oxygen attachment set of the EMO vapouriser to its inlet port. This attachment has an open-ended corrugated tube, which acts as a reservoir and a side tube. Feed the oxygen from the cylinder into this side tube. If necessary, this attachment can be made in a local workshop.

(2) Fix any piece of 2.5 cm corrugated tube, 20 cm or longer, to the inlet of your vapouriser and pass the tube from the oxygen supply down it.

(3) Push the tube from the oxygen supply well inside its inlet port. If it is only just inside the port, oxygen will escape. If you tape the tube in place, make sure the tape does not prevent air entering.

If you give oxgen to a patient in the ward, give him 2 to 3 litres a minute through a loosely fitting face mask. This will provide about 33% oxygen. Oxygen tents are extravagant and obsolete in adults, but are satisfactory in children.

10 Systems for inhalation anaesthesia

10.1 Making the gases go in the right direction

When a patient breathes spontaneously, he draws the mixture of air, anaesthetic vapour—and, when necessary, oxygen—through the vapouriser by himself. When you control his ventilation, you have to do this for him with a bag or bellows. Three valves are necessary to make the mixture of gases he breathes go in the right direction. The first valve (A in Figure 10-1) is an inlet valve on the bellows or bag to prevent the anaesthetic mixture going back into the vapouriser. The second is a non–return valve (B) to stop the patient rebreathing into the bag or bellows and accumulating carbon dioxide. The third is an expiratory valve (C) to let him discharge the mixture he has breathed into the air, without letting air in. Different systems arrange these valves in different ways, and in some of them valves A and B are in the vapouriser itself.

We shall start by considering valve C.

An expiratory spill valve of the Heidbrinck type is the simplest form of valve C. This is shown in diagrams 1, 2, and 3 in Fig. 10-1, and in more detail in Fig. 11-3. The Americans call it a "pop-off" valve. If you order an EMO outfit, it will be supplied with a valve of this type. It is also the only valve you need when you use the simplest (Magill) system on an anaesthetic machine of the Boyle's type. This expiratory spill valve has a flap, a spring to control it and a screw to tighten the spring. If your system has one, use it as described below..

A SAD STORY—not from Kenya! An anaesthetist was called to a hospital because several patients had "died on the table". He found that the anaesthetic assistant was assembling his equipment without including an expiratory valve in the system, so that the patients could not exhale! LESSON An understanding of the valves in Fig. 10-1 is critical!

A SIMPLE EXPIRATORY SPILL VALVE

If a patient is breathing spontaneously, screw the valve open. As he exhales, the outlet valve on the Oxford bellows (if you are using an EMO vapouriser) will close, the pressure will rise, and the flap of the expiratory spill valve will open.

If you are controlling the patient's respiration, screw the expiratory spill valve shut. Let him exhale by removing the mask from his face or by removing your finger from the tracheal connector (13.2). Removing the mask from his face each time he breathes is inconvenient, so most anaesthetists screw the expiratory spill valve partly shut, as described in Section 13.1.

10.2 Non–rebreathing valves

If the non–return valve B in Fig. 10-1 is a long way from the patient, as in Diagrams 2 and 3 in this figure, there is a large compressible dead space between his mouth and the valve. The largest part of this dead space is the corrugated tube that joins him to the bag. Because a large dead space makes breathing inefficient, valve B should be as close to him as possible, as in Diagram 4. This shows the non–return valve (B) and the expiratory valve (C) close together. A double valve like this has a very small compressible dead space, and is called a non–rebreathing valve.

If possible, always use a non–rebreathing valve when you use a vapouriser because: (1) You can change immediately from spontaneous to controlled ventilation and back again without changing the circuit or the valves. (2) You can easily control the patient's ventilation with one hand only. (3) The mask can remain on his face all the time during controlled ventilation, and there is no need to remove it each time he exhales. (4) There is less chance of error, which is useful at 3 a.m!

Non–rebreathing valves have no means of spilling any large excess gas supplied to the patient, by a plenum system (a system supplying gas under slight pressure). So you cannot normally use them with a machine of the Boyle's type, or when you supply the patient with an excess of pure oxygen. The pressure of gas tends to make the valves stick, so that the patient cannot easily exhale. The small volume of oxygen you add to enrich the gases from a vapouriser causes no problems, nor does the very slight plenum you may need to use with some arrangements for the AMBU "Paedivalve" (18.3).

NON–REBREATHING VALVES ARE FOR DRAW–OVER VAPORISERS
THEY ARE NOT FOR PLENUM SYSTEMS

You will need an adult non–rebreathing valve, like the AMBU E valve, and a smaller paediatric one, like the AMBU "Paedivalve", for children under 15 kg (18.1). Both these valves are made of three pieces of transparent plastic which screw together and hold two yellow rubber valve leaflets. As the patient breathes, you can see these leaflets opening and closing. You can also see his breath condensing inside the valve. The valve leaflets sometimes break, or are lost during cleaning, so keep spares.

Some models of non–rebreathing valve, including the AMBU E valve, are made in two types. *The anaesthetic type* is for controlled or spontaneous respiration with a draw–over vapouriser. The *resuscitation type* is only for resuscitating a patient who fails to breathe, and so has no expiratory valve (C). The resuscitation type of valve allows the patient to entrain (take in) air when he starts to breathe again spontaneously. The anaesthetic type allows only fresh gas to enter from the system, and is a one–way valve. If you mistakenly use a valve designed for resuscitation instead of one designed for anaesthesia, the patient will breathe only atmospheric air.

If you are getting an AMBU valve, the one you need is this.

- *VALVE, adult, non–rebreathing, anaesthesia type, for controlled or spontaneous respiration, with 22 mm male inlet cone, 22/15 mm patient cone, and 22 mm male outlet cone, complete with 4 spare leaflets, as the AMBU E valve, (AMBU) 21-00, or its equivalent two only.* There are several makes of non–rebreathing valve, AMBU is only one. There are also 6 different kinds of AMBU E valve, so get the right one. These valves are fragile, so keep a spare.
- *VALVE, simple expiratory spill-valve, Heidbrinck type with angled connector, 20 mm ISO cone fittings, two only.* This is the valve that is normally supplied with the EMO vapouriser.

VALVES

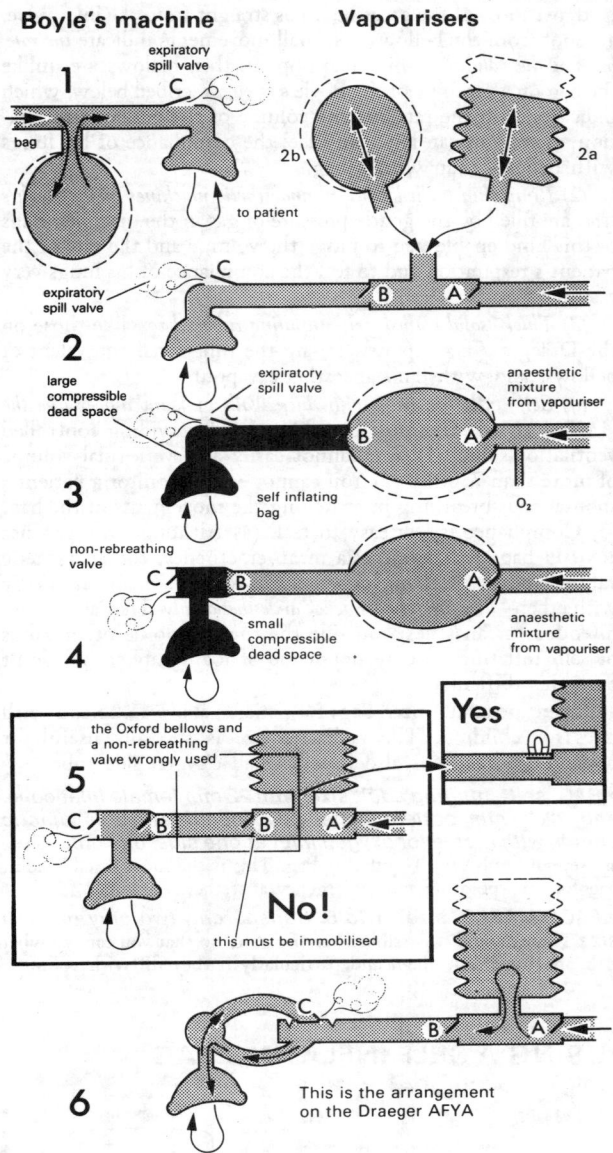

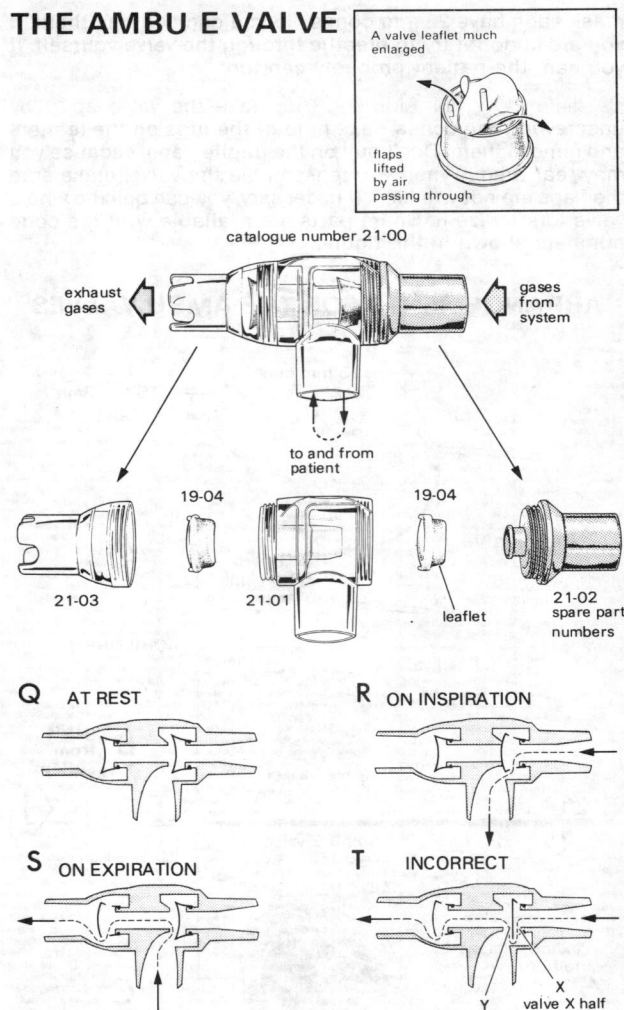

Fig. 10-2 THE AMBU E VALVE. The valve is in three pieces that unscrew and has two rubber leaflets.

Fig. 10-1 VALVES FOR ANAESTHETIC MACHINES. In this diagram anaesthetic gases from the Boyle's machine enter from the left, and those from a vapouriser enter from the right. The inlet valve A prevents the mixture from the bellows going back into the vapouriser. The non-return valve B prevents exhaled gases from the patient going back into the bellows, or into a self-inflating bag. Expiratory valve C allows gases from the patient to escape into the air.

(1) shows an anaesthetic machine of the Boyle's type with the gases entering from the left. It has a bag, and an expiratory spill valve of the Heidbrinck type.

(2) to (6) show arrangements for vapourisers with the gases (air and vapour) entering from the right.

(2a) is the arrangement for the Oxford bellows used with an expiratory spill valve, (2b) is that for the simpler Dräeger AFYA system. (3) is a self-inflating bag used with an expiratory spill valve. (4) is a self-inflating bag with a non-rebreathing valve. (5) is the Oxford bellows with a non-rebreathing valve, used in the wrong way without a magnet, and in the right way with one. (6) shows the more complex Dräeger AFYA system. Valve C in this particular system directs mixture round the circuit and also serves as an expiratory valve.

The compressible dead space between the patient and the non-return valve has been shown in a darker tone in (3) and (4). Note that it is much smaller in (4) than in (3).

USING NON-REBREATHING VALVES

These valves have three openings—

(1) An AMBU E valve has a 22 mm male cone on the opening which joins it to the circuit. The "Paedivalve" has a 15 mm male cone here, so it needs the ring shaped adapter shown in Fig. 10-3 to join it to the circuit.

(2) On the opening that connects to the patient, both valves have a 15 mm female cone surrounded by a 22 mm male cone. The 22 mm male cone will fit a mask and the 15 mm female cone will fit the adapter of a tracheal tube. Always fit the adapter of a tracheal tube straight into the "Paedivalve". This minimises the dead space. Don't use a catheter mount with a "Paedivalve", because this also has too much dead space, especially for small babies.

(3) The E valve has a 22 mm male cone round the opening to discharge the exhaust gases. Fit a length of corrugated tube here to carry these gases to the floor, as in Fig. 16-8. Leave the small exhaust cone of the "Paedivalve" open. The exhaust gases are of such a small volume in a child that there is no need to carry them away.

CAUTION! (1) Make sure the leaflets of these valves move during respiration. If you compress bellows slowly enough, it is possible to partly open leaflet "X", in Diagram T Fig. 10-2 without it blocking port "Y". The air in the bellows can then go through the valve without inflating the patient. Prevent this by starting to compress the bellows with a short sharp "attack" movement which will push leaflet "X" across to block port "Y". (2) Note that the opening for the gas inlet and the

73

mask each have 22 mm cones, so you can confuse them. If you are in doubt try to breathe through the valve yourself. If you can, the patient probably can too.

CARING FOR AN AMBU VALVE Take the valve apart by unscrewing the cones. Take hold of the lugs on the leaflets and remove them. Don't pull on the fragile flaps, because you may tear them. When you reassemble the valve, make sure the flaps are not wrinkled. If necessary, you can boil the whole valve to sterilize it. Spare parts are available with the code numbers shown in the figure.

ARRANGEMENTS FOR THE AMBU VALVES

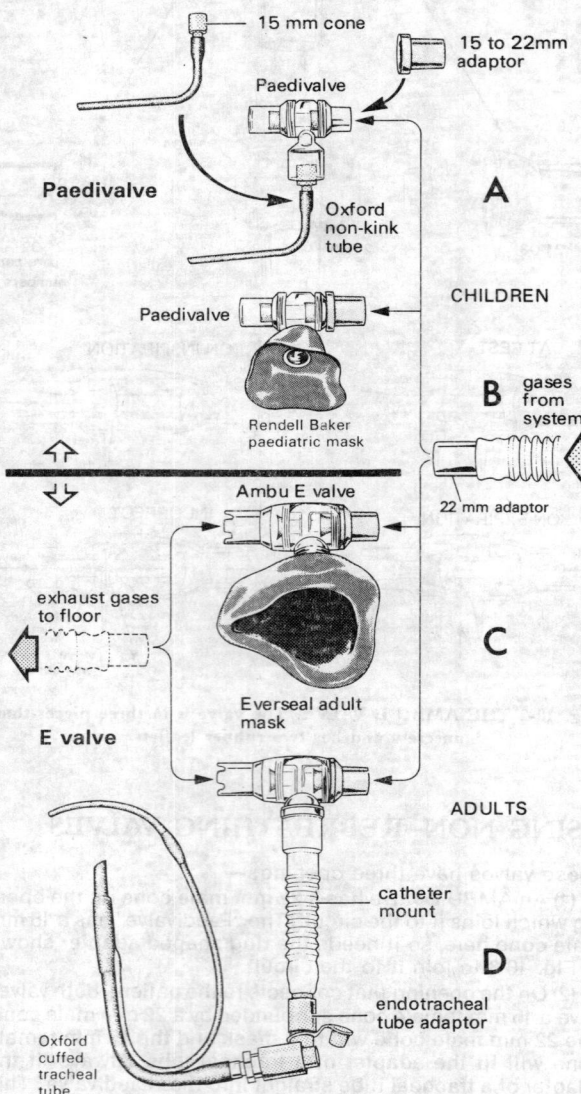

Fig. 10-3 ARRANGEMENTS FOR THE AMBU E VALVE. The "Paedivalve" is at the top of the figure and the E valve at the bottom. Note that in the Paedivalve the adaptor of the tracheal tube fits straight into the valve, without a catheter mount, which would increase the dead space dangerously.

CHANGE TO AN AMBU PAEDIVALVE AT 15 KG

10.3 Bellows and bags, etc.

You will need a bellows or bag to direct the anaesthetic gases through the system to the patient. Firstly, bellows.

(1) Bellows are fitted to most vapourisers, either to the vapouriser itself, or standing on a separate base, and are more durable, but less easy to use than a bag. A bellows but not a self-inflating bag, moves slightly as a patient breathes. Because he draws most of the gases he needs straight from the inlet valve, and not from the bellows, its small movements indicate *the rate, but not the volume* of his breathing. In this, bellows are unlike the bag on a machine of the Boyle's type, described below, which indicates both the rate *and* the volume of the patient's respiration. Also, you can less easily feel the compliance of his lungs with bellows than with a bag.

(2) Limp thin walled bags on anaesthetic machines of the Boyle's type. are filled by the gentle pressure of gas in the machine. Bags of this kind enable you to judge the volume and the rate of the patient's respiration and to feel the compliance of his lungs very easily.

(3) Thick, solid walled, self-inflating rubber bags, like those on the Dräeger Afya vapourisers, are the functional equivalent of bellows, and withstand anaesthetic vapours.

(4) Self-inflating bags with thick walls of foam rubber like the AMBU bag, are the most portable way of providing controlled ventilation. But: (1) You cannot easily achieve a tidal volume of more than 750 ml. (2) You cannot easily monitor a patient's spontaneous breathing by watching the movements of the bag. (3) Compliance is less easy to feel. (4) Although you can use AMBU bags for anaesthesia in an emergency, the anaesthetic vapour soon rots them, especially if you use them repeatedly with ether—*they are for emergency anaesthesia only.* They are mostly intended for anasthesia outside the theatre. Some other kinds of self-inflating bag are not made of foam rubber and don't have this difficulty

There are adult-sized bags for patients above 15 kg and small ones for children. The pediatric size is specially useful for neonates. Some bags also have a small oxygen side tube.

• *BAG, self-inflating adult size, with 22 mm female inlet cone, and 22/15 mm patient cone, ISO specification, in plastic pouch, with nipple for oxygen inlet at one side, one only.* There are several kinds of self-inflating bag. This is the most suitable adult bag for incorporating into emergency anaesthetic circuits.

• *FACE MASKS, sizes 1 to 5, transparent, two only of each size.* These should if possible be transparent, so that you can see what is happening inside them and particularly if they fill with vomit.

USING A SELF INFLATING BAG

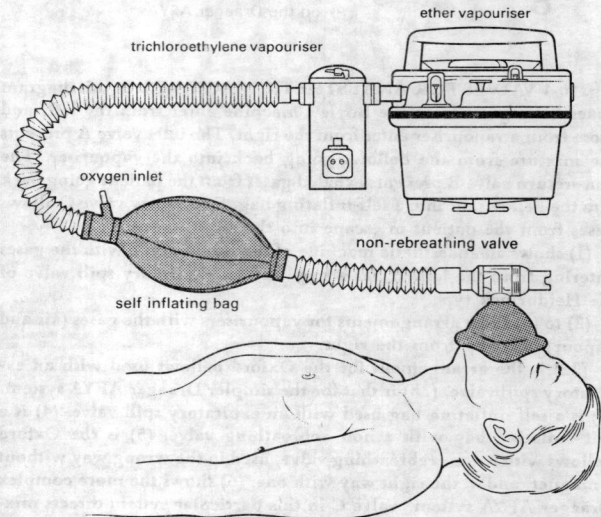

Fig. 10-4 ANAESTHESIA WITH ETHER, TRICHLOROETHYLENE AND A SELF INFLATING BAG. This is for emergency rather than for routine use, because ether soon rots the foam rubber of a self-inflating AMBU bag.

- HARNESS, for face mask, two only.
- TUBE, corrugated, anaesthetic, 12 mm × 100 cm, two lengths only. You will find a few extra lengths of corrugated tube very useful.

SELF–INFLATING BAGS OF THE AMBU TYPE

CHECKING THE BAG

The valve(s) in a bag can easily be removed, so check that the valves are present and working, before you use the bag. Make sure there is a spring–loaded plastic check valve in the oxygen inlet. Make sure that the large rubber bush at the inlet end of the bag is fitted with the metal socket incorporating the inlet valve. Fit the other end with a standard breathing tube outlet cone.

To check the bag, squeeze it and apply its outlet to the palm of your hand. Allow it to expand, and squeeze again. There should now be strong resistance with no air escaping anywhere.

CAUTION ! If you have checked a bag and feel it may not be working, disconnect the bag and blow down the tracheal tube or ventilate the patient mouth to mouth.

USING THE BAG

These bags are usually fitted with an inlet valve (A), but have no non–return valve (B), so always use the bag with a non–rebreathing valve. Fix the bag directly into the valve, or put some corrugated tube with female and male connectors between the bag and the valve.

If you are using the bag for resuscitation, as in Fig. 3-4, allow air to enter through the inlet valve.

If you are using the bag for anaesthesia, connect the inlet valve to a vapouriser through a length of corrugated tubing.

10.4 Draw–over vapourisers

All draw–over vapourisers follow the same principle. They have a chamber for ether, lined by a wick, through which air passes and picks up ether vapour. A control lever opens and closes ports to admit air to this chamber, or to by–pass it, depending on the concentration of vapour you want. While the ether is warm, the concentration of ether vapour is high. As ether evaporates it becomes colder, and the concentration of the ether vapour coming off it falls. The speed at which the air flows through a vapouriser also determines the concentration of the ether delivered. In older and simpler vapourisers the concentration of the vapour delivered varies greatly.

A modern vapouriser compensates automatically for changes in temperature, by means of: (1) a thermostat that also opens and closes a port, and (2) a water jacket that stabilises the temperature. A modern vapouriser can also compensate for changes in respiratory rate and volume, but only within certain limits, which vary with each model. With the best vapourisers you can choose the concentration of ether you want, from 0 to 20 per cent, regardless of variations in temperature and flow, and without making any further adjustment. You can thus give a smooth ether anaesthetic much more easily than you can with an anaesthetic machine of the Boyle's type, or with an open mask.

A vapouriser compensated for flow and temperature is comparatively expensive. With a little more skill you can readily use the simpler vapouriser in Fig. 10-5, which has only a basin of water to minimise changes in temperature, or you can make your own vapouriser as in Fig. 10-17. You will however have to rely more on the signs of ether anaesthesia in the patient, and less on the setting of the control lever on the vapouriser.

You cannot use a vapouriser designed for ether with any other agent, so if you are going to give halothane or trichloroethylene, you will need one or two accessory calibrated vapourisers. These also have a chamber for the volatile agent and a wick, but they do not need a water chamber, so they can be smaller. They too are usually designed for one agent only. In time, non–volatile substances in all inhalation agents accumulate in a vapouriser. So, from time to time, tip out the residual agent and swill it out with ether.

There are many makes of vapouriser for ether and other agents. We have been able to describe only some representative makes in the rest of this chapter.

DONT USE AN ETHER VAPOURISER FOR ANY OTHER AGENT

A SIMPLE VAPOURISER ASSEMBLY

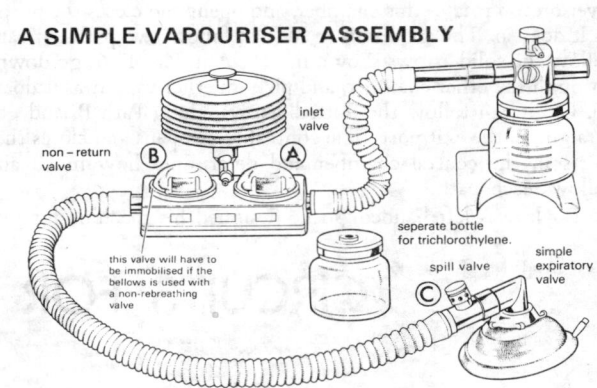

Fig. 10-5 A SIMPLE ETHER VAPOURISER. This vapouriser is not temperature and flow compensated and is more difficult to use then the EMO. There is no water jacket for the ether bottle, so to prevent the ether cooling, immerse it in water. The spare bottle is for trichloroethylene.

10.5 A simple vapouriser

The vapouriser in Fig. 10-5 is not very efficient, but is widely used. It has an ether bottle, a hood, and a control lever to vary the concentration of ether. To prevent the ether becoming too cold you can immerse the whole vapouriser in a basin of warm

THE MECHANISM OF THE EMO VAPOURISER

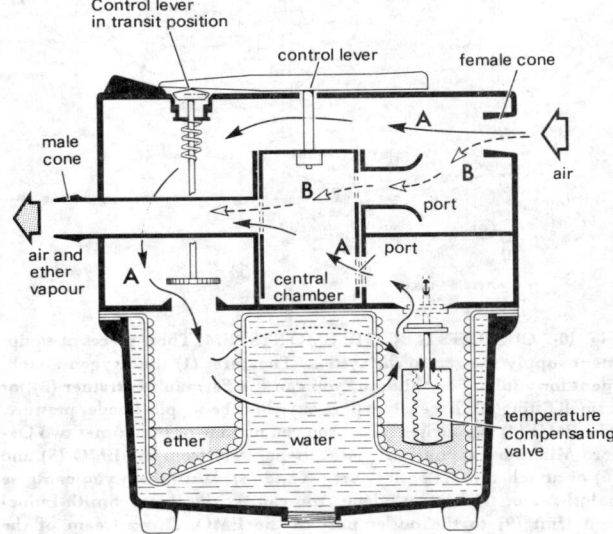

Fig.10-6 THE MECHANISM OF THE EMO. At the bottom of the vapouriser is a circular ether compartment, lined by a wick. Above is a central chamber with ports in it, controlled by a lever. This lever controls the proporion of the incoming air passing through the ether chamber, or going directly to the exit port.

water. The bellows resembles the Oxford bellows, and like it, has two valves. Note that it is supplied with a simple expiratory valve of the Heidbrinck type; if you want to use it with a non−rebreathing valve, you will have to find some way to immobilise the non-return valve (B).

10.6 The EMO vapouriser

The Epstein Macintosh Oxford, or EMO, is the most widely used vapouriser, and the one which has been most rigorously tested in service. Inside, it has a circular compartment filled with ether, and lined with a wick. Above this compartment there is a small cylindrical chamber with three ports in it. A control lever on top rotates this chamber, and opens and closes the ports as it does so. The air that is inside can follow two paths. It can follow the solid arrows shown in path A in Fig. 10-6, go down through the ether chamber, and pick up ether vapour as it does so. Or, it can follow the dotted arrows, along Path B, and go straight to the exit port. The control lever opens and closes the ports in the central chamber and determines how much air follows each path.

Boyle was left handed, so he designed his machine for his own convenience, with the gas flow from left to right. All subsequent machines of the Boyle's type have followed this pattern. As you will see from Fig. 10-6, the designers of the EMO broke this tradition, and designed it so that the gas flows from right to left.

The EMO can compensate for changes in the temperature of the ether, and for variations in a patient's respiratory rate and volume—but only within certain limits. If a child weighs less than about 15 kg, his breathing is so rapid and shallow that it cannot compensate adequately, so you have to use the special equipment in Section 18.3. The EMO can compensate for changes in temperature only between 15 and 30°C. If it is colder or hotter than this, you will have to warm or cool it. There is an indicator on top of the EMO to show you when this is necessary.

The Oxford bellows was the first bellows to be made for the EMO, and it is still the most useful one because it stands on its own base, so you can use it by itself. It was originally designed for use with an expiratory spill valve, so it has two valves in its base, an inlet valve (A) to admit gases from the EMO, and a non−return (outlet) valve (B) to prevent the patient rebreathing into the bellows. The non−return valve can be a danger (see

CIRCUITS FOR THE EMO SYSTEM

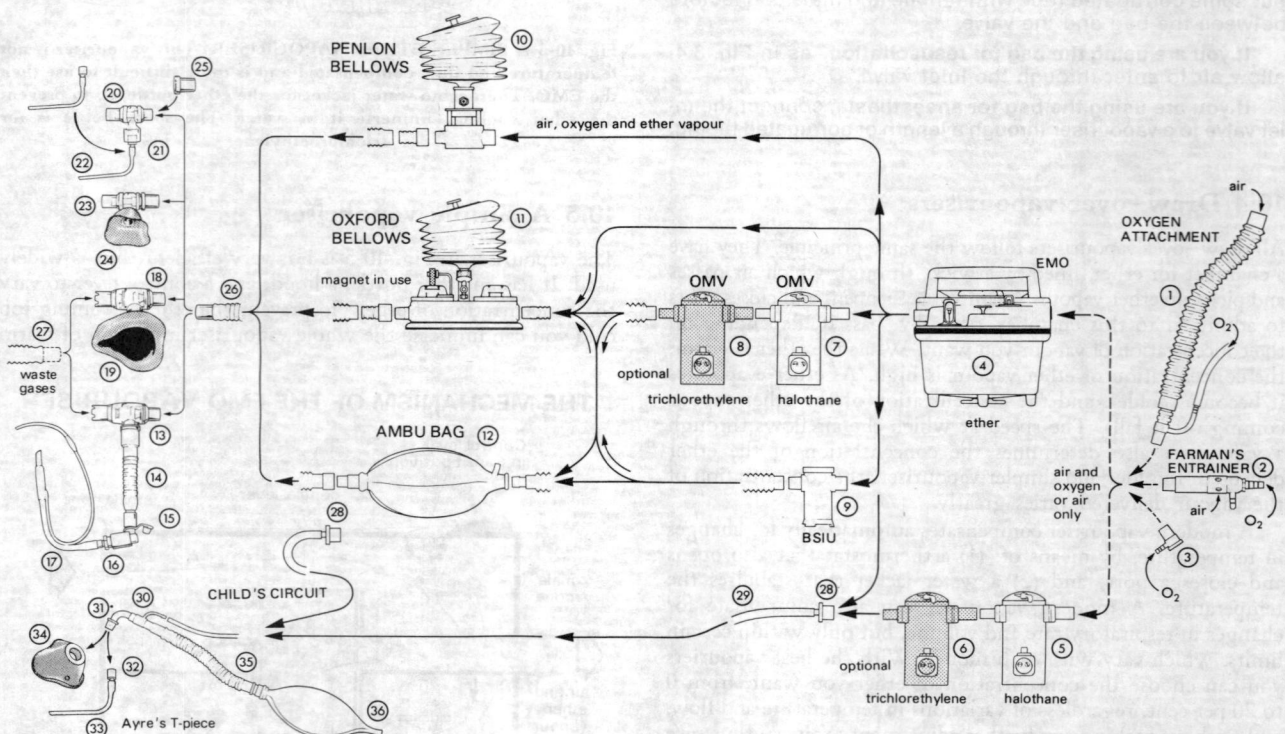

Fig. 10-7 CIRCUITS FOR THE EMO SYSTEM. Three pieces of equipment supply oxygen to the system. They are: (1) the oxygen attachment for adults. For children, you can use Farman's entrainer (2), or a small fitting (3) that enables pure oxygen to be supplied under pressure. The EMO (4) vapourises ether. You can use one or sometimes two Oxford Miniature vapourisers, either separately from the EMO (5) and (6) or attached to its outlet port (7) and (8). With them you can give halothane or trichloroethylene. You can fix the Bryce−Smith Induction Unit (9) to the outlet port of the EMO. Downstream of the vapourisers come the Penlon bellows (10) or the Oxford bellows (11) or the AMBU bag (12). The left of the figure shows the equipment that delivers the anaesthetic gases to the patient. This is shown in more detail in Fig. 10-3. There is an AMBU E valve (13), a catheter mount (14), a connector (15), an adaptor (16), and a Magill cuffed tracheal tube (17). Another AMBU valve (18) is shown fitted onto a mask (19). One AMBU "Paedivalve" (20), is connected straight to the adaptor (21) of a plain cuffed Oxford child's tracheal tube (22). Another AMBU "Paedivalve" (23), fits a Rendell−Baker child's mask (24). "Paedivalves" require a 15 mm female to 22 mm male adaptor (25) to fit them to the corrugated tube (26). A further piece of corrugated tubing (27) carries the exhaust gases from the AMBU E valve (but not the "Paedivalve") to the floor.

The bottom part of the figure shows the circuit for Ayre's T-piece. A fitting (28) takes gases from the EMO or the OMV through a gas hose (29) to the T-piece (30). This fitting (28) should be used on the output side of the bellows. You can attach the T-piece (30) via a connector (31) to an adaptor (32) and a tracheal tube (33), or to a Rendell−Baker face mask (34). 20 cm of 10 mm tube act as a reservoir (35). For older children you will need a 500 ml bag (36). *Drawn at the suggestion of John Farman.*

Fig. 10-8) if you use these bellows with a non–rebreathing valve, so there is a magnet to immobilise it. If you need the non–return valve, park the magnet out of use (as in N, Fig. 10-8). If you don't want the valve, put the magnet on an arm above the valve, so that it lifts the iron valve flap away from its seating and prevents it working (as in M, Fig. 10-8). If you are always going to use a non–rebreathing valve, and never going to use a Heidbrinck valve, you can unscrew the plastic cover of the outlet valve of your Oxford Bellows and remove the metal valve flap. You can then forget about the magnet.

There is a stopcock on the base of older models of the bellows. This is to admit oxygen when it is used for resuscitation. Oxygen dilutes the anaesthetic mixture if you add it here during anaesthesia, so add it earlier in the circuit in one of the ways described in Fig. 9-5. If your bellows has this tap, keep it closed. New models of the bellows have a safety valve, set at 60 cm of water. Should you ever want higher pressures, you can block it with your thumb.

Both the Oxford and the Penlon bellows described below deliver about 1300 ml at each stroke. Smaller paediatric bellows with a volume of 400 ml are available which fit onto the base of the standard bellows.

CHANGING OR REPLACING A BELLOWS UNIT Find the red plastic lock-nut on the central stem underneath the bellows. Screw it up 2 turns. Unscrew the knurled metal ring below it, and lift off the bellows. Check that there is a washer inside the central stem. Screw up the knurled metal ring, and screw down the red plastic lock-nut.

The Penlon bellows is the exact functional equivalent of a self–inflating bag and is designed to be mounted on an EMO. Unfortunately, if you place an Oxford Miniature Vaporiser between the EMO and the Penlon bellows, the combination tips over. One solution to this problem is to mount the Penlon bellows on a small board and to connect it to the EMO with a short breathing tube.

The Penlon bellows has an inlet valve (A) only, and no non–return valve (B) to prevent the patient exhaling into it, so you cannot use it with an expiratory spill valve; *you must use the Penlon bellows with a non–rebreathing valve.* Because it has no non–return valve, it does not need a magnet. Its oxygen inlet valve closes automatically, so it does not have a tap either.

The dangers of an extra valve with the Oxford bellows. If you use the Oxford bellows with a non–rebreathing valve, like the AMBU E valve, *there will now be two non–return valves of type B in Fig. 10-1.* Unfortunately, these valves do not always work together, and the non–return valve on the bellows can be very dangerous, unless you inactivate it with the magnet.

During spontaneous respiration there is no difficulty. But during controlled ventilation it can happen that the patient cannot exhale at all. Compressing the bellows to inflate his lungs pushes leaflet X over to obstruct port Y, as shown in diagram L, in Fig. 10-8 Pressing the bellows down to inflate him, only makes matters worse. In order to draw the flap back and let the patient exhale, a little air must pass back along the corrugated tube towards the bellows. This readily happens if you immobilise the non–return valve of the Oxford bellows, with the magnet, as in diagram M. *So always do this when you use a non–rebreathing valve* If however you use an expiratory spill valve, you will need the non–return valve, so don't inactivate it.

• **EMO PORTABLE OUTFIT, with 15/22 mm connections, one only.** This consists of (1) an EMO ether inhaler, (2) 2 male breathing tube connectors, (3) two female breathing tube connectors, (4) two 30 mm breathing tubes, (5) a head harness, (6) a connector mount, (7) 9 cm of plain connecting tube, (8) the Oxford inflating bellows, (9) a 105 cm breathing tube, (10) a Heidbrinck type expiratory spill valve, (11) an angle connector, (12) a facemask size 3, and a carrying case with tray. This is the basic EMO outfit and does not include a non–rebreathing valve. It needs minor modification to fit the needs of the anaesthetic system described here. The EMO outfit (without a non–rebreathing valve) is also available from UNICEF.

• **OXYGEN ATTACHMENT KIT, For EMO, each one only.** This

WHEN TO IMMOBILISE THE OUTLET VALVE

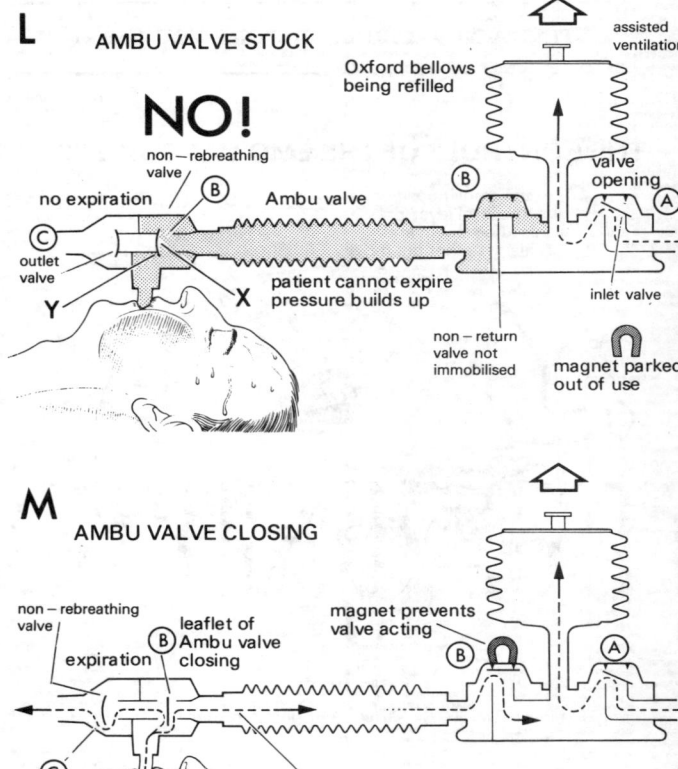

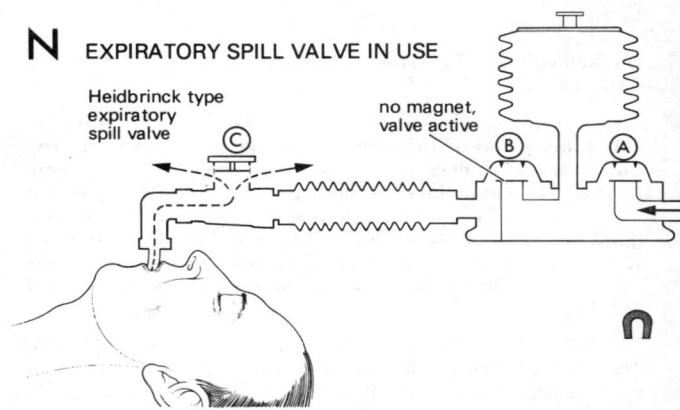

Fig. 10-8 WHEN TO IMMOBILISE THE NON–RETURN VALVE (B) OF THE OXFORD BELLOWS. L, if you don't immobilise the non–return valve (B) of an Oxford bellows when you are using a non–rebreathing valve, a high pressure can build up during controlled ventilation. So immobilise the valve, as in M. You will need it (N) when you are using a simple expiratory spill valve, so park the magnet out of use.

is the short metal tube that fits onto the inlet of the EMO. It has a side tube to admit oxygen, and is attached to a corrugated reservoir tube.

The EMO is not equipped with a flowmeter or with a pressure gauge, but you can easily use Wright's spirometer and a pressure gauge if you wish. Provided you follow the few simple rules listed below, you can assemble the EMO system in any of the ways shown in Fig. 10-7. *When you assemble a new circuit, test it to make sure the air flows towards the patient.*

TEST A NEW CIRCUIT BEFORE YOU USE IT

THE CONTROLS OF THE EMO VAPOURISER

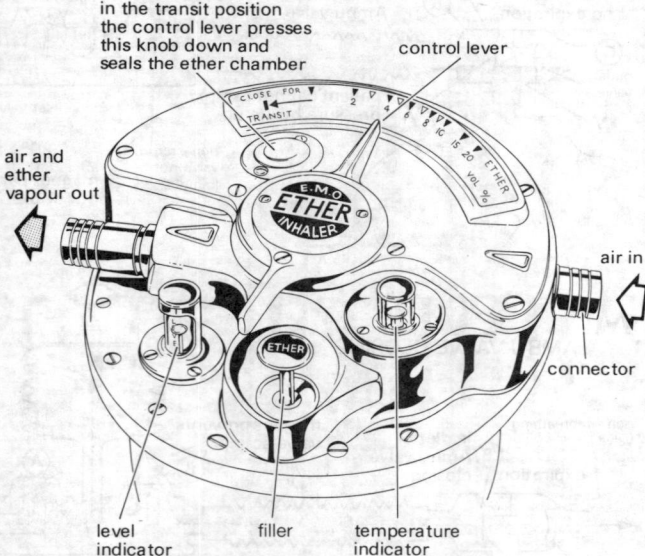

Fig. 10-9 THE CONTROLS OF THE EMO VAPOURISER. Gases flow from right to left, which is the reverse of anaesthetic machines of the Boyle's type.

USING THE EMO

RULES FOR ASSEMBLING ANY VAPOURISER SYSTEM
Unpack your EMO and check the items carefully against the parts list.

MALE AND FEMALE CONNECTORS The inlets to vaporisers and bellows are all female 22 mm sockets. The outlets are all male cones of the same size. Fit a female connector to one end of each long piece of corrugated tube, and a male cone to the other. The grooved part of the connector goes inside the rubber. Don't fit corrugated tubing directly to any major component. Instead, always use male and female connectors. They enable you to join and detach equipment rapidly.

COMBINATIONS OF VAPORISERS If you use an EMO with one or more OMVs (10.10), place the OMV with the more volatile agent upstream of the less volatile one. Ether is always furthest from the patient, then come halothane, chloroform and trichloroethylene in that order. If you put them in the wrong order, the less volatile agent will condense in the vapouriser downstream containing the more volatile agent.

BELLOWS AND BAGS Place these between the vapouriser(s) and the patient. Vaporisers are more accurate when used like this.

OXYGEN Add this upstream of the vapouriser as shown in Fig. 10-7.

THE MAGNET ON THE OXFORD BELLOWS This magnet immoblizes the iron non-return valve (B) of the EMO and is critical. Park the magnet out of use when you use a simple expiratory valve (10-8). Hang it on the arm above the non-return valve whenever you use a non-rebreathing valve.

FILLING AN EMO
WATER The water jacket of a new EMO is dry. Turn the indicator to "transit". Turn the EMO upside down, unscrew the filler cap, and fill it with 1,200 ml of cold distilled water. Under freezing conditions, fill it with car antifreeze containing 25% glycol, or it may be damaged. Check the water level at least each month.

If your EMO is an early model with an aluminium water jacket, change the water every 3 months. This is not necessary in later models with steel jackets.

ETHER Turn the indicator to "zero", hold the filler down and pour in the ether. 150 ml will bring the level indicator to "empty", and 300 ml more to "full". The level may fall again as the wicks soak up the ether. Don't overfill it, because the wicks will be covered, and no ether will evapourate.

CAUTION ! If you fill the vapouriser during use, turn the control indicator to "zero", or dangeroulsy high concentrations of ether will be delivered, as you pour in more ether.

Check that the filler knob returns to the closed position after filling. In new models of EMO, this happens automatically.

After use, turn the indicator to "transit". This will seal the ether chamber until the EMO is used again.

ROUTINE CHECKS
Check your EMO occasionally. If it fails to pass any of these checks, send it for servicing.

LEVEL INDICATOR With the ether compartment empty, slowly turn the EMO upside down. The level indicator should fall freely to the "full" position, and fall back again when the EMO is upright.

When refilling, check that the indicator responds to the volume of ether you add.

CLOSING MECHANISM AND FILLER Turn the control lever to the transit position. Connect the outlet of the bellows to the inlet of the EMO. Block the outlet of the EMO. Apply gentle pressure on the bellows and open the ether filler. No air should escape through the filler, or through the top of the closing mechanism.

Now open the control indicator to "10". Close the filler and press on the bellows. No air should leak through the filler.

SAFETY RELEASE VALVE This is in the closing mechanism. Put the Oxford bellows in its normal position on the outlet of the EMO. Set the control lever at "2". Block the inlet port of the EMO and check that operating the bellows draws air in through the safety valve.

TEMPERATURE COMPENSATOR At normal room temperatures (20 to 25°C), the metal top of the compensator, and its black band should be visible. Above 30°C the red band will begin to show. If only the metal top, and not the black band can be seen between 20°C and 30°C, the compensator is faulty and must be replaced. If you are in doubt, check the vapouriser by filling it with ice cold water, then with hot water.

DIFFICULTIES WITH THE EMO
Is the inlet port of the EMO blocked?

If you are using the Oxford bellows and a simple expiratory spill-valve of the Heidbrinck type, make sure the magnet is parked out of use.

If you are using the Oxford bellows and an AMBU E valve, check that the yellow valves of the AMBU E valve are the right way round, that it works properly and that the magnet is suspended over the non-return valve of the Oxford bellows.

If the rotor has stuck, you have probably left your EMO standing idle too long, or you have not emptied out the ether container often enough. Empty the water, refill it with hot water, apply penetrating oil to the rotor, leave it for several hours, and try to free it. If this fails, return the EMO the agent.

If the ether level indicator fails to rise, when you add ether, but not when you turn it upside down, the float is broken. Fit a new one. If the indicator is caught at any point, and will not move when the EMO is inverted, the indicator float may be caught by a frayed wick. Remove the indicator, trim the wick, and replace the indicator.

If the concentration of the ether delivered by the EMO is too low make sure that there is no leak in the circuit, particularly round the face mask. Make sure that the ether chamber is not overfull. Check the temperature compensator, and replace it if necessary. Make sure that the relief valve on the closing mechanism has not stuck.

If the red band of the temperature indicator of the EMO shows the EMO is too hot, and the ether chamber is shut off. Cool it. (1) Keep it in a cool place, below 30°. Or, (2) put it in a refrigerator for an hour before you use it. Or, (3) set the dial at 20% ether. Pump vigorously with the bellows, and leave the filler knob open. This effective but wasteful method evapourates some of the ether, and in doing so cools the rest. Or, (4) refill the water jacket with cool water, tap water is usually cool enough.

If neither "black" nor "red", show on the indicator, the EMO may be too cold. Either leave it in a warm room for some hours, or refill it with water at 25° C. If the indicator still fails to appear, the temperature compensator has failed because of metal fatigue, and you must not use the EMO. An indicator lasts about 10 years. Replace it every five years.

If the EMO delivers too much ether you may have left the filler cap of an old model open.

If the patient does not become anaesthetized : (1) The mask may not be fitting tightly round his face, so he is breathing round the edge of the mask. Listen to the expiratory valve. If he is exhaling through the valve, it will make a noise. (2) There may be too much ether in the EMO. (3) The temperature compensator may have failed. Check it as described above. (4) The release valve on the closing mechanism may have stuck open.

THE DRÄGER AFYA ETHER VAPOURISER

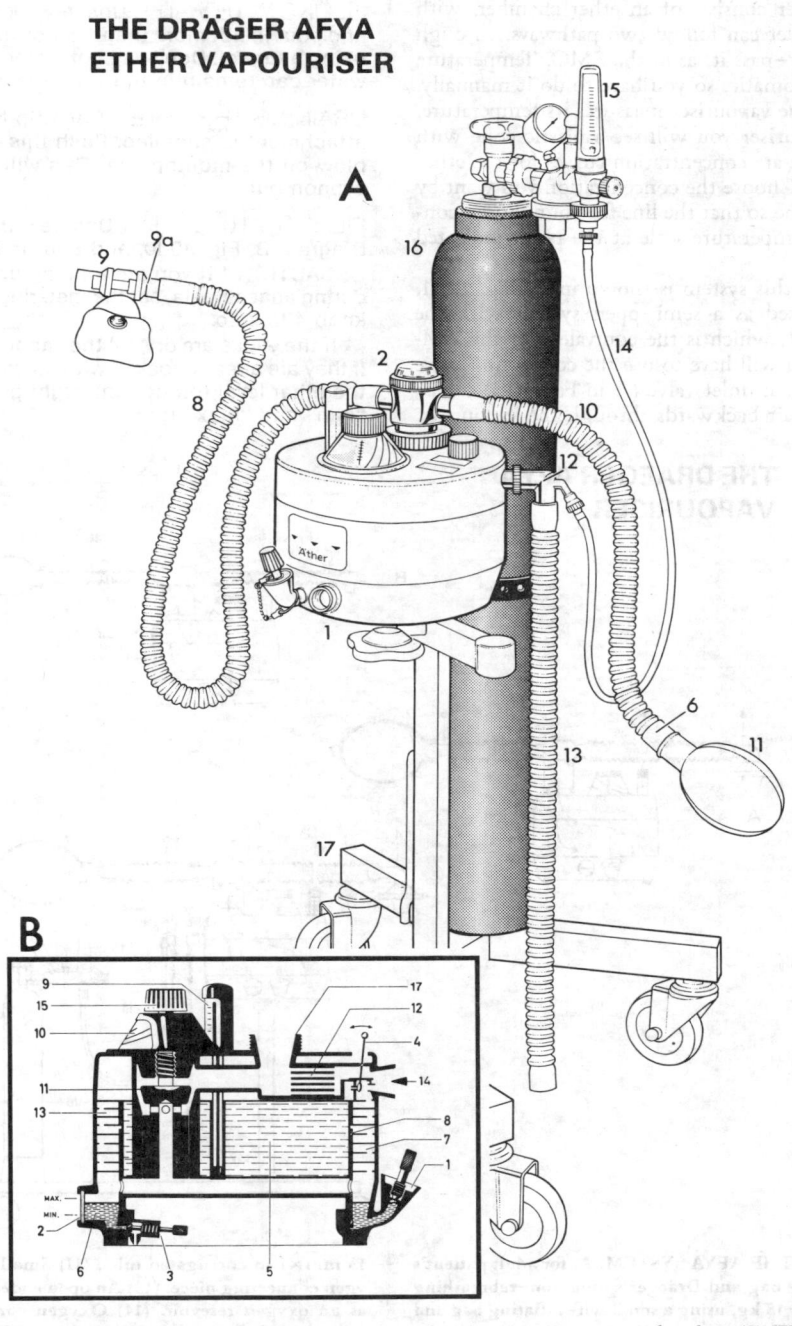

Fig. 10-10 THE AFYA ETHER VAPOURISER. A, the vapouriser on its trolley, with an oxygen cylinder. For the numbers of the various parts on the larger figure, see Fig. 10-11. Diagram B, a cross sectional view. (1) The filler funnel with screw plug. (2) Ether sight glass. (3) Ether drain valve. (4) ON/OFF knob. (5) Water jacket. (6) Ether chamber. (7) Vapouriser chamber. (8) Wick. (9) Thermometer. (10) Concentration adjustment scale. (11) Metering cone. (12) By-pass control. (13) Pressure compensation chamber. (14) Air inlet. (15) Concentration control knob. (17) Connection for breathing system.

If the ether concentration appears to be higher than normal to start with, but then drops rapidly during use the temperature compensator is not operating.

10.7 The Dräeger AFYA system

This well—made vapouriser is in increasing use and can be used for all ages of patient, including neonates. In its simplest form it consists of a drawover vapouriser, a self—inflating bag, and a non—rebreathing valve. If you wish, you can add an oxygen attachment, a sphygmomanometer, and a pair of gauges, one for airway pressure and another for tidal volume and minute volume. One of its disadvantages is that it is difficult to use with an accessary vapouriser for halothane or trichloroethylene, like the OMV.

The AFYA vapouriser consists of an ether chamber, with a wick. Air from the inlet can follow two pathways, through the ether chamber, or by—pass it, as in the EMO. Temperature compensation is not automatic, so you have to do it manually. A thermometer inside the vapouriser measures its temperature. On the top of the vapouriser you will see a plastic cone with some curved lines. These are concentration curves for the ether vapour being delivered. Choose the concentration you want by turning the metering cone so that the line for your chosen concentration crosses the temperature scale at the point indicated by the thermometer.

The easiest way to use this system is shown in A, Fig. 10-11. This shows it being used as a semi—open system with the non—rebreathing valve 4, which is the equivalent of the AMBU E valve. With it you will have to use the connecting valve 2 in Fig. 10-11. This has an inlet valve (A in Fig. 10-1) which prevents you squeezing air backwards through the vapouriser.

You can use this semi—open system for patients who are breathing spontaneously, or for controlled ventilation in patients of any age. For adults use the large bag and the large tubing. Or, for children or less than 15 kg you can use the AMBU "Paedivalve", the small bag and the small tubing.

Another way of using the system is shown in the upper part of Fig. 10-12. Change the connecting valve 2 for the valve chamber 18. On top of this fit the gauges for the airway pressure and tidal or minute volume. The inspiratory and expiratory valves are part of this system, so connect the system to the patient with a Y-piece without any valves. You will find this system useful for training purposes.

THE AFYA SYSTEM

FILLING WITH WATER Unscrew lock nut (16) marked "water" and pour in not more than 1.5 l of water at room temperature using a funnel. Don't use hot water. Close the filler port. The water can remain in the vapouriser indefinitely.

DRAINING THE WATER Don't tip it out. A special draining attachment is supplied. Push this into the water inlet, and blow on the mouthpiece. This will start to make the water syphon out.

FILLING WITH ETHER Unscrew the ether filler screw 1 in Diagram B, Fig. 10-10, and pour in ether.

CAUTION ! If you are topping up the reservoir with ether during anaesthesia, set the metering knob 15 and the ON/OFF knob 4 to zero.

If the wicks are dry, fill the vapouriser with 370 ml of ether. If they are already soaked with ether, fill it with 270 ml. Monitor the ether level through the sight glass. Keep it between the "min" and "max" marks.

THE DRAEGER AFYA VAPOURISER

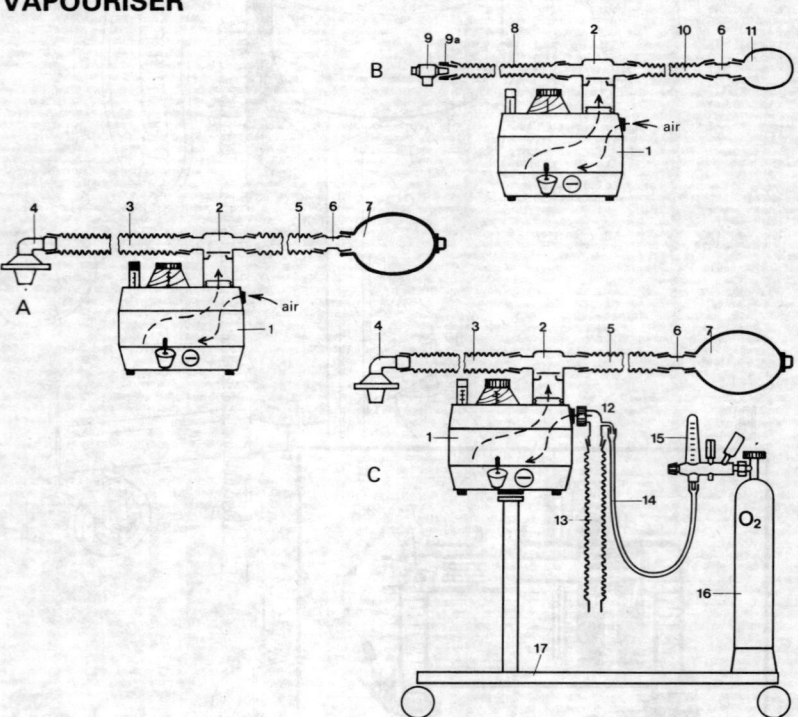

Fig. 10-11 CIRCUITS FOR THE AFYA SYSTEM. A, for adult patient's using a large self—inflating bag and Dräeger's own non—rebreathing valve. B, for children under 15 kg, using a small self—inflating bag and a "Paedivalve". C, as A, but this time on a trolley with an oxygen supply and a resevoir tube. (1) The vapouriser. (2) Connecting valve, (3) and (5) 22 mm by 1 m corrugated tube. (4) Non—rebreathing valve. (6) Connector for self—inflating bag. (7) Large self—inflating bag. (8) 13 mm × 1 m corrugated tube. (9) "AMBU Paedivalve". (9a) Adaptor. (10) 13 mm × 1 m corrugated tube. (11) Small self—inflating bag. (12) Oxygen connecting piece. (13) An open ended corrugated tube which acts as an oxygen resevoir. (14) Oxygen connecting tube. (15) Pressure reducer with flowmeter. (16) Oxygen cylinder. (17) Trolley. (18) Valve chamber with expiratory control valve. (19) Inspiratory valve. (20) Expiratory valve. (21) Pressure relief valve. (22) Meter for tidal and minute volume. An oxygen driven bronchial aspirator (27) can be attached to the system.

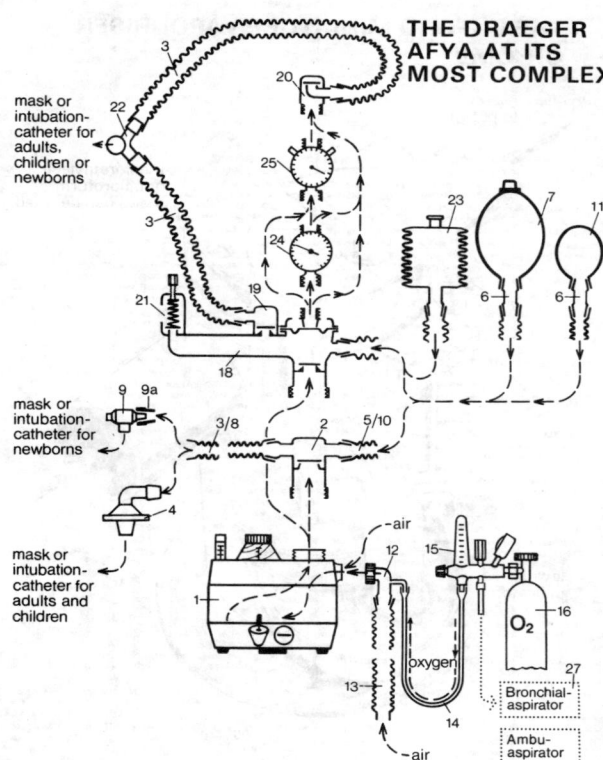

Fig. 10-12 THE AFYA SYSTEM AT ITS MOST COMPLEX. The numbers are the same as in Fig. 10-10.

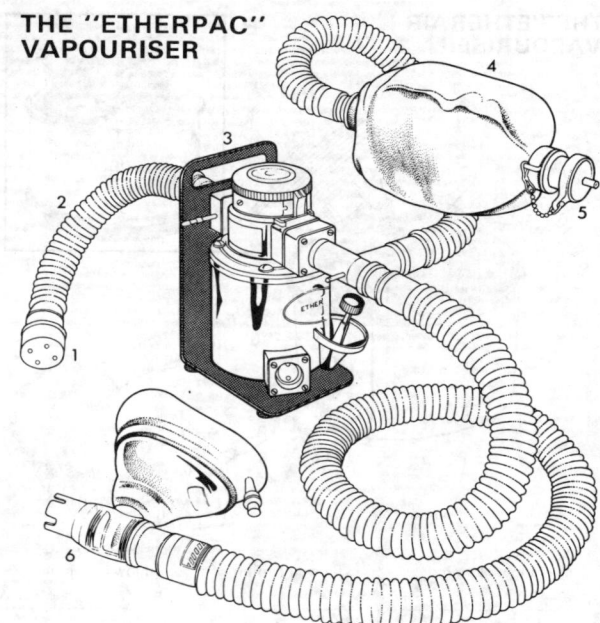

Fig. 10-13 THE "ETHER-PAC" VAPOURISER. (1) Air inlet with protective head. (2) Oxygen economiser tube. (3) Inlet valve (A) inside here. (4) Self–inflating bag. (5) Cap to close the open end of the bag. (5) Non–rebreathing (AMBU E) valve.

ROUTINE CHECKS Check your AFYA system occasionally. Is the vapouriser water compartment full of water? Check that the valve discs are in place and not damaged. They should move when you press the breathing bag. No air should escape from the inlet port when you do this. If air does escape, send the vapouriser for servicing.

DIFFICULTIES WITH THE AFYA VAPOURISER

If the metering cone has stuck you have probably left it standing idle too long or not emptied out the ether container often enough. Non-volatile substances accumulate in a vapouriser and make its metering cones stick. Send it for servicing.

If the patient does not become anaesthetized, the concentration of the ether delivered is too low. Make sure that: (1) There is no leak in the circuit, particularly round the face mask. (2) The ether chamber has not run dry. (3) The connecting valve 2 or the valve in valve chamber 18 is not damaged (Figs. 10-11, and 10-12). (4) The relief valve 21 may have been set too low, and may be allowing too much anaesthetic gas to escape. Increase the setting.

If the thermometer shows a temperatures higher than 28°C or less than 16°C, the wrong concentration of ether will be delivered. If the temperature is 30°C, the concentration of the ether delivered will be about 10 per cent higher than it should be. For temperatures above 30°C, fill the vapouriser with cold water. Use the draining attachment described above to change the water without emptying out the ether.

If the temperature is below 16°C, fill the vapouriser with warm water between 16 and 28°C.

If too much ether is delivered: (1) Check that you have not left the filler screw 1 Diagram B in Fig. 10-10 partly open, so that too much air is being sucked through the vapourizing chamber during spontaneous breathing. (2) Is the vapouriser tilted more than 45°?

If no gas flows when you press the breathing bag, check that all valves are correctly assembled. Replace damaged valve discs and seats or complete valves.

10.8 The "Ether–Pac" and "Fluo–Pac" vapourisers

These are handy, robust, light, easily portable, comparatively inexpensive, popular little vapourisers, one for ether only, and the other for halothane only. The "Fluo–pac" is the equivalent of the OMV (10-10). If you want to use both agents on the same patient, you can join an "Ether–pac" and a "Fluo– Pac" together. Both are adequately flow and temperature compensated. At the low flow rates, needed for children, the vapourisers deliver a lower concentration of both ether and halothane than the control knob indicates. Other vapourisers (including the EMO) behave in the same way, and it is perhaps a safety factor, rather than a disadvantage. The "Ether–pac" holds only 115 ml of ether, so you have to refill it more often than other vapourisers.

10.9 The Loos "Etherair" vapouriser

This is a compact, portable ether vapouriser with a water jacket. The Mark Two model is not fully temperature compensated, but instead has thermometers for the ether and water. As you will see from the graphs, setting A of the control knob represents an ether concentration of about 5%. Setting E will deliver 25 % ether (more than is necessary) if the vapouriser is warm (25°C) but if it is cold (15°) you will have to turn it up to "max" to get this concentration. This vapouriser is supplied with an expiratory spill valve and a non–return valve that fit together. When you want to use the non–return valve, screw the spill valve shut. When you want to use the spill valve, replace the non–return valve by an angle piece.

10.10 The Oxford Miniature Vaporiser (OMV)

If you are going to use halothane, trichloroethylene, or chloroform (11.8) you will need calibrated vapourisers for them. Most vapourisers are for one agent only, but you can use this

THE "ETHERAIR" VAPOURISER

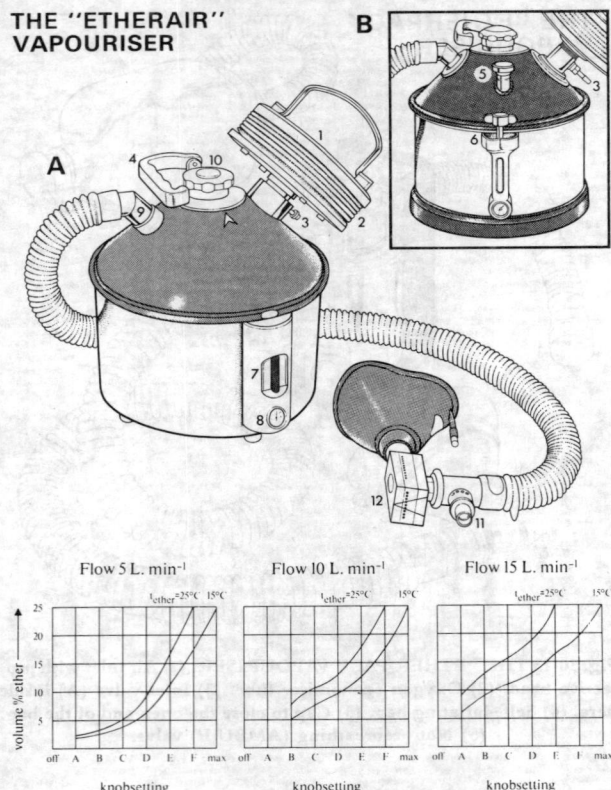

Fig. 10-14 THE LOOS "ETHERAIR" VAPOURISER. A, the Mark One. B, the Mark Two. (1) Inlet valve. (2) Bellows. (3) Oxygen inlet. (4) Handle. (5) Ether thermometer. (6) Ether filler. (7) Ether level gauge. (8) Water thermometer. (9) Outlet port. (10) Control knob. (11) Expiratory spill valve. (12) Non–rebreathing valve.

THE OXFORD MINIATURE VAPOURISER OR 'OMV'

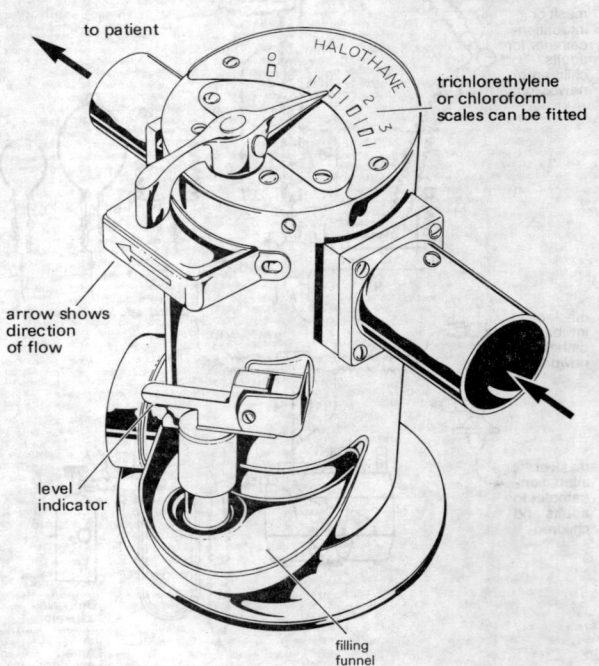

Fig. 10-15 THE OXFORD MINIATURE VAPOURISER OMV. This is the older model, the newer one, the "OMV 50" is similar, but holds 50 ml, has an easier filling arrangement, and a sealed water jacket. *Kindly contributed by John Farman.*

one for all three. This beautiful little vapouriser is flow compensated, but it does not need to be temperature compensated, because so little halothane evapourates that it cools very little. The OMV is made in two versions—one with right to left flow for use with ether vapourisers, and one with left to right flow for use with machines of Boyles type. If you use the wrong one, the controls will be at the back.

The OMV has a water–filled base, a control lever, and a scale that is calibrated for halothane. The rules for using these scales are easy. Induce the patient with either halothane or chloroform at 1%. If you are using relaxants, maintain the patient at 0.5 %. Never give him more than 1% of halothane if he is having thiopentone or ether. Never give more than 2% chloroform (11.8).

One of the disadvantages of both halothane and trichloroethylene is that neither of them will stimulate the patient's respiration enough for him to breathe adequately with air alone. So he needs continous extra oxygen if he is respiring spontaneously. But if he is paralysed, you can control his ventilation with sufficient vigour to make oxygen unnecessary, except for special purposes.

• *VAPOURISER, Oxford miniature, "OMV Fifty" right to left flow, with halothane scale as standard, and scales for trichloroethylene and chloroform, two vapourisers only.* A second and even a third vapouriser are useful, so that one can be used for trichloroethylene, and the other for chloroform.

USING THE OXFORD MINIATURE VAPOURISER (OMV)

The newer version of this vapouriser (the OMV 50) has a reservoir holding 50 ml.

If you have one of the older models, keep the water jacket full. Examine the water level every three months, and refill it with a syringe and needle. There is no need ever to open the water jacket of an "OMV 50".

If you use the OMV with an ether vapouriser, fit it on the downstream side, as in Fig. 11-5.

If you use Farman's entrainer, or any plenum system, turn the vapouriser off before refilling it or the pressure in the system will expel the halothane.

CLEANING This is only 5 minutes, work every 3 months, and will prevent the vapouriser sticking. Turn it upside down over a sink, to drain the residual halothane out of the inlet and outlet ports.

Put a cork in one of the ports. While the vapouriser is still switched full on, pour 50 ml of ether into the other port, and put a cork in that also. Turn the vapouriser upside down, shake it and work the control lever. Remove the cork, pour away the ether, and then repeat the whole process twice more. Finally, turn it full on, and blow air through with the bellows until you can no longer smell any ether coming from it.

TO CHANGE AGENTS, clean it as above, and then pour in the new agent.

DIFFICULTIES WITH THE OMV VAPOURISER

If you do not have one of the special conversion scales which can be supplied with the vapouriser, use the approximate scale in Fig. 11-6.

If the control level sticks, accumulated thymol is probably responsible. This is added to halothane to stabilize it. In time this accumulates in the OMV, colours the halothane yellow or brown, and makes the control lever stick. Shake out the halothane, and rinse the vapouriser out several times with ether. Finally, set the control lever to 3%, and blow air through it until you can no longer smell ether in the air coming through it.

RINSE OUT YOUR OMV WITH ETHER EVERY THREE MONTHS

10.11 An uncalibrated vapouriser (the Bryce–Smith Induction Unit or BSIU)

This simple little vapouriser delivers a single measured dose of halothane and is a way of assisting the induction of ether. It has a small chamber, and a baffle assembly that directs air onto a wick which can absorb halothane. You cannot use it for continous anaesthesia, or with trichloroethylene or chloroform. There are no controls and no water reservoir. The disadvantage of the BSIU is that it is holds too little halothane for a very large adult, and it can give a child an overdose.

• *VAPOURISER, uncalibrated, for halothane only, Bryce–Smith, one only.* If you have a calibrated vapouriser, like the OMV, you won't need it. Use it as in Section 11.6.

THE BRYCE-SMITH INDUCTION UNIT

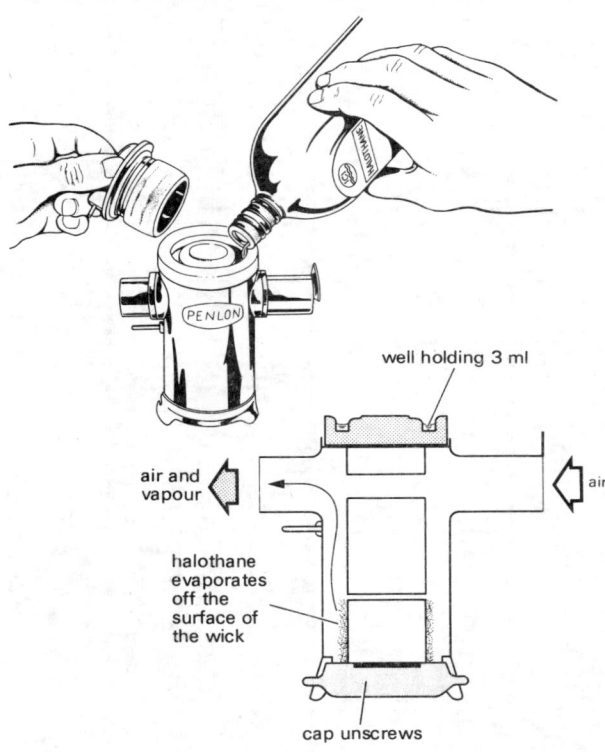

Fig. 10-16 THE BRYCE–SMITH INDUCTION UNIT. This allows you to give a single measured dose of halothane as an induction agent. Kindly contributed by John Farman.

10.12 The "Cyprane" vapouriser

The vapouriser in Fig.11-7 is only for trichloroethylene and is mainly for obstetrics, as described in Section 11.7. It is not thermocompensated, and is not graduated, except with the words "max" (1.5% trichloroethylene), and "min" (0.5%). It has a key that allows you to lock it in any position within this range. Although the 'Cyprane' vapouriser is designed to be used on its own, you can, if necessary, plug it into the inlet port of the EMO. Or, you can plug it into the AMBU bag and use it with muscle relaxants. It is designed to be held in a mother's hand, and is deliberately made so it does not stand up on its own. If necessary, support it in a tin.

• *VAPOURISER, trichloroethylene, hand held, "Cyprane" pattern, one only.*

10.13 An improvised vapouriser

Although the pioneer approach is appealing, rag–and–bottle methods have little place in district hospital anaesthesia, now that modern equipment is available. But there may be times when you have to improvise. You can give chloroform on the corner of a towel (11.8), and if you don't have a mask, you can give a child open ether with a tea strainer. In an adult, you can use a 'chimney' made from two tins (11-4).

The improvised vapouriser described below produces concentrations of vapour within the anaesthetic range, and has been used for many major operations. In some parts of the world it is a standard piece of anaesthetic equipment.

AN IMPROVISED VAPORISER

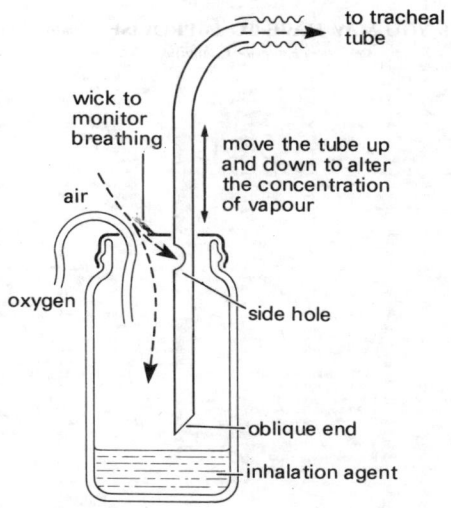

FIG. 10-17 USING AN IMPROVISED VAPORISER. You can make this from an old coffee jar, and some pieces of tubing. *Kindly contributed by Tom Boulton.*

AN IMPROVISED VAPORISER

Find a glass jar about 7.5 cm in diameter and 13 cm high. The size is important. It should be about the size of the bottle on an anaesthetic machine of the Boyle's type.

Punch two 1.25 cm holes in the lid, and insert a 1.25 cm plastic tube through one of them. Cut the end of this obliquely, so that fluid is less likely to be sucked through it. Cut a wide hole in the tube, in such a position that you can lift it above the lid to reduce the vapour concentration, if necessary.

Fix a piece of cotton wool at one edge of the open hole. Each time the patient breathes it will move, and allow you to monitor his ventilation.

Add oxygen through a tube fitting loosely in the open hole. Fill the jar about 4 cm deep with ether, trichloroethylene, or halothane. Use the jar with a non–rebreathing valve, and an Oxford bellows or a self inflating bag, or attach it straight to a tracheal tube, after you have intubated a patient under open ether.

CAUTION! This vaporiser is dangerous if it is knocked over. It is much safer if you use it with an Oxford bellows.

ETHER. When the ether gets cold so that the vapour concentration falls, gently agitate the bottle, or put it in a bath of warm water.

YOU MAY HAVE TO IMPROVISE

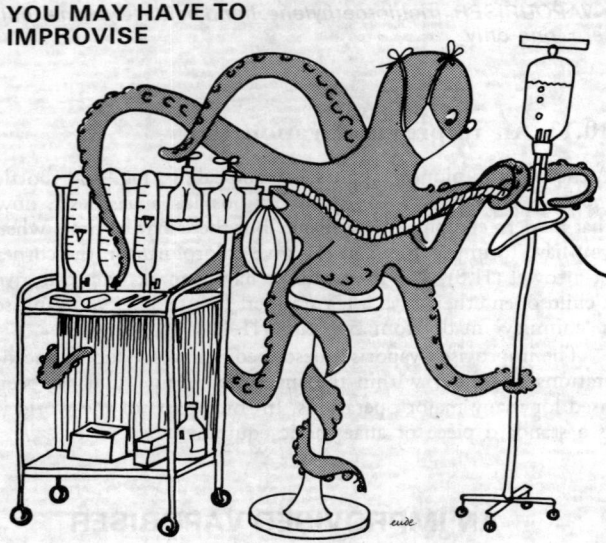

Fig. 10-18 YOU MAY HAVE TO IMPROVISE. *Kindly contributed by Ende de Glanville.*

TRICHLOROETHYLENE If necessary, gently agitate the bottle to increase the concentration.

HALOTHANE Tie the bottle firmly to a trolley leg to keep it still, agitation produces a dangeroulsy high concentration.

11 Inhalation agents

11.1 Ether as an anaesthetic agent

Ether has some very useful properties. Unlike halothane, which depresses a patient's respiration, ether in the concentrations you normally use, stimulates his respiration and his circulation, and in doing so encourages its own absorption. This makes it possible for you to use air as the carrier gas in a fit patient, whereas with most other anaesthetic agents, including halothane, you must add oxygen. Even if you are giving the patient so much ether that his respiration is depressed, his cardiac function is still fairly good, so ether has a wide safety margin. It is certainly the safest inhalational anaesthetic if you are not an expert. It is also the only agent described here that you can give in a sufficient concentration to relax a patient's muscles enough for major abdominal surgery and still be safe. All the other inhalation agents need the help of relaxants.

Ether does have some disadvantages: (1) Induction is slow and unpleasant if you use it alone. (2) It is highly inflammable in air. (3) It is explosive when mixed with oxygen or nitrous oxide (9.1), but fortunately not with air. (4) Nausea and vomiting are common postoperatively. (5) It has such a low boiling point that it is not satisfactory at altitudes over 2,000 metres, although it has been used up to 3,500 metres. If you do have to use ether at high altitudes, add oxygen because of the decreased partial pressure of oxygen at these altitudes.

11.2 The stages of ether anaesthesia

When you give any inhalational anaesthetic, you must know at any moment how deeply anaesthetized your patient is. The signs of anaesthesia are easier to recognise with ether than with any other anaesthetic. The stages that follow apply only to ether. Relaxants abolish many of them, and premedication with opioids or atropine may modify them. Other inhalational anaesthetics, such as halothane, behave differently.

Stage one, Analgesia The patient gradually loses the sensation of pain. His eyes move and his pupils remain their normal size. His muscle tone, breathing, and pulse are normal. This stage ends as he becomes unconscious. You can use ether analgesia like this:

ETHER ANALGESIA

INDICATIONS (1) Obstetric analgesia. (2) To supplement local anaesthesia in minor surgery. (3) To help a patient cough effectively in chest physiotherapy.

MEHOD Give the patient the face mask, and ask him to take deep breaths when he has pain. Give him 2 to 3% ether, and take care not to give him so much that he reaches the second stage.

Stage Two, Delirium This stage begins as the patient loses

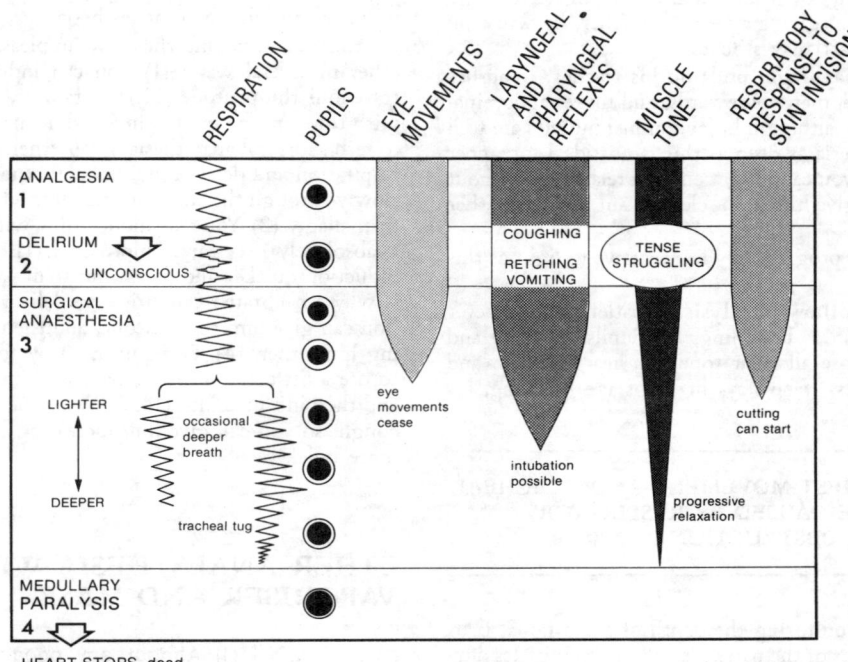

Fig. 11-1 THE STAGES OF ANAESTHESIA. It is usual to divide surgical anaesthesia into several planes, but to make things simpler we have not done so here. Other anaesthetics produce different signs. *Adapted from Atkinson, with kind permission.*

consciousness and becomes excited, he struggles and is difficult to control. His abdominal muscles contract during expiration. He breathes irregularly, and he may hold his breath. He loses his eyelash reflex, his eyes move about, and his pupils dilate, but they still react to light.

Try to get him through this stage quickly, because he may vomit, or develop laryngeal spasm, especially if he stays in it too long.

Stage Three, Surgical Anaesthesia It is usual to recognize 4 planes in this stage, but it is easier to recognise only two, light and undesirably deep surgical anaesthesia.

Light surgical anaesthesia. As the patient enters this plane from the stage of delirium, his breathing becomes regular again. Every 2 to 3 minutes he takes a deeper breath. These occasional deep breaths also occur in deep surgical anaesthesia. They are normal, and are not a sign that anaesthesia is becoming lighter.

His pupils start small, but they gradually dilate as anaesthesia deepens. His eyes stare straight ahead and stop moving. He no longer moves about, and his muscles lose some of their tone. The contractions of his abdominal muscles during expiration become weaker and weaker before they disappear. His chest and abdomen move together when he breathes. His pulse is fast and full, and his blood pressure normal.

Don't try to insert an airway or to intubate a patient until he reaches this stage. Most operations not requiring much muscular relaxation can be done in this stage of anaesthesia, and it should seldom be necessary to take him to the next stage.

Undesirably deep surgical anaesthesia. The patient's intercostal muscles become progressively paralysed, so that the movement of his his chest lags behind that of his diaphragm. Eventually, his chest moves in completely the opposite way. It falls during inspiration and rises during expiration—paradoxical chest movement. The peripheral part of his diapharagm, which is supplied by his intercostal nerves, becomes paralysed, and only its central part continues to work. Its contractions become jerky. With each sudden inspiration his diaphragm pulls on his intercostal muscles, his supraclavicular fossae, and his mediastinum, including his trachea. This sharp downward movement of his trachea with each breath is called "tracheal tug". You will also see it in upper airway obstruction and after giving sub—paralytic doses of muscle relaxants. It is an inefficient way of breathing, and a dangerous sign. Treat it by making sure that the upper airway is clear, and turn down the ether. If you fail to recognise tracheal tug, and go on giving the patient ether, he will stop breathing, and his heart may stop too.

As the patient's diaphragm pulls on his trachea, it pushes the contents of his abdomen downwards, and makes abdominal surgery difficult. Thus, although his abdominal muscles are well relaxed, ether anaesthesia as deep as this is not ideal for upper abdominal surgery. If you cannot get enough relaxation without causing tracheal tug, give him a muscle relaxant and light ether anaesthesia.

The pupils become progressively less reactive to light as this stage advances.

Stage Four, Medullary paralysis. A patient should never reach this stage. He stops breathing, his pupils are fixed and dilated, his muscles lose all their tone, his heart is slow, and his blood pressure falls. If he stays in this stage too long, his heart stops and he dies.

PARADOXICAL CHEST MOVEMENT AND TRACHEAL TUG CAN BE CAUSED BY RESPIRATORY OBSTRUCTION

A useful way of monitoring the depth of anaesthesia, is to observe the contractions of the patient's abdominal muscles during expiration. As ether (or halothane) anaesthesia deepens, these contractions weaken, as if his spinal cord was being progressively paralysed from below upwards. As soon as you can no longer see or feel his abdomen contracting during expiration, and his eyes have stopped moving, he is ready for surgery and, if necessary, for intubation. So put your hand on his abdomen, or watch it. If it is still tight during expiration, he is probably too light for surgery. Note that the abdominal wall of a fully conscious patient does not contract like this, and that relaxants abolish all contractions.

11.3 Ether with a vapouriser

Ether with a vapouriser is the recommended method of inhalation anaesthesia for a district hospital.

You have first to induce a patient, or make him unconscious. To do this you have to give him as much ether as he will take, so that it is taken up and distributed to his body. Your success in doing this will depend on how well he is breathing and on how much ether he will tolerate. He should, if possible, breathe a high concentration, but unfortunately ether is irritant, and too much will make him cough, gag and hold his breath. So you will have to give him as much ether as he will take without letting him do these things. Induction like this with ether alone is safe, but it is slow and it may be difficult. The secret of success is to induce the patient slowly; take 20 minutes over it if necessary. This may not be practical in a long operating list, but it is the safest way for an inexperienced anaesthetist to induce an occasional case.

But as soon as the patient is asleep and his cough reflex is depressed, you can give him progressively more—up to 20%—ether vapour, if necessary, so that he reaches the stage of surgical anaesthesia quickly. Having done this, you need only give him as much ether as he needs to maintain the depth of anaesthesia that you require, about 6 to 8%.

Ether is very soluble in water and is distributed by blood to the tissues. The brain has a high blood flow and takes up ether rapidly, so that the patient goes to sleep. During this early part of the anaesthetic, the concentration of ether in other tissues is lower than that in his brain. If, at this stage, the concentration of ether in his alveoli, and thus in blood, falls for any reason, ether will leave his brain and be distributed elsewhere in his body. This will make him wake up. So try to avoid unnecessary interruption in the delivery of ether to his alveoli during induction, for example by breath holding, which will greatly influence the depth of anaesthesia.

You can overcome the slow, unpleasant induction of plain ether in several ways: (1) You can induce a patient with intravenous thiopentone (12.1), ketamine, or diazepam. But even with thiopentone induction an adult man may take 20 minutes to reach surgical anaesthesia under ether. Thiopentone depresses respiration and delays the uptake of ether, so that he only goes slowly through the stage of delirium, which is the difficult part to manage. (2) You can induce him with halothane (11.6) or, if absolutely necessary, chloroform (11.8). These agents make induction quicker and pleasanter than with ether alone, which is why a calibrated vapouriser to deliver them is so useful. (3) You can give him thiopentone, and then halothane, before giving him ether. (4) The quickest way to induce the patient is to use a little thiopentone, paralyse him with suxamethonium and then intubate him (14.2). When he is paralysed, he cannot cough, so you can give him increasing concentrations of ether more quickly.

ETHER ANAESTHESIA WITH A VAPORISER AND MASK

INDICATIONS (1) Almost any occasion when a general anaesthetic is needed. (2) Ether is safest general anaesthetic for an inexperienced anaesthetist.

If the patient is a child, go to Section 18.4.

HOLDING THE MASK WITH ONE HAND

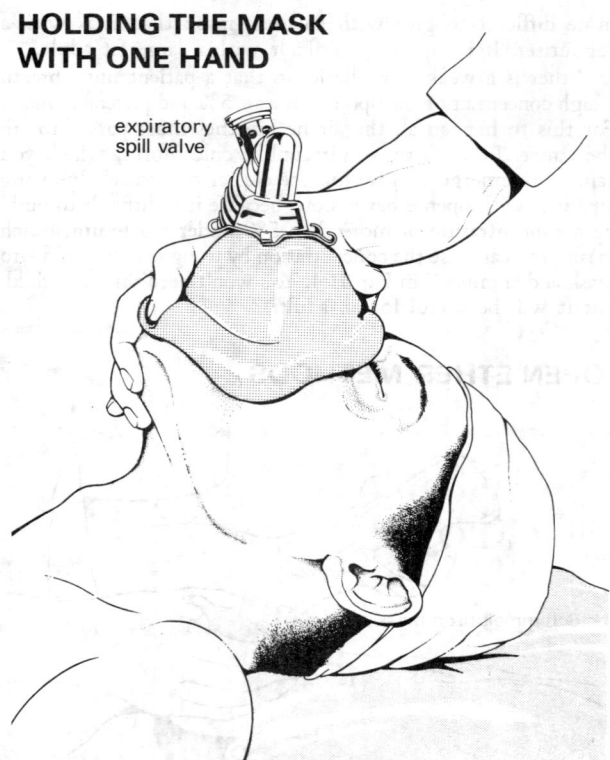

Fig. 11-2 HOLDING THE MASK WITH ONE HAND. *After Brenda Vaughan.*

CONTRAINDICATIONS Respiratory infection. A cold is only a relative contraindication.

EQUIPMENT An ether vapouriser, a bellows or self-inflating bag, a non-return valve, a mask, tubing, equipment for tracheal intubation (13.2), a sucker, and a table that can tip.

DRIP A patient who is having any general anaesthetic should *always* have a drip up, or an open vein, especially if he is critically ill, the procedure is major, or you expect it to last a long time. This is one of the "ten golden rules of anaesthesia" in Section 3.1.

PREMEDICATION Always give atropine when you give ether, to reduce respiratory secretions (2.7). If the patient is likely to be anxious, give him diazepam. Don't give him an opioid with ether, or with any inhalational anaesthetic, because it will depress his respiration, slow induction, and weaken his pharyngeal reflexes.

INDUCTION WITH ETHER ALONE

In this method we assume you are using an EMO vapouriser. With other systems you will have to modify the method slightly.

Pump the bellows a few times, with the ether control indicator set at zero per cent. This will blow air through the system, and remove any ether remaining in the breathing tubes from the previous patient.

Hold the mask about 10 cm above the patient's face. Slowly raise and lower the bellows with the ether control set to 2%. He may object to this by coughing and holding his breath. If he does, reduce the concentration.

Keep talking to him and encouraging him while you gradually lower the mask onto his face. At the same time steadily increase the concentration of ether to 6%. Make sure there is a good fit between the mask and his face. The advantages of a good vapouriser are lost if air leaks in. As soon as there is no leak, the patient's own respirations will move the bellows, so stop pumping. Don't try to inflate him.

During the next 10 minutes steadily increase the concentration of ether to 15% in a robust adult. Don't increase the concentration suddenly, or he will cough. *Increase it about 1% each time he has taken six clear breaths* without swallowing or breath-holding.

If he coughs, reduce the percentage, wait, and try again more slowly. You may take 15 minutes to reach 15% ether, but the time is well spent.

As ether reaches the patient's brain, he will pass through the stages of analgesia and delirium described in Section 11.2. He sleeps, he loses his eyelash reflex, he stops struggling, he breathes regularly, and he looks straight ahead.

CAUTION ! Don't let the surgeon start until you are ready.

MAINTENANCE After breathing 15% ether for about 10 minutes, the patient will probably have reached the stage of light surgical anaesthesia. His abdominal muscles no longer contract during expiration. Insert an oral airway and the operation can start. Reduce the ether concentration to 6%. For abdominal operations, this may not keep him relaxed enough. He may need 15% ether until his peritoneum is closed. These higher concentrations will relax his muscles, but he will recover consciousness more slowly. During long operations, you can usually reduce the ether concentration to about 4%.

Keep anaesthesia smooth and even. Keep the patient a little deeper than the operation requires. Difficulties are more likely to arise because anaesthesia is too light than because it is too deep.

If you want to intubate the patient, wait until his abdominal muscles no longer contract during expiration.

If he struggles and is difficult to control and his eyes move about, anaesthesia is too light. Re-induce him steadily. Don't suddenly give him a high concentration of ether, or he may start to cough.

If his pupils become steadily larger, his chest falls on inspiration, and a "tracheal tug" develops. he is too deeply anaesthetized. Turn the control lever to "air" or disconnect the vapouriser altogether until anaesthesia lightens.

Turn off the vapouriser about 5 minutes before the end of the operation. By the time the last stitches are put in, anaesthesia will be lighter. After a long operation you can usually turn off the ether 15 minutes before the last stitch, for example when the surgeon is closing the abdomen after a laparotomy.

HOLDING THE MASK WITH TWO HANDS

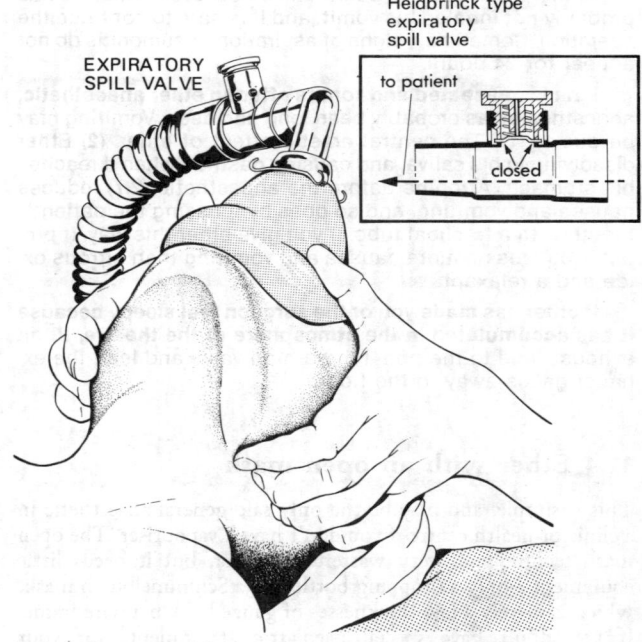

Fig. 11-3 HOW TO HOLD THE MASK WITH TWO HANDS. *After Brenda Vaughan.*

Turn the patient into the recovery position (4-5); don't send him back to the ward until he is safe to be left alone. He should be able to talk and be breathing quietly and well. He should have warm hands and a good pulse. If the operation allows it, he should be able to lie on his side and stay there.

OTHER INDUCTION METHODS FOR ETHER

Thiopentone (12.1), halothane (11.6), trichloroethylene (11.7), and chloroform (11.8) are described elsewhere.

KETAMINE Give 1 mg/kg. Use ketamine and diazepam in the same way as thiopentone. It is much safer than thiopentone for shocked patients.

DIAZEPAM Give 0.25 mg/kg. The patient will need less ether and relaxant after diazepam.

DIFFICULTIES WITH ETHER

If the patient holds his breath during induction, or there is laryngeal spasm, you may have given him too much ether too quickly, or given it irregularly, or there may be a poor fit between the mask and his face. This is one of the difficulties that intravenous induction, followed by a relaxant and intubation, will prevent. Give a few breaths of air and continue more slowly.

If laryngeal spasm develops during the operation, anaesthesia is probably too light, so stop all surgery and deepen it until he breathes normally (3.2). Give him oxygen.

If he stops breathing: (1) You may be giving him too much ether. (2) His respiratory tract may be obstructed. (3) He may be holding his breath. (4) His heart may have stopped (3.5). Resuscitate him immediately.

If secretions accumulate in his throat, you may have forgotten to give him atropine, or given it at the wrong time, or given him ether too quickly. If you have forgotten to give him atropine, give it. Sucking him out will only remove the secretions temporarily. You have three alternatives: (1) Continue ether anaesthesia, sucking him out as necessary. (2) You can change to halothane. (3) If you do need relaxation, give suxamethonium, suck him out and intubate him.

If he vomits while you are anaesthetizing him with ether, he will probably do so during the stage of delirium, while anaesthesia is light. The longer he stays in this stage, the more likely he is to vomit (16.2). Fortunately, his laryngeal reflexes will probably still be competent, so quickly tip him head down, turn him onto his side if this is possible, and suck him out. If his breathing, pulse, and colour are normal, he has probably not inhaled his vomit, and it is safe to continue the operation. Sometimes, signs of aspiration pneumonitis do not appear for 24 hours.

If he is nauseated and vomits after an ether anaesthetic, anaesthesia has probably been long and deep. Vomiting may be due to: (1) The central emetic effect of ether. (2) Ether dissolving in his saliva, and causing gastritis when it reaches his stomach. Atropine before the anaesthetic (2.7) reduces nausea and vomiting, and so does by-passing the patient's mouth with a tracheal tube. If you give ether this way, it probably causes no more nausea and vomiting than nitrous oxide and a relaxant.

If ether has made you or the surgeon feel sleepy because it has accumulated in the atmosphere of the theatre, fit an exhaust tube to the non-rebreathing valve and lead the exhaust gases away to the floor.

11.4 Ether with an open mask

This is simple, and may be the only safe general anaesthetic in a clinic or health centre if you don't have a vapouriser. The open mask technique is very wasteful of ether, but it needs little equipment—only a dropping bottle and a Schimmelbusch mask, which is merely a few thicknesses of gauze held in a wire frame. If you don't have special paediatric attachments for your vapouriser (18.2), this is one of the safest inhalation anaesthetics for a child. Unfortunately, a smooth ether anaesthetic is much more difficult to give with an open mask than it is with a vapouriser. It is especially difficult with a large fat adult.

Ether is a weak anaesthetic, so that a patient must breath a high concentration of vapour—at least 5% and preferably more. For this to happen all the air he breathes must pass through the gauze. Ether is thus quite unlike chloroform, which you can, in an emergency give, on the corner of a towel. Inducing a patient with open ether is slow, because it is difficult to build up a concentration of more than 5% under a Schimmelbusch mask. You can raise the concentration by using the "to-and-fro mask and chimney" in Fig. 11-4. You won't need this for a child, but it will be useful for an adult.

OPEN ETHER METHODS

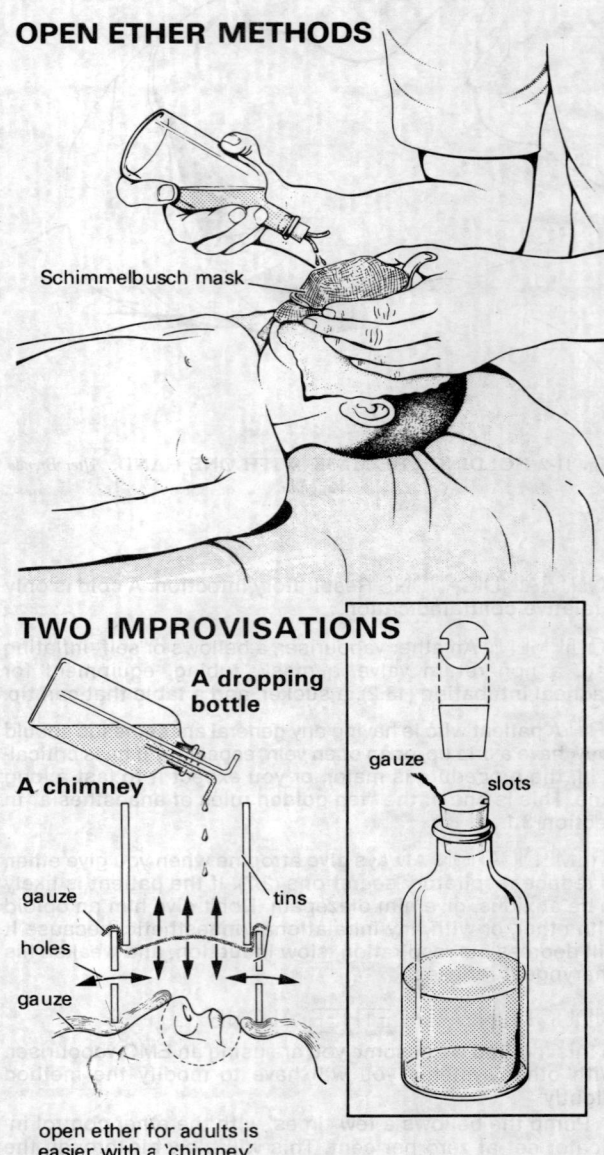

Fig. 11-4 ETHER WITH AN OPEN MASK. Ether is one of the safest anaesthetics for children. To get enough ether into an adult, you will find a "chimney" helpful. *Partly after Tom Boulton with kind permission.*

OPEN ETHER

INDICATIONS A patient of any age, but especially a young child.

EQUIPMENT

You must have the emergency equipment for any general anaesthetic, especially a sucker and a table that will tip.

BOTTLES Either use a special dropping bottle, or make one (11-4).

MASKS If possible, prepare two masks. If you have no infant mask, use a wire mesh tea strainer. Place 6 or 7 layers of gauze over the masks, depending on the size of their mesh. You should be able to see light through the full thickness of the gauze, otherwise air will not pass through it easily enough.

AIRWAYS If the patient's respiration is obstructed, try an oral airway, If you place it correctly, you can feel or hear air going in and out of his lungs at each breath. If there is no improvement, remove it and try to find and rectify the cause.

TWO-AND-FRO MASK AND CHIMNEY You may find this useful in an adult. Make it with two tins that fit into one another, and three (not more) layers of gauze. In longer operations it is useful to have some side holes in the lower tin. For shorter operations, seal these with adhesive strapping.

METHOD USING A MASK
Take a piece of gamgee tissue, or several layers of gauze and cut a hole for the child's nose and mouth.

Hold the mask above the gamgee, and drop ether onto it. Never place the mask directly on the face of a conscious patient, or he will feel suffocated. Wait until his eyelash reflex has gone, and then put the mask on his face.

Drop ether steadily onto the mask. Be patient. Drop it all over the mask. Don't pour it on so fast that it makes him cough. As soon as he begins to tolerate the ether, drop it on faster.

Listen to every breath. Correct any respiratory obstruction. If the patient coughs, or holds his breath, stop dropping on the ether until he breathes regularly again.

Drop the ether on more slowly when surgical anaesthesia is reached.

Keeping the patient at the right depth of anaesthetisa will not be easy. Most anaesthetists like to err on the side of being just too deep. If the patient becomes too light, regaining control will not be easy.

CAUTION ! (1) Don't give stronger concentration of ether for longer than is necessary, or anaesthesia will become too deep. The signs of ether anaesthesia in children are the same as those in adult. An additional sign is that a baby relaxes his grip as he becomes anaesthetized. (2) Keep the ether out of his eyes.

When the mask becomes so cold that it is covered with frost, change it for a fresh one.

One of the difficulties is that there may be so much ether vapour in the atmosphere of the theatre that it will make you sleepy. Minimise this by placing two layers of lint on the mask after you have poured on the ether. Remove and replace it each time you pour on more ether. This will minimise its escape.

If oxygen is available, and the operation is a long one, lead a fine tube under the mask and give him 250 to 500 ml per minute.

CAUTION ! Ether in air is inflammable. Adding oxygen makes it explosive, so take the precautions described in the next Section.

INTUBATION If you want to intubate the patient, continue the anaesthetic for 10 to 15 minutes before doing so. Wait until his abdominal muscles no longer contract during expiration, indicating that he is now deep enough to intubate. Intubating a small child with open ether is easier than intubating an adult.

CAUTION ! Don't try to intubate too early.

MAKING INDUCTION EASIER Induction will be easier and pleasanter if you drop 3 ml of halothane or trichloroethylene slowly onto the mask from a glass or nylon syringe. Some disposable plastic syringes dissolve in these liquids. Then, drop ether rapidly and evenly over the mask.

11.5 Fires and explosions with ether

Unlike the other inhalational agents discussed in this chapter, ether is inflammable, and under some circumstances it explodes. But, provided you take reasonable precautions, you can avoid these dangers.

Two or three per cent of ether vapour in air will not burn, because as soon as it escapes from the vapouriser circuit it is diluted beyond the limit of inflammability. Even if it is not diluted, it will only burn quite slowly. But ether will become explosive if you add as little as one litre a minute of oxygen. Nitrous oxide also makes ether explosive. The risks of flames and explosions are greatest close to the expiratory valve, so keep all sources of flame and sparks, and particularly diathermy, away from it. Lead the expired gases away to the floor with a piece of corrugated tube attached to the non-rebreathing valve, as in Fig. 16-8. If possible, lead them out of the room. If you have to use diathermy with ether, arrange a fan to blow the ether vapour away from it. Inflammable vapours are also commonly ignited by the static electricity produced by rubbing together two non conductors, particularly in a very dry atmosphere. So, where possible, all anaesthetic equipment should be made conductive, so as to lead any electric charges to earth. Theatre boots and the wheels of trolleys should also be conductive, and all electrical equipment made spark-proof.

Fortunately, explosions are very rare. You can even use diathermy with ether but only provided: (1) You don't use oxygen with the ether. (2) You don't use diathermy for procedures involving the lung, chest wall, neck, face, eye, or oral cavity. (3) You keep diathermy more than 25 cm away from the expiratory valve or the end of the tube that is used to carry away waste gases.

11.6 Halothane

This is an expensive and powerful anaesthetic—as little as 2 to 4% will anaesthetize a patient, whereas he may need up to 20% of ether vapour. But: (1) Halothane is a poor analgesic, so that the patient is apt to move with the stimulus of surgery if he is only lightly anaesthetized. (2) Halothane depresses respiration, which becomes progressively more shallow, so that the he must have additional oxygen. (3) If you are inexperienced, you cannot give a sufficient concentration of halothane alone to relax a patient's muscles enough for major surgery and still be safe. If you want muscle relaxation, you must use relaxants. In this respect halothane is quite unlike ether.

Because halothane is so powerful, you can easily give too much, so follow these rules carefully:

(1) If you are using halothane with any other agent, such as trichloroethylene, don't give more that 1% halothane. After 20 or 30 minutes with trichloroethylene, 0.5% halothane may be enough. Only if halothane is the sole agent is it safe to give more that 1%.

(2) *Always give halothane with a calibrated vapouriser*, such as the OMV (10.10).

(3) Watch the postion of the control lever of the halothane vapouriser carefully. It can easily be moved up to 4% by mistake. When this happens a patient can rapidly become deeply anaesthetized without the characteristic changes in his respiration that ether produces and that therefore make ether so safe.

(4) Know what agent you are giving. Halothane is so much more powerful than trichloroethylene that you can kill a patient if you think you are giving him trichloroethylene and you have filled the vapouriser with halothane by mistake.

HALOTHANE IS A VERY POWERFUL ANAESTHETIC

Halothane is very useful: (1) It is a good induction agent for ether, and if you use it in small quantities like this it is cheap. (2) You can use halothane with air alone in fit patients for short operations that take less than 15 minutes. If you use it for longer periods, the patient must have oxygen. (3) You can use halothane with relaxants, intubation, controlled ventilation and oxygen.

(4) Because halothane is a weak analgesic, and trichloroethylene such a good one, you can give them together by joining two vapourisers (for example, two OMVs) in series. Incoming air goes first into the halothane vapouriser, and then into the vapouriser containing trichloroethylene. This combination is useful for most operations, except those on the abdomen, or inside the thorax. *Don't try to mix two agents in the same vapouriser!*

Most signs of halothane anaesthesia differ from those of anaesthesia with ether. But the sign of a patient's abdomen ceasing to contract, as anaesthesia becomes deep enough for surgery, is the same for both. This sign is however much less obvious with halothane, because halothane depresses respiration instead of stimulating it as light ether does. Halothane will also depresses the circulation, so take the patient's blood pressure regularly, and reduce the concentration of halothane if this falls. Monitor him carefully, and don't give him more halothane than is necessary.

The principle of the method that follows is to give thiopentone; as soon as the patient is asleep, to give him halothane and to increase the halothane concentration to 1%, then to give him ether as soon as he is breathing halothane smoothly, and finally to stop the halothane.

HALOTHANE INDUCTION AND ETHER MAINTENANCE

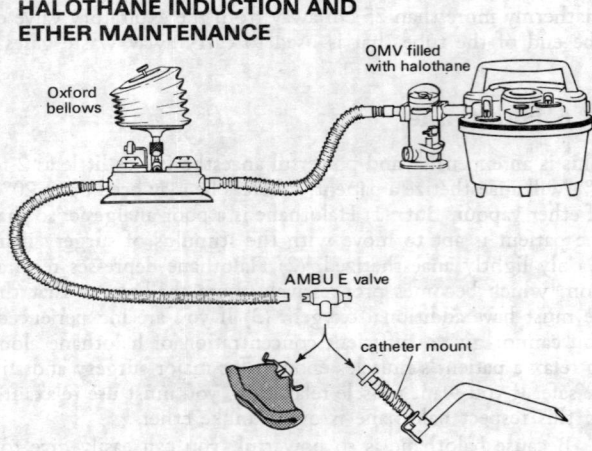

Fig. 11-5 A CIRCUIT ARRANGED FOR HALOTHANE INDUCTION AND ETHER MAINTENANCE. *Kindly contributed by Michael Wood.*

A METHOD FOR HALOTHANE

You will need an ether vapouriser and another vapouriser for halothane. The following instructions mention only halothane, but you can use trichloroethylene or chloroform in the same way.

PREMEDICATION Give the patient atropine (2.7).

OXYGEN If possible, give him oxygen at 1 litre a minute for maintenance.

INDUCTION WITH THIOPENTONE Give him thiopentone as usual (12.1). As soon as he is asleep, put the mask on his face. When he starts breathing, after the apnoea caused by the thiopentone, increase the concentration of the halothane from zero to 1%. If you have given him a sleep dose of thiopentone, you may need 2 or 2½% halothane. This will allow you to give ether quickly, and you can soon turn off the halothane.

As soon as the patient is breathing smoothly and regularly with halothane, set the ether concentration to 2%, and slowly increase it by 1% every third breath with halothane or chloroform, or about every tenth breath with trichloroethylene, as long as respiration is smooth, without breath-holding or coughing. If he breathes irregularly, increase the ether more slowly.

As soon as he is breathing 10% ether smoothly, reduce the concentration of the halothane slowly during five minutes. Don't reduce it too quickly, or its effect may have gone before he is sufficiently anaesthetized with ether. If that happens, he will cough.

INDUCTION WITHOUT THIOPENTONE Proceed exactly as with ether alone (11.2), except start with the control indicator on the vapouriser set at zero. Slowly increase the concentration of the halothane. As soon as the patient is breathing halothane smoothly, slowly and steadily increase the concentration of the ether. As soon as he is breathing 10% ether steadily, slowly reduce the concentration of the halothane.

INDUCTION USING THE BRYCE–SMITH INDUCTION UNIT (BSIU) You can use this with or without thiopentone. The depression on the top of the BSIU holds approximately 3 ml, which is the dose of halothane for an adult. Unscrew the wick, fill the well with halothane, stand the wick in the well to absorb the halothane, and replace the wick in the unit. The unit is now "on", and will deliver 2% halothane for about 4 minutes. It is "off" when all the halothane has evaporated. The BSIU is satisfactory only with halothane.

As soon as the patient is breathing well with the halothane alone, cautiously increase the concentration of the ether.

CAUTION ! The BSIU is adapted to the needs of the average adult, and not to very large adults or children.

MAINTENACE Maintain the patient on halothane alone (with added oxygen) or on ether. Don't try to give him a mixture of both.

CAUTION ! The scale in Fig. 11-6 applies only to the OMV, which can be filled with any of these three agents. Don't try to fill other vapourisers with agents that are not intended for them.

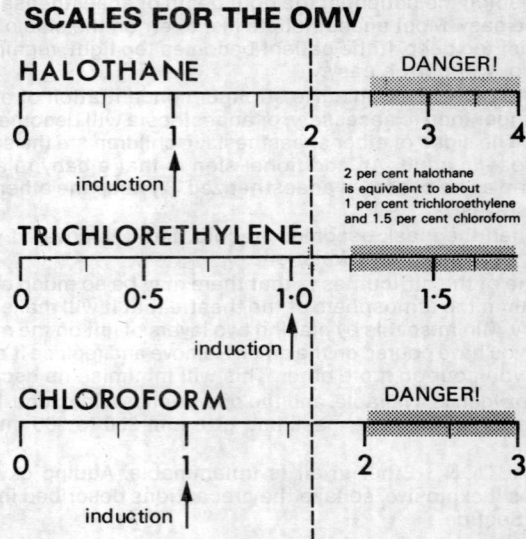

Fig. 11-6 SCALES FOR THE "OMV". The OMV is calibrated for halothane, and has clip-on scales for trichloroethylene and chloroform. If you do not have these scales, you can use this chart. For example, the dotted line shows that 2% on the halothane scale corresponds to 1% of trichloroethylene and about 1.5% chloroform. *Kindly contributed by John Farman,*

11.7 Trichloroethylene

This is a powerful analgesic, but a poor anaesthetic—the reverse of halothane. It is cheap, safe and non-inflammable. It is easily transported, and unlike ether, you can use it at high altitudes. Don't confuse trichloroethylene with *tetra*chloroethyelene, which is used to treat hookworms. If you cannot get anaesthetic grade trichloroethylene, use the best technical grade. You can give it with a calibrated vapouriser (such as the OMV), or with a "Cyprane" vapouriser (11-7).

Use trichloroethylene as: (1) An induction agent for ether (11.3) with or without thiopentone. Induction takes longer than with halothane, but is cheaper. (2) A general analgesic for minor operations and during labour. A mother can inhale it for a short period at a time, only when she needs it, at any stage in labour. It is thus much more satisfactory than the routine use of pethidine. But, if you are not careful, she can easily be sedated excessively with trichloroethylene, and it tends to prolong labour. (3) As a general anaesthetic for continued anaesthesia.

Trichlorethylene analgesia If a patient is co-operative, and the mask fits well, and you control the vapour concentration carefully, you can use trichloroethylene in the stage of analgesia to reduce fractures and dress wounds. You can also use it for minor cutting operations, such as incising abscesses. But it is not ideal, and local anaesthesia is safer. Although a patient's pharyngeal and laryngeal reflexes are largely preserved by trichloroethylene, if you use it to the plane of analgesia, they are not completely preserved. So: (1) Starve the patient first. (2) Anaesthetize him on a tipping table. (3) Have suction ready. Trichloroethylene analgesia without these precautions is dangerous, especially if you are tempted to give a bit too much and so reach the stage of anaesthesia.

You can also use trichloroethylene to provide paramedicatiom (5.2) for local anaesthesia with lignocaine (provided you don't use adrenaline with the local anaesthetic). If you use trichloroethylene like this, remember that it is easier to control an awake patient with firm comforting words than a disoriented one in the second and excited stage of anaesthesia.

TRICHLOROETHYLENE ANALGESIA

FOR MINOR OPERATIONS Start with the "Cyprane" inhaler near the minimum and fairly quickly move to the maximum position. The patient will probably move about and may need to be held down, but he will recover rapidly and will probably not remember the operation. If he coughs start again from the lowest concentration he can tolerate.

CAUTION ! (1) Take the full anaesthetic precautions (3.1). (2) Don't use it after the failure of a block containing adrenaline, because of the danger of cardiac arrest.

IN LABOUR give trichloroethylene like this.

If you use a calibrated vapouriser, like the OMV, use it as you would in the theatre, but watch the concentration carefully—never give more than 1%.

If you use the Cyprane inhaler, set it to half way between "Maximum" and "Minimum" (about 1%) and lock it with the Allen key provided.

Ask the mother to hold the inhaler in her hand and to give herself as much as she needs. As anaesthesia becomes deeper, she will drop the inhaler from her lips, so that she becomes less deeply anaesthetized. Never let anyone else hold the inhaler for her, or she may inhale too much.

In the second stage of labour, ask her to take three deep breaths from the inhaler each times she "bears down".

CAUTION ! Mothers who have been given trichloroethylene must not be later anaesthetized using a soda lime absorber (9.1).

Trichloroethylene anaesthesia Trichloroethylene has some disadvantages as an anaesthetic, but you can overcome most of them: (1) It produces short sharp respirations. (2) It is a weak anaesthetic, and so does not relax a patient's abdominal muscles. (3) Used alone, it does not reduce the patient's reflexes enough for intubation, so spray his cords with lignocaine before you pass the tube. (5) In concentrations above 1% it causes bradycardia.

You can overcome limitations (1) and (2) by combining trichloroethylene with ether, and using two vapourisers in series. Ether will stimulate the patient's respirations, so that he does not need any extra oxygen.

You can overcome the weakness of trichloroethylene's anaesthetic effect by: (1) Combining it with halothane, using two vapourisers in series. Neither of these agents stimulates the patient's respirations, so he will need extra oxygen. Or, (2) you can combine trichloroethylene anaesthesia with relaxants, intubation, and controlled ventilation. You can use this combination on almost any patient, however sick. Trichloroethylene is not inflammable, so this is a good method for chest operations in which diathermy is used.

Because trichloroethylene will not relax a patient's abdominal muscles: (1) You cannot use it alone for abdominal surgery (2). It does not produce the signs of abdominal muscle relaxation, which are so useful for judging the depth of ether anaesthesia.

If the patient's heart slows, intravenous atropine will reverse the bradycardia. Trichloroethylene also causes ectopic beats, especially in higer concentrations. So: (1) always use an inhaler, (2) don't give more than 1%, and, *(3) don't give it by open drop methods, except in the gravest emergencies, because these can deliver dangerously high concentrations.*

**NEVER GIVE MORE THAN 1%
TRICHLOROETHYLENE
DONT GIVE IT BY OPEN DROP METHODS**

THE CYPRANE INHALER

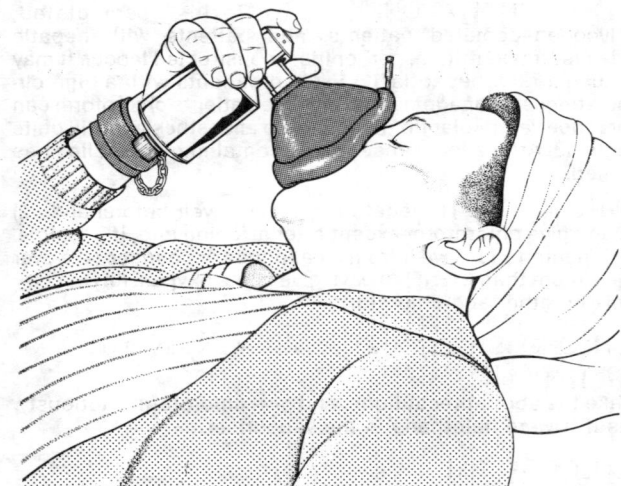

Fig. 11-7 TRICHLOROETHYLENE ANALGESIA used in labour with the "Cyprane" vapouriser. A mother cannot give herself too much trichloroethylene because the vapouriser will drop from her face as she becomes sleepy.

11.8 Chloroform

Chloroform is controversial largely because it was discovered long before the correct way of using it was known. Despite its bad reputation, we have included it here because: (1) It may be very useful in an emergency and under difficult conditions. (2) It is being used in some parts of the world, so it should be used correctly. (3) It is a very effective induction agent and is only a tenth the price of halothane. (4) Some hospitals have used it for years without ill effect. (5) Some respected anaesthetists use it regularly. Many equally respected ones condemn it. If you are using it, and have nothing else, here are the rules for minimising its dangers.

Chloroform is more powerful even than halothane, so it will induce a patient very quickly indeed, and you can overdose him only too easily. It is also a better analgesic than halothane. Besides being very cheap, chloroform is non—flammable and easily transported—a small bottle will anaesthetize many patients. But: (1) It is so powerful that you can easily overdose a patient and cause cardiac and respiratory depression—*during induction, and even when anaesthesia seems to be very light.* (2) Chloroform has a toxic action on the heart and the liver, particularly if you use it for maintaining anaesthesia, so avoid doing this. Use it for induction only, for which it is very effective, and quickly follow it up with ether. It has been well said that chloroform is 'fatally easy to give and easily fatal".

If necessary, you can use chloroform *in a vapouriser* as a substitute for halothane to settle a patient after thiopentone and atropine, and before ether when you have taken all the precautious listed below.

Inducing a patient with *open* chloroform needs great skill, because struggling, breath holding, or a trace of hypoxia all greatly increase the risk of cardiac arrest. It is almost non−irritant, so you can overdose a patient very easily. Induction is so much safer and easier with a vapouriser that you must use one. The open method is only for use in the direst emergency.

CHLOROFORM

INDICATIONS (1) As an induction agent, when given in a calibrated vapouriser. (2) In emergencies when there is no other anaesthetic agent or equipment.

CONTRAINDICATIONS (1) Toxic, emaciated, glycogen−depleted patients, and patients with hepatic disease, malnutrition, peritonitis, or obstructed labour. It may cause a fatal hepatitis. (2) Excited patients with a high circulating level of adrenaline. In these patients chloroform can produce ventricular fibrillation while anaesthesia is still quite light. (3) After a local anaesthetic containing adrenaline has failed.

PRECAUTIONS (1) Sedate the patient well beforehand. (2) Don't give chloroform except after atropine and, if possible, thiopentone. (3) Give it from a calibrated vapouriser. (4) Never give more than 2%. (5) Always give some oxygen. (6) Don't try mixing ether and chloroform.

CHLOROFORM FROM A VAPORISER AS AN INDUCTION AGENT FOR ETHER

Take the above precautions, and give chloroform cautiously, as if it were halothane in the vapouriser.

CHLOROFORM IN DESPERATE EMERGENCY

Give it with a Schimmelbusch mask, with a not more than 6 layers of gauze. Cover the mask with a layer of cloth. Apply the mask loosely with your thumb under the rim, to allow the patient to breathe some air round it.

Drop chloroform slowly and evenly on the mask—not more than 30 drops a minute.

Pay great attention to the airway. If possible lead additional oxygen under the mask.

CAUTION ! (1) Don't apply the mask closely to the patient's face. (2) Don't let the chloroform fall onto his face or his eyes, or it will burn them. (3) Make sure that there is no sudden noise or other disturbance during induction. (4) You have to saturate a mask with ether, you only have to dampen it with chloroform.

If you don't have a Schimmelbusch mask, you can use the corner of a towel.

11.9 Ethyl chloride

Ethyl chloride is another controversial agent. The common modern view is that it now has no place in anaesthesia. Some anaesthetists, however, particularly those working in out−of−the−way places and difficult environments have used it without mishap all their working lives. Nonetheless: (1) It is not a satisfactory local anaesthetic when sprayed on the tissues. (2) It is dangerously powerful—the margin between clinical anaesthesia and cardiac and respiratory arrest is small.

Its main use is as an induction agent for ether—a patient becomes unconcious in ½ to 2 minutes and recovers 2 or 3 minutes after you stop giving it. Induction is so rapid that he is not excited and does not struggle. Induction will be much more difficult, but he will be much safer if you induce him with ether alone. Ethyl chloride is particularly convenient (and dangerous) in children. Never use it if you can possibly use ketamine or some safer anaesthetic method instead.

ETHYL CHLORIDE

INDICATIONS *If possible, use some other agent!* In an emergency you can use ethyl chloride: (1) As an induction agent for open ether, or ether from a vapouriser, when no OMV inhaler for halothane is available. You can spray a little into the inlet of a vapouriser. It is convenient for children, say from 5 to 7, who are too apprehensive to tolerate local infiltration, and too small for you to find a vein easily. In a desperate emergency you can use it for adults. (2) For momentary operations only as the sole agent.

CONTRAINDICATIONS (1) Cardiac disease. (2) Gravely ill patients. (3) As the sole agent in any operation lasting longer than a minute or two.

METHOD Give the child atropine (2.7). Ethyl chloride is supplied in a cylindrical container that will deliver it in drops, or as a spray. Drop it onto a Schimmelbusch mask, listening carefully for every breath. *You must hear every one.*

If the patient holds his breath, remove the mask and begin again.

CAUTION ! (1) The great danger is that the patient will hold his breath, while you continue to pour on the ethyl chloride. If he does so, he may suddenly inhale a high concentration, with the result that his breathing or his heart may stop—so you must hear every breath. (2) Be sure to maintain a perfect airway—he must not become anoxic.

As soon as he starts to breathe freely, stop the ethyl chloride, and drop on plenty of ether. Don't pour it on too lightly, or he will react to the irritant vapour and rapidly lighten.

CAUTION ! (1) Always give atropine first. (2) Don't try to use ethyl coride in a vapouriser; always give it on an open mask. (4) As soon as the patient is asleep, change to ether rapidly, either on the mask, or from a vapouriser. (5) Use the very minimum. You will need between 3 and 20 ml. (6) Circulatory failure follows respiratory failure very quickly. (7) Don't use ethyl chloride as the sole agent for more than momentary operations.

ETHYL CHLORIDE IS A PARTICULARLY DANGEROUS GENERAL ANAESTHETIC IN UNSKILLED HANDS

12 Thiopentone

12.1 Thiopentone as an induction agent

Thiopentone is a useful induction agent, especially for ether when combined with suxamethonium, but if you don't use it carefully, it is also a dangerous agent. It has a very small safety margin in a sick patient and can kill him if he is shocked, severely anaemic, in cardiac failure, or if his respiration is obstructed. Although inducing a patient with thiopentone looks so easy, it is in fact more dangerous than a struggle to induce him with ether alone. Thiopentone alone is not an easy induction agent for ether. By the time the patient has overcome the respiratory depression of thiopentone, he may be awake, and gagging with ether again. If possible thiopentone should be followed by suxamethonium and intubation, as in Section 13.3. Failing this, induction with a non—irritating agents, such as trichloroethylene, halothane, or chloroform will be safer than with thiopentone alone, especially if you are not very skilled.

Thiopentone weakens the reflexes that protect a patient's airway, so that if he vomits, he may inhale his vomit. Thiopentone is only slowly destroyed in the body, so that if you give repeated doses, he becomes more and more drowsy. He is more likley to stop breathing suddenly than with ketamine, or to vomit. Also, his blood pressure is more likely to fall.

So, whenever you use thiopentone, be prepared for its serious side effects. While anaesthesia is light: (1) The patient may have laryngeal spasm. (2) He may vomit. When anaesthesia is deeper, (3) he may regurgitate, (4) his blood pressure may fall, or (5) his respiration may become depressed.

Don't give thiopentone, or any other general anaesthetic, unless you follow "the ten golden rules" in Section 3.1. In particular, you must have suction immediately available and working. The patient must be on an operating table or a trolley that can tip head down. You must give him atropine. He must have been starved, and you must have the equipment ready for cardiopulmonary resuscitation (3.1).

One of the most valuable features of thiopentone is that it shortens the time necessary to induce patients, and so enables you to work through an operation list much faster. Use it: (1) To induce anaesthesia that you will continue with other agents. (2) With pethidine, as described in Section 8.8, for procedures that you are sure will be very short. (3) To treat convulsions. *Never try to do an operation that needs continuous muscle relaxation, such as removing an the appendix, using only thiopentone!* And, never use a thiopentone drip. This does have some special uses in anaesthesia, particularly for neurosurgery, but is not suitable for the circumstances for which we write.

EUGENIA (25) was to have a Caesarean section and needed blood. The pathologist kindly brought a bottle of blood to the theatre. The surgeon said "Just give her the thiopentone for me, will you". The pathologist did so—all 20 ml of a 2.5% solution, rapidly (he knew something about blood but, at that time, very litle about thiopentone). Cardiac arrest was immediate. The surgeon did a quick midline incision, incised the patient's diaphragm, massaged her heart and restarted it. She recovered completely.

ACHMAD (31) a capable and dedicated water engineer, developed appendicitis in a remote province. He was anaesthetized using intermittent thiopentone only, and died on the table.

HANS–JURGEN (85) was to have a very large inguinal hernia repaired. His history had not been taken properly, and he was not examined. Induction with thiopentone and ether by the assistant (who was drunk at the time) was stor-

my. He coughed and gagged because the percentage of ether he was given was raised too quickly. This was dealt with by injecting more and more 5% thiopentone, until he had been given a total of 1,500 mg. His heart stopped, and the doctor was called to resuscitate him—unsuccessfully. LESSONS (1) Give a patient only just enough thiopentone to get the effect you want. (2) When he coughs while being induced with ether, don't give him more thiopentone. Instead, reduce the concentration of ether and then slowly increase it. (3) The maximum dose of thiopentone for an unpremedicated 60 kg adult is about 500 mg. It is dangerous to exceed this dose. (4) Use thiopentone as a 2.5%, not 5% solution. (5) If induction is likely to be difficult, or your assistant unskilled, do it yourself. (6) If an important member of staff is unable to perform his duties, postpone the operation. (7) If you diagnose cardiac arrest promptly, you can usually treat it successfully. (8) Never use thiopentone alone for any operation lasting more than a minute or two, especially if it requires muscular relaxation.

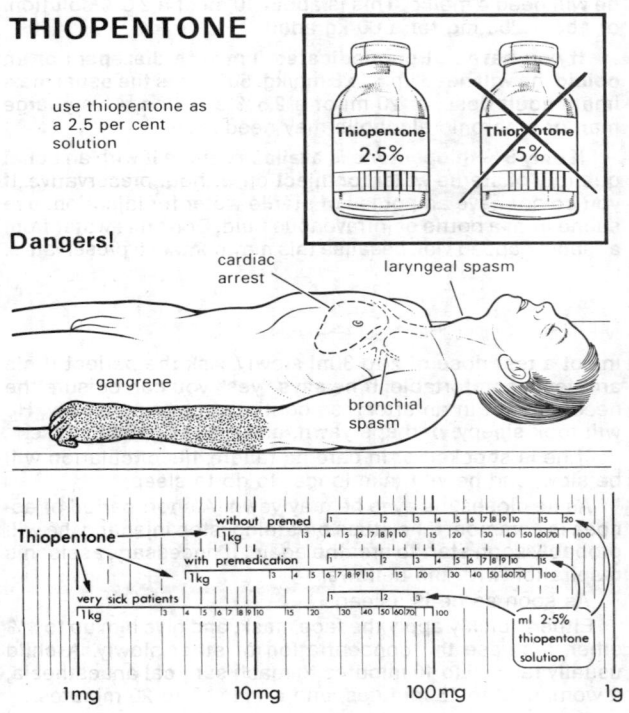

Fig. 12-1 THE EFFECTS OF THIOPENTONE. Use a 2.5% not a 5% solution, be aware of the dangers, especially respiratory depression, and adjust the dose to the needs of the patient.

THIOPENTONE INDUCTION, FOLLOWED BY ETHER FROM A VAPOURISER

INDICATIONS A fit patient with none of the contraindications listed below.

CONTRAINDICATIONS (1) Hypovolaemia, caused by haemorrhage or dehydration. You can use very small doses indeed, but ketamine is better, either for induction or as the total anaesthetic. (2) Upper airway obstruction, or any operation around the throat or neck that might precipitate laryngeal spasm. (3) Bronchial asthma. (4) Severe anaemia. (5) Barbiturate hypersensitivity, (6) Porphyria. (7) Inability to follow any of the "ten golden rules for safe anaesthesia" listed in Section 3.1.

ATROPINE Be sure to give the patient atropine. This is essential.

DOSE OF THIOPENTONE

CAUTION ! (1) Check the quantity of drug in the ampoule. Some ampoules contain 0.5 g and others 1 g. (2) Always use it as a 2.5% solution and check the solution for precipitate.

Give just enough thiopentone to send the patient to sleep and get the effect you want, as described below. This is better than giving a fixed dose. You will probably find that he will need doses in the following range:

If he is hypovolaemic or very sick, try to avoid using thiopentone. Instead, use ketamine or diazepam. If you have to use thiopentone, he will need 1 to 2 mg/kg. This is about 3 ml of a 2.5% solution for an adult. His circulation is slow, so he will take longer to go to sleep.

If you have premedicated him with diazepam or an opioid, he will need 4 mg/kg. This is about 10 ml of a 2.5% solution, or about 250 mg for a 60 kg adult.

If you have not premedicated him with diazepam or an opioid, he will need up to 6 to 8 mg/kg. 500 mg is the usual maximum adult dose, or 20 ml of a 2.5% solution. A very large man or a chronic alcoholic may need more.

If only 5% thiopentone is available, dilute it with an equal quantity of sterile water for injection without preservative. If you do not have ampoules of sterile water for injection, use saline from a bottle of intravenous fluid. Don't use water from a rubber capped vial, because this may contain a preservative.

METHOD OF USING THIOPENTONE

Inject a test dose of 2 to 3 ml slowly. Ask the patient if his arm feels comfortable. If he says "yes" you can be sure the needle is not in an artery, so continue injecting slowly. He will look sleepy, perhaps yawn, and his eylids will close.

If he is shocked or in cardiac failure, his circulation will be slow, and he will take longer to go to sleep.

As he closes his eyes he may yawn. A short period of apnoea is common. If he stops breathing, stop injecting; he will probably soon start to breathe again. If necessary, assist his respiration with the bellows.

As soon as he is asleep:

Either, quickly apply the face mask, and give him up to 4% ether. Increase the concentration of ether slowly. A child usually takes 5 to 10 minutes to reach surgical anaesthesia, a woman 10 to 15 minutes, and a man 15 to 20 minutes.

Or, give him suxamethonium and intubate him, as in Section 13.2. As soon as he is intubated you can give him ether, starting with a low concentration and quickly increasing to 15%. He will not cough or gag.

12.2 Dangers and disasters with thiopentone

"The patient stops breathing" A short period of apnoea is common, even if you have given thiopentone correctly. If you give the patient too much or if you give it too quickly, his breathing will stop, and perhaps his heart also, particularly if he is very sick. This really is a disaster, especially if you don't control his ventilation quickly and effectively, or you fail to restart his heart. So always give thiopentone slowly, and don't exceed the doses in Fig. 12-1.

If the patient stops breathing, the first thing to do is to inflate him with a bag and mask, and then, if apnoea is prolonged, to quickly intubate him, if you have not done so already.

"He feels an intense pain radiating down his arm" If the needle comes out of the vein and thiopentone goes into the tissues, little serious harm will be done. It will cause a painful haematoma and occasionally an ulcer. The particular danger with thiopentone is injecting it into an artery by mistake. So stop injecting if the patient feels pain—your needle may be in an artery. Don't take the needle out. The artery will go into spasm, and then it will be very difficult to put it back, in order to inject the sequence of drugs that may prevent gangrene.

INTRA-ARTERAL THIOPENTONE

PREVENTION Always take the following precautions.

(1) If possible, use veins on the back of the patient's hand or forearm. Even the vessels on the back of his hand are not completely safe, because his digital arteries may lie close to the surface.

(2) Feel the chosen vessel carefully to make sure it does not pulsate.

(3) Use 2.5% thiopentone, not the dangerous 5% solution.

(4) Don't inject a vessel on the medial side of the front of his elbow, because this is one of the more likely places for an aberrant artery.

(5) Always ask the patient if he feels pain down his arm as you start to inject. If he has severe pain, the needle is probably in an artery, and you have given him an intra-arterial injection. Keep the needle in. Stop injecting thiopentone, and proceed immediately with the regime below for an intra-arterial injection.

TREATMENT When the needle is still in the artery, inject 2,500 units of heparin into it. If there are no contraindications, continue with a normal regime of systemic heparin for the next 24 hours.

Continue the operation and the anaesthesia, preferably by inhalation.

Meanwhile inject chlorpromazine 25 mg into the artery. This is a good substitute for phentolamine in relieving spasm.

Then inject hydrocortisone 100 mg intra-arterially to reduce the local inflammation.

Finally, inject 3 ml of 2% procaine or lignocaine. This will also reduce the spasm.

Block the patient's stellate ganglion, or his brachial plexus (6.17).

If the needle has come out before you have given all the necessary drugs, and the patient has no radial pulse and his hand is cold, wrap his hand in a moist cloth to keep it cool. Refer him urgently for arterotomy, and thrombectomy.

13 Controlled ventilation and intubation

13.1 Controlled or intermittent positive pressure ventilation (IPPV)

This is one of the most useful procedures in anaesthesia: (1) You can ventilate a patient after you have deliberately paralysed him with a relaxant. (2) If his respiration should stop accidentally, you can keep him alive until it starts again. Controlled ventilation is also useful in many other situations, both in anaesthesia and in general medicine.

IPPV requires air or oxygen under pressure. This can come from a bag or bellows or a ventilator, but the most instantly available source is your own lungs; so, in an emergency, be prepared to use them, as described in Section 3.4. Even so, never anaesthetize anyone without having a bag or bellows available, in case his breathing does become inadequate or stop and you need to control it.

You can use a non–rebreathing valve, or a simple expiratory spill valve of the Heidbrinck type. As we saw in Section 10.1, controlling a patient's ventilation is much easier with a non–rebreathing valve, because you can change from spontaneous to controlled ventilation without adjusting the valve, and the mask can remain on the patient's face all the time.

You have first to blow air into the patient's lungs—inspiration. Then you have to allow air to escape spontaneously—expiration. Besides enabling the patient to ventilate his lungs, these movements also assist his circulation. During normal inspiration, the reduced pressure inside his thorax sucks air and blood into it, and so increases the venous return to his heart. When you control ventilation, with a bag or bellows, you force air into his lungs. This raises the pressure in his thorax and reduces the return of blood to his heart. Compensate for this *by keeping inspiration short and gentle, and allowing twice as long for expiration.* If you don't allow a patient enough time to exhale, the pressure in his thorax will become too high, and impede the return of blood to his heart. So watch his chest, or put a hand under the drapes, and *don't inflate his lungs until they have emptied.* Make sure his chest expands adequately during inspiration. Follow this rhythm with the bellows—DOWN—UP—PAUSE—DOWN—UP—PAUSE. DOWN blows up his lungs. UP during one second fills the bellows. PAUSE during 2 or 3 seconds gives him enough time to exhale.

Start the DOWN movement sharply, so that it moves leaflet "X" in Diagram T, Fig.10-2 across to block port "Y". If you fail to do this, you can empty the bellows through the expiratory valve without inflating a patient's lungs.

A healthy adult takes about 12 breaths a minute, each of about 500 ml. Simple anaesthetic systems have no flowmeter to measure the volume of air going through them, so you will have to judge this clinically. If you under–ventilate a patient seriously, he will become cyanosed. If you are giving him oxygen, he will accumulate carbon dioxide, which will cause tachycardia, hypertension and ectopic beats. Moderate over–ventilation is usually not harmful, but it may cause some fall in his blood pressure, and it can also quickly lead to regurgitation. A chest that is moving well is usually being ventilated adequately.

Don't make the mistake of ventilating a patient too rapidly. *Twelve to 16 breaths a minute of adequate volume are usually enough.* Controlled ventilation can continue for weeks if it is done properly. Moving a bellows is easier if you rest your elbow on the trolley, and pronate and supinate your forearm, as in Fig. 13-2.

BIG SLOW BREATHS ARE BETTER THAN SHORT FAST ONES

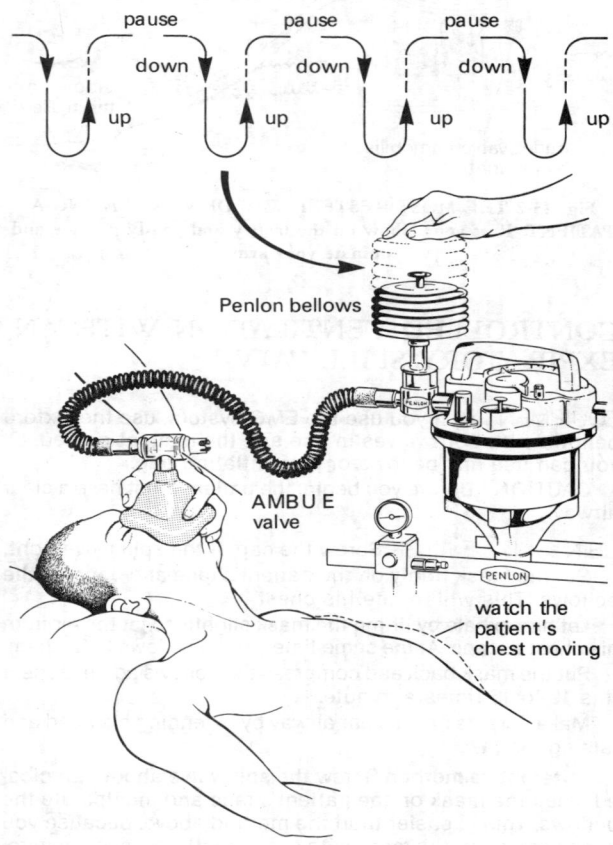

Fig. 13-1 CONTROLLED VENTILATION WITH THE PENLON BELLOWS AND THE AMBU E VALVE. When you push the bellows down you inflate the patient. Be sure to pause at the top of the stroke so that he has enough time to exhale.

Remember that whenever you control a patient's respiration, there must be: (1) A clear airway from the bellows to his lungs. (2) An airtight seal between the mask, if you are using one, and his face. If you try to ventilate him forcibly when his airway is obstructed, you will blow up his stomach with air. A mask is not ideal, he may regurgitate suddenly and inhale his stomach contents as he does so. Prevent this by passing a *cuffed* tracheal tube. If controlled ventilation is prolonged, always pass one. In an adult, controlled ventilation is not satisfactory with a non–cuffed one. A child is different, because if you choose the right size of tube, you can make a non–cuffed one seal itself into his trachea. Or, safer, you can allow a small leak and still be able to ventilate him enough.

Controlled ventilation with a simple expiratory spill valve. Although you can do this, it is much less convenient than ventilating with a non–rebreathing valve. You can do it in two ways. (1) You can lift the mask off the patient's face, or your finger from the tracheal connector, each time you want him to exhale. For this you will need to use both hands, one for the mask and one for the bellows. (2) You can set the valve partly closed to let him expire and use a high minute volume. Like this, you only need one hand.

THE MOST RESTFUL WAY OF VENTILATING A PATIENT

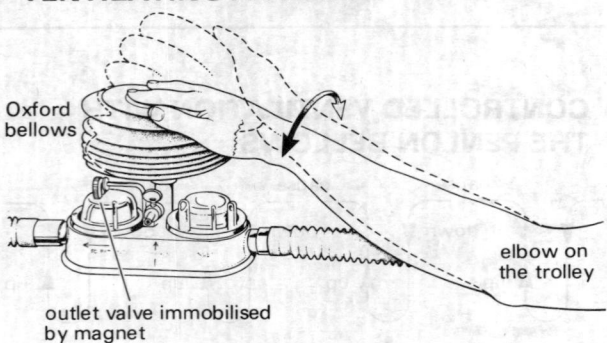

Fig. 13-2 THE MOST RESTFUL WAY OF VENTILATING A PATIENT. Rest your elbow on the trolley and gently pronate and supinate your arm.

CONTROLLED VENTILATION WITH AN EXPIRATORY SPILL VALVE

EQUIPMENT (1) If you use the EMO system, use the Oxford bellows with both valves in use and the magnet parked. (2) You can use any bellows or self-inflating bag.

CAUTION ! Before you begin, the patient must have a clear airway.

USING A FACE MASK Screw the cap of the spill valve tight.

Put the mask firmly on the patient's face and depress the bellows. This will inflate his chest.

Let him exhale by lifting the mask slightly to let the air from his chest escape. At the same time, lift the bellows to fill them.

Put the mask back and compress the bellows again. Repeat this 12 to 16 times a minute.

Make sure he has a clear airway by extending his head and raising his jaw.

Alternative method Screw the spill valve about half closed, keep the mask on the patient's face and manipulate the bellows. This is easier than the method above, because you don't need to lift the mask with each breath, but each inspiration contains a higher proportion of expired air (rebreathing). This is a useful for preoxygenation, but it is not suitable for longer term ventilation.

USING A TRACHEAL TUBE Remove the cap of the tracheal connector. Close it with your finger each time you inflate him. Then remove your finger and let him exhale.

GIVE HIM TIME TO EXHALE
START INSPIRATION SHARPLY
KEEP HIS AIRWAY CLEAR
DON'T VENTILATE TOO FAST

CONTROLLED VENTILATION

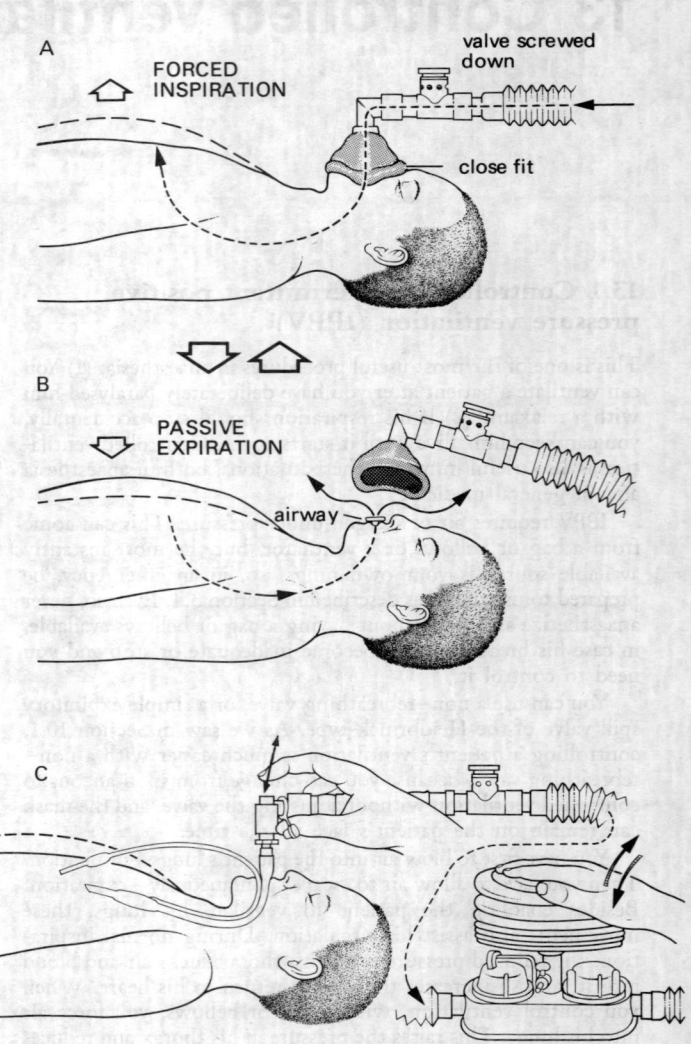

Fig. 13-3 CONTROLLED VENTILATION WITH AN EXPIRATORY SPILL— VALVE. Screw the valve down, inflate him, and then lift the mask off his face to let him exhale.

13.2 Tracheal intubation

Putting a tube through a patient's larynx into his trachea is the best way of making sure that air reaches his lungs and that foreign materials do not. It is one of the most useful anaesthetic skills, and is essential for safe and reliable anaesthesia. The more difficult the circumstances, and the less help you have, the more important it is for you to be able to intubate a patient immediately after you have induced him intravenously. One of the few disadvantages of passing a tracheal tube is that it may make his patient's throat sore for a few days afterwards, but this is a small price to pay for such a great increase in safety.

Intubation, with controlled ventilation if necessary, is invaluable on many occasions: (1) It is the best protection against the dangers of a full stomach, and it is often impossible to be sure that a patient's stomach is not full. (2) It is the best way of preventing his airway being obstructed by his tongue, or by blood and secretions from his upper respiratory tract. A tracheal tube is essential if a patient needs an operation on his nose, teeth, or jaws, and it minimises the danger of his inhaling blood, pus or teeth. (3) Intubation is essential if a patient's intestine is obstructed, or if a mother is being given a general anaesthetic for Caesarean section. (4) It is particularly useful if you are giving ether, because it makes induction easier and prevents ether dissolving in a patient's saliva and causing post–operative vomiting. (5) It is life–saving if paralysis spreads too high in subarachnoid or epidural anaesthesia. (6) It is an effective way of minimising the dead space between a patient's alveoli and a non–rebreathing valve. (7) It is the safest way of controlling ventilation after you have given a patient a muscle relaxant. (8) It allows you to operate on him in any position, even face downwards if necessary, as in Fig. 16-8. (9) It keeps the anaesthetic apparatus away from the operation site when you are operating on his head, eyes, or thyroid. (10) It can maintain his airway in spite of almost any anatomical deformity. (11) If you have to induce a patient yourself and then operate, intubation will help to safeguard his airway regardless of the skill of your anaesthetic assistant. (13) If a patient has oedema of his glottis, intubation is safer than an immediate tracheostomy. (12) Intubation is essential when prolonged respiratory failure requires control of a patient's ventilation. (13) It is useful in coma (S 63.1), in cardio–respiratory arrest, and in cases where the patient needs extensive bronchial toilet, in head injuries and in severe chest injuries (S 65.1)

INTRODUCING THE LARYNGOSCOPE

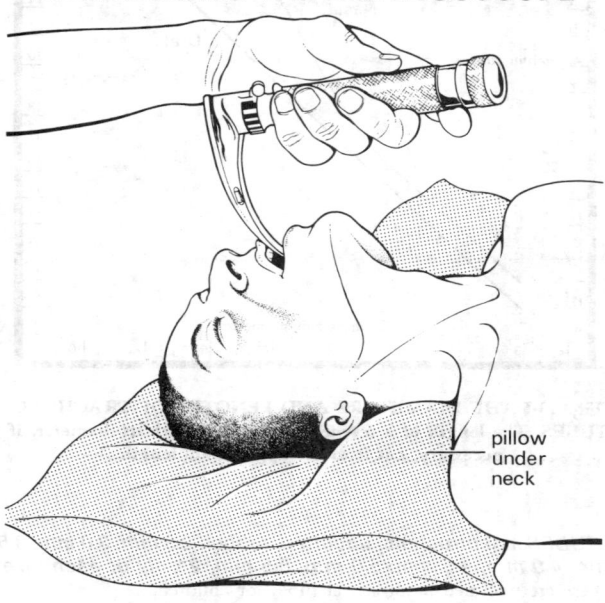

Fig. 13-4 INTRODUCING A LARYNGOSCOPE. *Kindly contributed by John Farman.*

Because intubation makes a general anaesthetic so much safer, some anaesthetists instruct their assistants to intubate every patient who undergoes general anaesthesia.

Before you can intubate a patient, his jaw muscles should, if possible, be relaxed and his laryngeal reflexes abolished. You can achieve this by:

(1) Deep general anaesthesia, for example, with ether. *Don't try to intubate a patient under trichloroethylene, thiopentone, ketamine, or diazepam alone.* They will not relax his jaw and his cords sufficiently, and trying to pass the tube will cause severe laryngeal spasm.

(2) Light general or dissociative anaesthesia, such as ketamine, combined with a short–acting relaxant, such as suxamethonium.

(3) Local anaesthesia, such as 4% lignocaine sprayed onto the larynx and down the trachea.

(4) If a patient is unconscious or semiconscious because of cardiac arrest or a head injury, you may be able to take advantage of his condition and pass a tracheal tube without any anaesthesia, or only a little lignocaine over the back of his tongue.

"Awake intubation" is described in Section S 52.1. Unfortunately, intubation is sometimes impractical if a patient has a maxillofacial injury (S 62.1).

Don't try to intubate a patient under long–acting relaxants, such as alcuronium. Relaxation takes longer to become established after these agents, and may not be complete enough. You will take too long to see his vocal cords, and to pass a tube through them. If you are not quick enough, he may die while you are trying to intubate him. Only expert anaesthetists should attempt intubation under long–acting relaxants.

DON'T TRY TO INTUBATE UNDER LONG–ACTING RELAXANTS

You will need some equipment to join a tracheal tube to the anaesthetic system.

Firstly, a tracheal *adaptor* has to fit into the tube. Tracheal tubes range in size from 1.5 mm to 10 mm, so you will need a set of adaptors of different sizes, all with 15 mm male cones. The male cone of these adaptors fits into the female cone of a non–rebreathing valve. Because this would bring the valve inconveniently close to a patient's mouth, it is easier to join the adaptor to a *connector*, the connector to a *catheter mount*, and the catheter mount to the non– rebreathing valve.

A connector bends the flow of gases coming out of the patient's mouth about 90°. At one end it has a 22 mm male cone combined with a 15 mm female cone. This enables it to fit a face mask, or a tracheal adaptor. At the other end it has a 15 mm male cone that fits into the corresponding female cone of the catheter mount.

A catheter mount is a 9 cm rubber tube. At one end it has 15 mm female cone that enables it to fit the connector. At the other end it has a 22 mm female cone, which fixes onto the non–rebreathing valve. A catheter mount enables you to take this valve away from the patient's mouth to a more convenient place at the side of his face.

Children are different A tracheal adaptor should always fit straight into a paediatric non–rebreathing valve such as an AMBU "Paedivalve", without using a connector or a catheter mount. Either of these, and particularly a catheter mount, will increase the dead space dangerously in a small child. This is the space between a child's alveoli (where respiratory exchange takes place) and the external air. The larger this dead space is in relation to his tidal volume (the volume of air moving in and out at each breath), the less efficient will his breathing be.

Some of the alternative equipment you may meet is shown in Fig. 13-5. Some connectors swivel and others have a suction port, through which you can suck out a tracheal tube.

Here are more details of the equipment you will need.

• *LARYNGOSCOPE HANDLE, large, American hook–on fitting, to take D type cells (also called U2 or R20) and No. 8 ANC threads, 2 only.* This is shown in Fig.13-4, and takes the larger and more commonly available D cells. With a hook–on fitting there is no screw pin on the handle to get lost. A spare laryngoscope handle is essential. When you use one hold it in your left hand with the handle uppermost.

• *BLADE, Laryngoscope, Macintosh, large and extra large, hook–on fitting, to take the standard bulb, one only of each size.* An extra large blade, rather than the standard one, which is not included in this list, is particularly important in countries, such as parts of East Africa, where some people are very tall and have long necks. The tip of the blade goes in the vallecula between the base of a patient's tongue and his epiglottis. The side of the blade pushes his tongue to the left. Make sure you at least wash the blade before using it on someone else.

• *BLADE, laryngoscope, Seward or Robertshaw, child, hook–on fitting, to take the standard bulb, one only.* The blade on a child's laryngoscope should be straight. A Macintosh children's blade is much too deep.

97

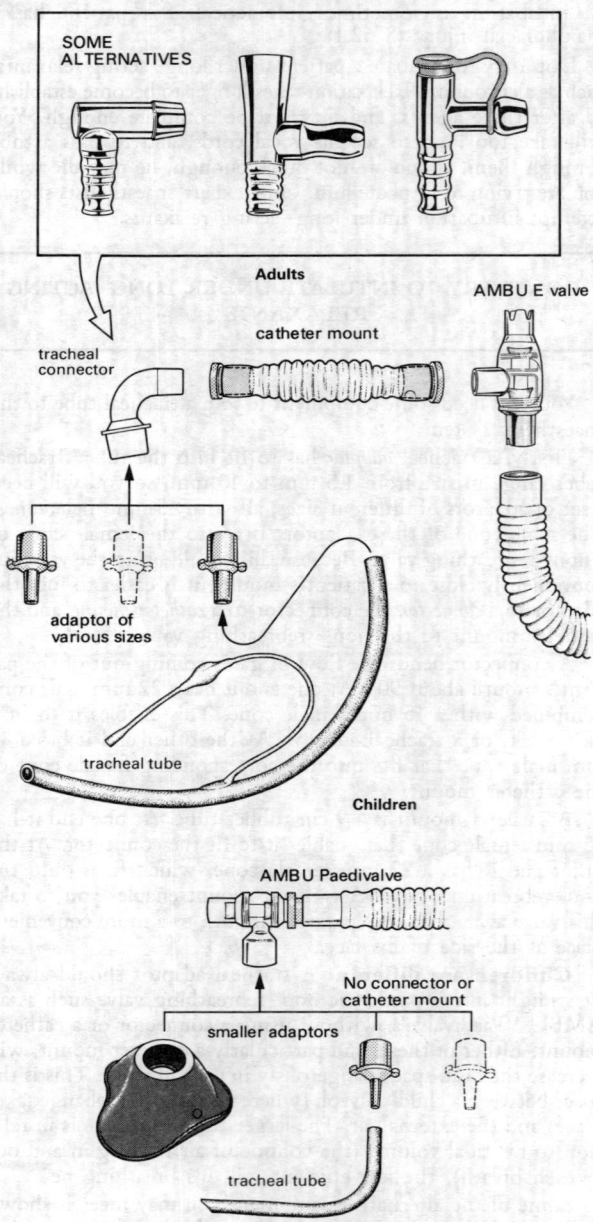

Fig. 13-5 FITTINGS FOR TRACHEAL TUBES. You will need a set of adaptors to fit various sizes of tracheal tube. The adaptor fits into a connector, and the connector fits onto a catheter mount, which fits onto a non-rebreathing valve. *Kindly contributed by John Farman.*

- BULB, spare, for laryngoscope, 3 volt, No. 8 ANC thread, *six only*. Alas, there is as yet no agreement about which bulb should become the standard one.
- TUBES, orotracheal, with cuff, Magill, red rubber, (a) 7mm, 5 only, (b) 8 mm, 10 only, (c) 9 mm, 10 only, (d) 10 mm, 5 only. These are the standard Magill cuffed tracheal tubes for older patients with a trachea larger than 7 mm. They have a cuff that you can blow up to seal the tube in the trachea, a pilot tube for inflating the cuff, and a balloon to show the cuff is inflated. You can boil and reuse them many times.

Test all cuffed tubes before you use them: (1) Make sure they don't leak. (2) Exclude an excessive bulge in any part of the cuff, which may cause undue pressure on the mucosa. (3) Look down them to make sure they are not blocked.

Magill tracheal tubes are always sold uncut, so cut them to the lengths shown in Fig. 13-6. If they are too long, they will kink. The best length allows the adaptor to lie between the patient's teeth, or, if it is a nasotracheal tube, in his nose.

- TUBES, orotracheal, plain without cuffs, Oxford non-kink, (a) 3 mm, 3 only, (b) 3.5 mm, 3 only, (c) 4 mm, 3 only, (d) 4.5 mm, 3 only, (e) 5 mm, 3 only, (f) 5.5 mm, 3 only, (g) 6 mm, 5 only. These are smaller tracheal tubes for children whose tracheas are not large enough for a cuff. Below the age of 10 the narrowest part of a child's respiratory tract is his cricoid ring, just below his larynx. If you choose a tube of the right size it will seal itself here, without the need for a cuff. "Non-kink" is a relative term, and any rubber tube that is not reinforced can kink.
- TUBES, nasotracheal, cuffed, rubber, 6 mm, 7 mm, 8 mm, and 9 mm, 6 only of each size. Pass these cuffed tubes through a patient's nose into his trachea. They are firm enough to maintain their curve, but not hard. They have a sharper bevel than oral tubes.

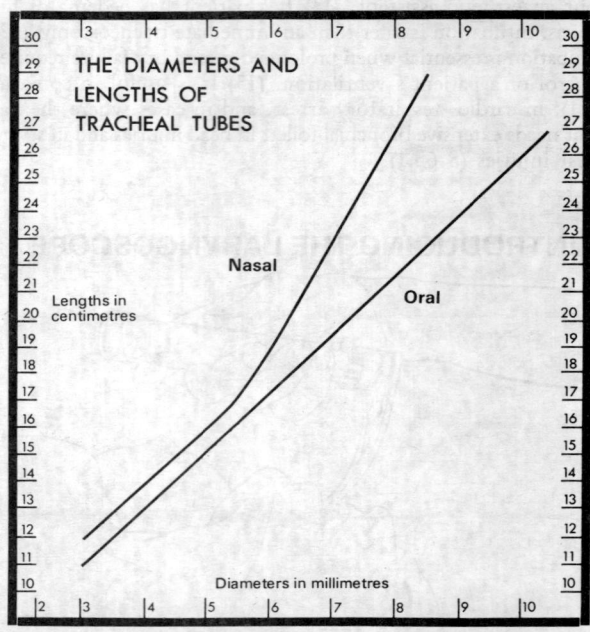

Fig. 13-6 THE DIAMETERS AND LENGTHS OF TRACHEAL TUBES. The length of a tracheal tube varies with its diameter. If necessary, cut it to the appropriate length.

- TUBES, nasotracheal, uncuffed, rubber, 2.5 mm, 3.0 mm, 3.5 mm, 4.0 mm, 4.5 mm, 5.0 mm, 5.5 mm, 2 only of each size. These are uncuffed nasotracheal tubes for children.
- ADAPTORS, tracheal, plastic, 3 mm to 10 mm, with 15 mm male cone fitting, 2 sets only. Tracheal tubes have to be fitted to something; This is a set of plastic adaptors with standard 15 mm ISO cones. There is one adaptor for each size of tube. Alternatively, you can order tracheal tubes with their adaptors already fitted.
- CONNECTOR, tracheal, angled, 15 mm female at one end combined with 22 mm male cone at the other end. This connector joins the adaptor to the catheter mount. The 22 mm male adaptor will also fit a facemask. When you want to suck out a tracheal tube, just disconnect the adaptor.
- CATHETER MOUNT, connecting tube, 9 mm, with 15 cm female cone and 22 mm female cone, plain, anti-static, one only. This is a short length of rubber tube to connect an adaptor to a non-rebreathing valve in an adult only.
- INTRODUCER, for adult tracheal tubes, malleable plastic, Portex type, two only. If you have difficulty passing a tracheal tube, put this introducer inside the tube and bend it to the shape you want. An introducer will often make a seemingly impossible intubation easy. Gum elastic bougies soften in the tropics, so plastic ones are better. If you use a metal introducer, its tip must not protrude beyond the end of the tracheal tube, or it may injure the mucosa of the larynx. If necessary, you can use any suitably shaped malleable rod.
- INTRODUCER, for infant and child tracheal tubes, chrome, two only.
- FORCEPS, anaesthetic, Magill, adult size, one only.

- *FORCEPS, anaesthetic, Magill, child size, one only.* Use these for difficult intubations, for packing the pharynx when there is likely to be bleeding, and for passing nasotracheal tubes under direct vision. You will need a small pair if you are going to intubate children.
- *CATHETERS, Tracheal, suction, plastic, 8 Ch, 12 Ch, 20 Ch, 10 only of each size.* Pass these catheters down a tracheal tube: (1) to make sure it is open and not kinked or blocked, and (2) to suck secretions out of the trachea. Suction catheters are essential. You can also use the larger ones to suck out a patient's pharynx. The outside diameter of the suction catheter should not be more than half the inner diameter of the tracheal tube. Sterilise suction catheters between patients. You can if necessary use a urethral catheter, or a child's feeding tube, or the tubing from an old drip set.
- *BRUSHES, for cleaning tracheal tubes, small, medium and large six of each size.*
- *SPRAY, Macintosh, oral, with malleable rubber covered tube, one only.* Use this to spray 4% lignocaine onto the larynx when you pass a tracheal tube under local anaesthesia.

DONT INTUBATE UNLESS YOU HAVE SUCTION CATHETERS

HOW TO USE A LARYNGOSCOPE

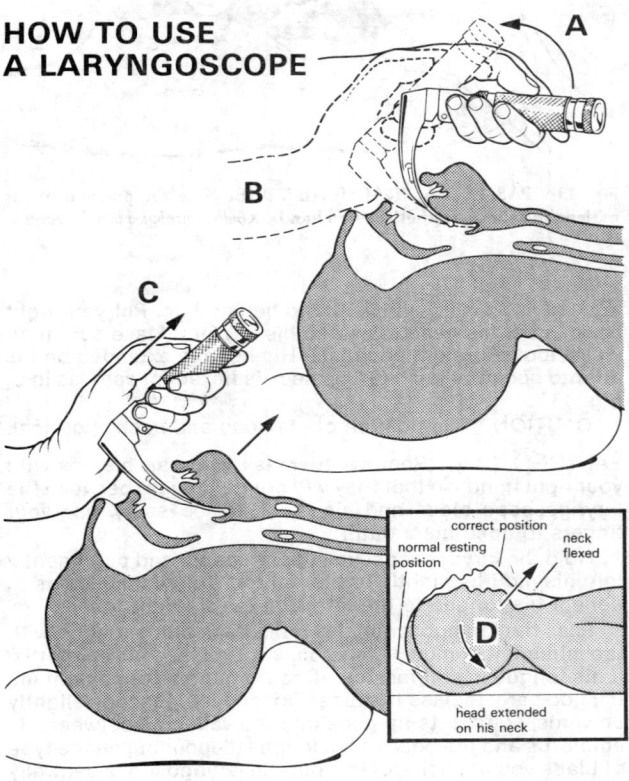

Fig. 13-7 HOW TO USE A LARYNGOSCOPE. A, insert the laryngoscope with your wrist straight, then extend your wrist. (B). Finally, lift the patient's jaw forwards (C). The secret of success is to have the patient's head extended on his neck before you begin (D) and to have his neck flexed forwards (E). Arrange the pillow under his neck and shoulders so that you can achieve this. This has been likened to the position of "sniffing the morning air". *Kindly contributed by Nigel Pereira.*

13.3 How to intubate

You will learn how to intubate more easily by practising it under the supervision of an expert than from reading books. Take every opportunity to let a skilled anaesthetist show you how to do it. The best time to start learning is at the end of a long operation, when a patient is deeply anaesthetized. When you can do this easily, try to intubate earlier and earlier. Don't try to intubate under relaxants until you can intubate confidently under ether. Intubation under relaxants is a useful skill, because it shortens the time needed for induction, and enables you to intubate a patient within 5 minutes of starting the anaesthetic.

Death from anoxia is the great danger! If there is only air in a patient's lungs, you have one minute only in which to intubate him. If his lungs are full of pure oxygen, you have longer, at most two minutes in a fit patient and less in one with anaemia or heart disease. So *always* preoxygenate a patient first (9.3). If you fail to pass the tube the first time, give him more oxygen before trying again. Be safe and give him two more breaths of oxygen when he has not had any for one minute. Ask an assistant to keep a hand on his pulse while you do so, and to warn you if it slows, or becomes feeble.

There are some other difficulties. One, which even expert anaesthetists often cannot avoid, is to pass the tube into the patient's oesophagus. You can also pass it so far down that it reaches one of his bronchi. Another danger is injuring his teeth.

If you fail to intubate a patient, you are in trouble and we give you a "failed intubation drill" later. Failure to intubate nearly always occurs just when you least want it to happen—in emergencies, during Caesarean sections, in patients with full stomachs, and when you have no help. Expect it in the "goofy" type of cartoon character with a receding jaw and prominent upper teeth, and also in a patient with a small mouth, disease of his temporomandibular joints or his cervical spine. Anticipating the problem often solves it. Preoxygenate the patient, give him a small dose of suxamethonium, and apply cricoid pressure. Or, if a full stomach is not a problem, induce him with ether or halothane, and then do a laryngoscopy after spraying with lignocaine blind.

THE SAFE PERIOD OF APNOEA WITHOUT EXTRA OXYGEN IS ONLY ONE MINUTE

LARYNGOSCOPY

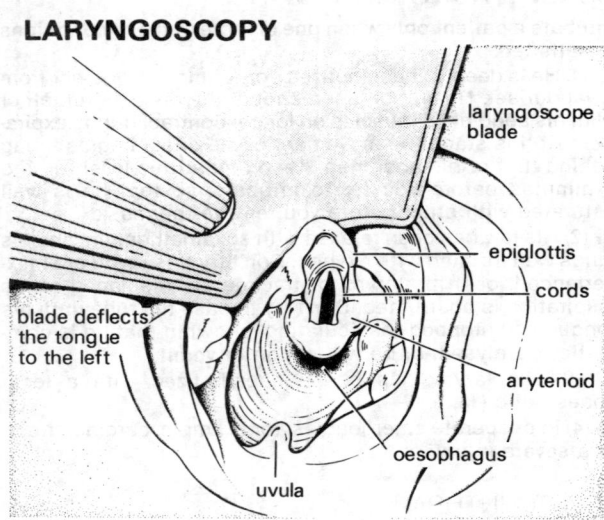

Fig. 13-8 A VIEW OF THE LARYNX. The blade of the laryngoscope is anterior to the patient's epiglottis. The blade has deflected the tongue to the left. *Kindly contributed by John Farman*

INTUBATION DURING ANAESTHESIA

INDICATIONS These are further discussed in Section 13.2, and include: (1) The patient with a full stomach (16.1). (2) To make controlling a patient's ventilation easier after you have given him a relaxant. (3) Caesarean section (16.6). (4) Intestinal obstruction. (5) Operations on the mouth and nose. (6) A patient who has to be turned into some unusual position. (7) As a means of minimising postoperative nausea and vomiting in patients who are being given ether. (8) Spinal anaesthesia that has ascended too high. (9) Patients with severe head and chest injuries who have difficulty maintaining their airways.

(10) Intrathoracic operations. (11) Some anaesthetists intubate almost all patients receiving a general anaesthetic.

WHEN TO EXPECT DIFFICULTY If you are inexperienced, you would be wise not to try to intubate patients with: (1) very receeding jaws, (2) maxillofacial injuries, (3) tumours of the jaw.

EQUIPMENT A laryngoscope, with detachable blades for adults, infants, and children. A set of tracheal tubes, an introducer, a 10 ml syringe to inflate the cuff, a pair of artery forceps to clamp the pilot tube, tape to fix the tracheal tube in place, a set of tracheal adaptors, a tracheal connecter, a catheter mount, Magill's tracheal forceps, a mouth gag, oropharyngeal airways, a syringe with a plastic tube attached to it to act as a spray, 4% lignocaine, and suction catheters in appropriate sizes.

Check all the equipment before starting. Make sure that the light on the laryngoscope is bright and steady.

CHOOSING THE RIGHT TUBE AND CHECKING IT An adult man will take a 9 or 10 mm tube, an adult woman will take a 9 mm tube, but sometimes only an 8 mm or 7 mm one. Use the largest size that will pass easily through the larynx. A tube that is too small makes breathing difficult, especially in children. The right tube for a child is about the size of his little finger.

Have one or two extra sizes smaller and larger than the size you think you will use. Oxford tubes are supplied ready cut; shorten Magill tubes as in Fig. 13-6.

Fit the largest adaptor that will go into the tube. It must stretch the tube, otherwise it will slip out. If it won't slide into the tube easily, wet it with spirit or water.

Hold the tube straight, hold it up to the light and look through it to make sure that there are no cockroaches or other foreign bodies inside it.

Blow up the cuff with a syringe. If it does not expand evenly, or herniates over the end of the tube, choose another tube.

CONDITIONS FOR INTUBATION

Intubate a patient only when one or more of these conditions is satisfied:

(1) He is deeply anaesthetized, for example with ether from a vapouriser. He will be deep enough if you give him ether until his abdominal muscles no longer contract during expiration. At this stage the movement of his chest begins to lag behind that of his abdomen. Keep him at this level for 2 to 3 minutes before you try to intubate, so that he is well saturated with ether before you remove the mask.

(2) His jaw has been relaxed with suxamethonium, and his lungs well inflated with oxygen. Don't try this if you are inexperienced, or if his larynx or trachea are displaced or his respiration is obstructed. Don't try to pass the tube until his tongue has stopped fasciculating, showing that he is completley paralysed, or he will cough or vomit.

(3) His larynx has been anaesthetized with a local anaesthetic (13.5).

(4) In desperate emergencies, for example, cardiac arrest, or a severe injury.

HOW TO INTUBATE

Start by checking the patient's teeth. Remove any dentures, and avoid any loose teeth. You must account for any missing ones.

If he has a nasogastric tube, aspirate it, leave it in place, and intubate using cricoid pressure (16.5).

Lubricate the tip of the laryngoscope blade and the end of the tracheal tube with water or jelly.

Place a large pillow under his neck and shoulders, and ventilate him with oxygen.

You have 20 or 30 seconds in which to intubate him. You cannot be looking at your watch to measure the time. So it is a good rule to hold your own breath while you intubate. If you become distessed from too much carbon dioxide, or too little oxygen, he will too, so ventilate him with oxygen for a minute or two before you try again.

PREOXYGENATION Let him breathe pure oxygen through the mask for 2 or 3 minutes (9.3).

PASSING A TRACHEAL TUBE

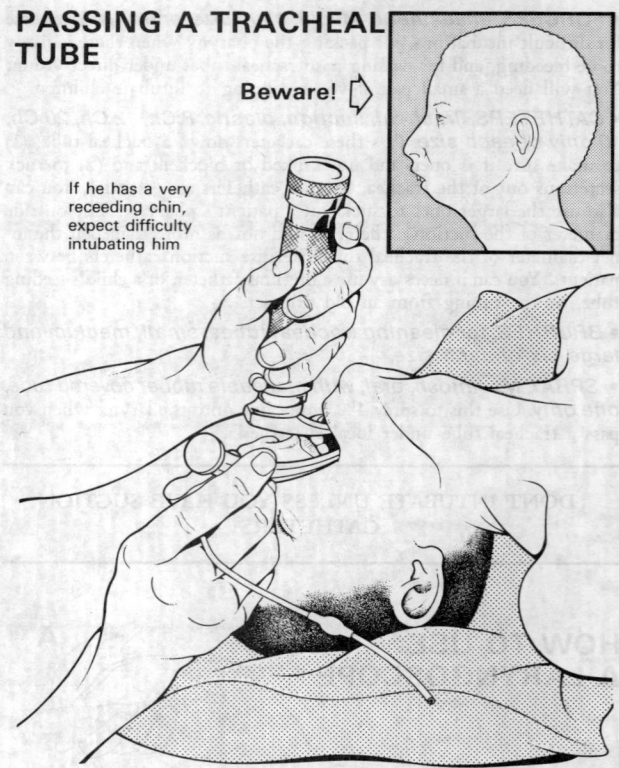

Beware!

If he has a very receeding chin, expect difficulty intubating him

Fig. 13-9 PASSING A TRACHEAL TUBE. Note the position of the patient and the anaesthetist's two hands. *Kindly contributed by John Farman.*

POSITION OF HIS NECK Stand behind him. Put your right hand under his head to extend his occiput. Make sure that: (1) He looks straight ahead. (2) His head is extended on his atlanto-occipital joint. (3) His neck is flexed forward, as in C, Fig. 13-7.

CAUTION ! The postion of his head and neck is critical.

LARYNGOSCOPY Remove the mask, and part his lips with your right hand, so that they will not get caught between the laryngoscope blade and his teeth. If necessary, use your fingers to open his mouth.

Hold the laryngoscope in your left hand, and put it gently into his mouth, slightly to the right of the midline, so as to deflect his tongue to the left. Aim for his right tonsil.

Pass the laryngoscope down the back of his tongue with the minimum of muscle tension, until you see his epiglottis. If his tongue is still fasciculating from the suxamethonium, it is too early to pass the tube. Tip the laryngoscope slightly upwards, so that its tip goes into the vallecula between his epiglottis and the base of his tongue (depending on the type of blade you are using). Now put the laryngoscope centrally in his mouth. Then *pull along the line of the handle,* so as to lift his tongue and his epiglottis out of the line of vision, so that you can see his larynx.

CAUTION ! Take care not to damage any of the patient's soft tissues. Treat his teeth gently, don't use them as a fulcrum, and don't dislodge them. You usually need very little force, if you pull in the right direction. But you may need considerable force; if you pull in the line of the handle, and away from his teeth, this is safe.

Provided there are no contraindications, spray 3 ml of 4% lignocaine onto his cords (13.5). This is the dose for an adult, reduce it proportionately in children.

PASSING THE TUBE If the patient's cords are relaxed and not moving, so that his glottis is open, pass the tube between them. Pass it from the right side, level with his premolar teeth. Don't pass it centrally, because this will prevent you seeing his cords. Make sure that the upper end of the cuff goes beyond his cords. This is the best guide as to how long the tube should be.

If you cannot see the patient's cords, ask an assistant to press gently on his larynx.

If there is a loud noise, his cords have closed and gone into spasm. Don't try to intubate between closed cords. Instead, quickly laryngoscope him, and if there are any secretions in his throat, suck them out. But don't push the sucker into his cords, because this will make his spasm worse.

Replace the mask and give oxygen. Eventually, the spasm will stop. As it does so, quickly pass the tube. Don't try to screw it in!

If you fail to pass the tube, give the patient several breaths of oxygen before you try again. This is especially important if you have to give him another dose of suxamethonium, or if you have paralysed him with a long acting relaxant.

SECURING THE TUBE When the tube is in position in his trachea, gently remove the laryngoscope, and insert an oral airway. Its metal end will act as a mouth prop, and stop him biting the tracheal tube and blocking it.

Use a piece of 5 cm ribbon gauze (or a piece of bandage) to tie the tube in place. Take a half hitch round the tube, pull it tight and tie it behind his neck. If you don't, the weight of the non-rebreathing valve and the corrugated tubing may pull it out of place. Do not release your grip from the tracheal tube until it is firmly secured.

Connect the adaptor, the connecter, the catheter mount, the non-rebreathing valve and the vapouriser. Give him oxygen. If he does not breathe, or if holds his breath, inflate his lungs from the bag or bellows. If you have no bellows, blow down the tube.

CAUTION! If you don't tie the tube in, it can easily slip out.

INFLATING THE CUFF Fix a 10 ml syringe to the end of the cuff tubing. At the same time blow air into the patient's lungs with the bellows or bag. You will hear air bubbling out between the tracheal tube and the wall of his trachea. Blow air into the cuff with the syringe until you can no longer hear or feel this bubbling. Two to 5 ml are usually enough. Clip the cuff tubing with a haemostat.

Listen to both his lungs to make sure that air is entering equally on both sides, and the tube has *not* passed into his right main bronchus. If the air entry is diminished on either side, pull the tube out 1 cm and listen again.

OTHER PROCEDURES FOR INTUBATION

INTUBATING WHILE GIVING OPEN ETHER Intubation improves the efficiency of open ether. You can pass a tube as soon as the patient is sufficiently anaesthetized. Remember to secure the tube under the mask, or it may disappear down his mouth!

OPERATIONS ON A PATIENT'S NOSE, MOUTH OR THROAT After joining up the adaptor to the catheter mount, use a laryngoscope and Magill's forceps to pack a length of ribbon gauze soaked in saline (not liquid paraffin) loosely round the tracheal tube. Preferably, don't use a piece of bandage, because this has loose threads.

CAUTION! Remember to remove the pack before pulling out the tube!

MAKING SURE A TRACHEAL TUBE IS PATENT Detach the adaptor from the connecter, and quickly pass a suction catheter down it. If it goes down freely, the tube is patent, if it meets resistance, it is blocked or kinked.

SUCTION THROUGH A TRACHEAL TUBE Preoxygenate the patient. Use a *sterile* catheter less than half the internal diameter of the tracheal tube, and suck him out as in Fig. 13-10. Don't use a catheter that is too large, or you will collapse the lung and make him hypoxic.

SUCKING OUT A TRACHEAL TUBE

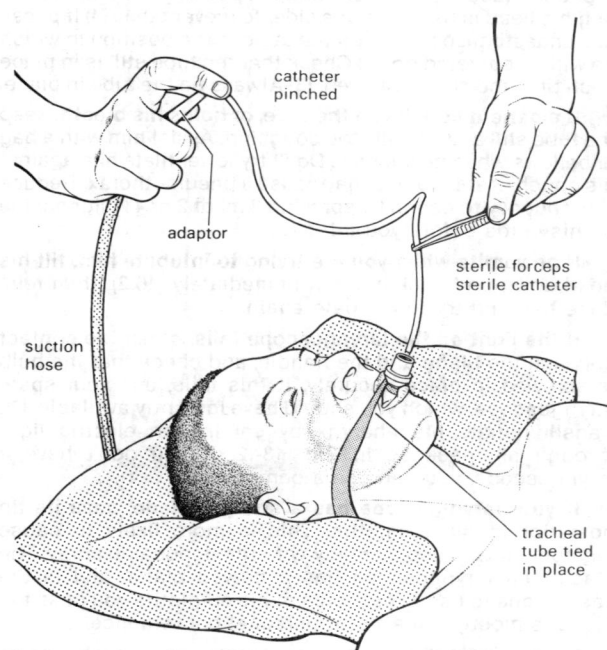

Fig. 13-10 SUCKING SECRETIONS FROM A TRACHEAL TUBE. First, preoxygenate the patient. (1) Attach the catheter to the suction tube without contaminating the patient's end. (2) Pinch the catheter before turning on the suction. (3) Pick up the catheter with sterile forceps or gloves, as shown here. (4) Pass the catheter down the tracheal tube to the carina. (5) Unpinch the catheter and put the forceps back in the sterile holder. (6) Withdraw the catheter through the tracheal tube, rotating it and twisting it in your fingers as you do so. (7) Place the catheter in a disposal container *Kindly contributed by John Farman.*

USING AN INTRODUCER

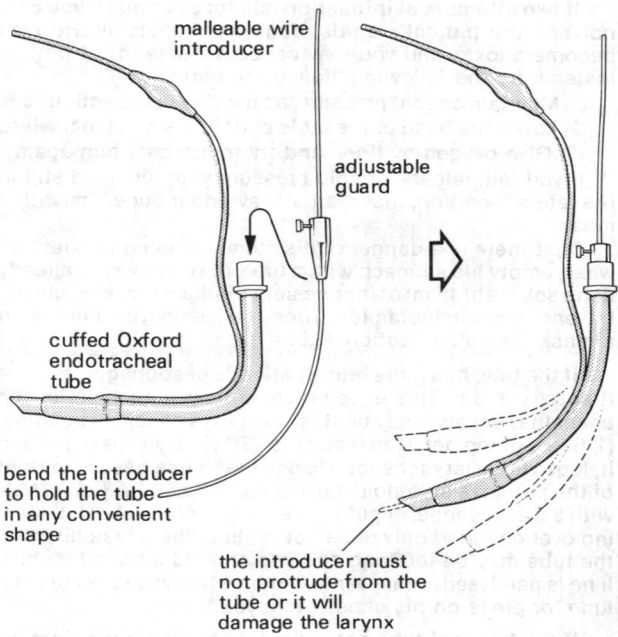

Fig. 13-11 USING AN INTRODUCER. If a tracheal tube has an inconvenient shape, you may be able to improve it by passing an introducer down it and bending this to the shape you want. A "hockey stick" shape is usually best. A plastic introducer is better and can project beyond the end of the tube. *Kindly contributed by John Farman.*

EXTUBATING A PATIENT

Do this while the patient is still lightly anaesthetized.

If you can hear secretions in the tube, or his trachea, first pass a suction catheter down inside the tube. Rotate it from side to side and suck as you remove it.

CAUTION ! Examine his larynx with a laryngoscope before you remove the tube. Under direct vision suck out any secretions which have collected around it. If you forget to do this, they will be inhaled immediately you remove the tube.

Give the patient extra oxygen for 2 or 3 minutes. Make sure he has an oral airway in position. Then, deflate the cuff and gently remove the tube.

If he holds his breath, or laryngeal spasm develops, lift his jaw, and give oxygen under a face mask, until he settles.

If he is likely to bleed from his mouth, don't remove the tube until he is lying on his side in the recovery position and preferably until he is conscious (4-5). This will allow blood to drain from his mouth.

CLEANING THE EQUIPMENT AFTERWARDS Wash the tracheal tubes and catheter mount after extubation and soak them in cetrimide or chlorhexidine. Scrub the laryngoscope blade in this solution. Rinse them and dry them in a towel. Although boiling the tracheal tube and catheter mount is better, it shortens their life.

DIFFICULTIES WITH INTUBATION

If you have no cuffed tubes, pack a gauze tape soaked in saline round a plain tube. Don't use paraffin or vaseline because it may be inhaled and cause a lipoid pnuemonitis.

If his anatomy makes intubation difficult, use an introducer to increase the curvature of the tube. Wet the introducer well, so that you can withdraw it easily. If it is metal, it must not project beyond the end of the tube. If it is plastic, let it protrude 4 cm. Slide the tube with the introducer inside it close behind the epigottis.

Intubation can be difficult if the patient has a short neck, a receeding jaw, or large upper teeth. If you can see his cords easily, you can usually pass a tube, provided it is well curved, and not too large.

If two attempts at intubation fail, for example, if you cannot see the patient's cords, don't try repeatedly. He may become anoxic, and you may cause oedema of his glottis. Instead: try the following "failed intubation drill".
(1) Maintain cricoid pressure, as described in Section 16.5.
(2) Lower the head of the table and tilt his head to the left.
(3) Give oxygen by IPPV, and try to intubate him again.

If you fail, release cricoid pressure with his head still in the lateral position, insert an airway and induce him with a mask.

Or, if there is a danger of his stomach being full, let him wake, empty his stomach with a tube, (if you have not already done so), instil 15 ml of magnesium trisilicate, or give him intravenous metaclopramide. Then reanaesthetise him using a mask. See also Section 16.6.

If the tube has gone into a patient's oesophagus, remove it and try again. This is common, and even an experienced anaesthetist can easily do this, so always check its position: (1) See it going between his cords. (2) When you have passed it, look with a laryngoscope to see that it has passed in front of the patient's arytenoid cartilages. (3) *Listen over both his lungs* with a stethoscope, or put your ear against his chest. Listening over one lung only does not exclude the possibility that the tube may be too long and has entered a main brochus. If he is paralysed, either ventilate him while you listen to each lung, or press on his chest while you listen.

If the tracheal tube has gone into the patient's right, or occasionally his left, main bronchus, slowly withdraw it with the cuff deflated until his breath sounds are equal on both sides, of his chest. Then reinflate the cuff. A tracheal tube which is too long can easily reach a bronchus. It is uncommon with an Oxford tube, but it can happen, especially in a small baby. Diagnose bronchial intubation by listening to both sides of the chest after intubation, to make sure that air entry is equal on both sides, top and bottom. If the tube is in a bronchus and you don't diagnose it, the patient will become cyanosed, because his underventilated lung will continue to be perfused with blood while it slowly collapses. He will retain carbon dioxide, and the speed and depth of his respirations will increase. If he is breathing spontaneously, this will exhaust him.

AN IMPROVISED LARYNGOSCOPE

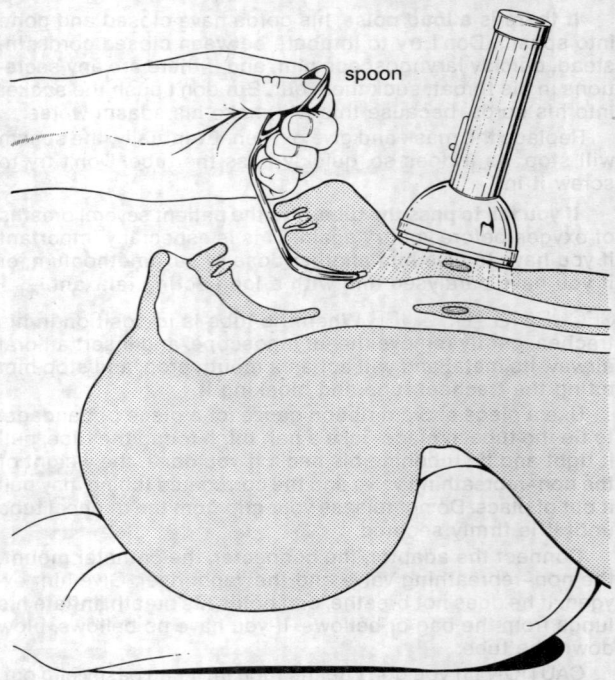

Fig. 13-12 AN IMPROVISED LARYNGOSCOPE *Kindly contributed by Peter Bewes.*

If the tube slips out, reinsert it. This can easily happen, especially in a child, if you do not tie the tube in place. It can also easily slip up into a patient's pharynx, or down into his bronchus (usually the right one), especially if he is moved, or if his head is turned to one side. To prevent this: (1) If possible, anaesthetize a child on the table in the position in which he will be operated on. (2) Check that the tube still is in place each time the child is moved. (3) Always tie the tube in place.

If a patient coughs on the tube, or holds his breath, keep the tube still and he will stop coughing. Assist him with a bag or bellows when he inspires. Don't try to ventilate him against his cough. If you do, you may cause a pneumothorax. Reduce his tendency to cough by spraying 3 ml of 2 or 4% lignocaine on his cords before you intubate.

If he vomits while you are trying to intubate him, tilt his head down and suck him out immediately (16.2), then reinduce him and try to intubate again.

If the light on the laryngoscope fails, clean the contact between the blade and the handle, and check that the bulb is screwed in place securely. If this fails, use your spare laryngoscope, which you should have instantly available. Or, transilluminate his pharynx by shining an electric light through his neck as in Fig. 13-12. If you don't have a laryngoscope, you can use a bent spoon.

If your laryngoscope has a straight blade, pass its tip posterior to his epiglottis. This is more likely to cause laryngeal spasm, so be ready with the lignocaine spray. The Macintosh laryngoscope has a curved blade, and is the easiest one to use. Which side of his epiglottis you pass the blade is mostly a matter of personal convenience.

If the patient has a sore throat or a husky voice postoperatively, reassure him. It will soon probably pass off. More serious traumatic complications include dislodged teeth and laceration or ulceration of anything touched by the tube or the laryngoscope. So be careful.

ALWAYS LISTEN TO BOTH SIDES OF THE CHEST WHEN YOU HAVE PASSED A TRACHEAL TUBE

13.4 Intubating through the nose

If a patient needs an operation on his mouth or throat, it is useful to be able to intubate him through his nose, so that the tube is out of the way of the operation. Passing a tube through his nose is more difficult than passing one through his mouth. So become good at oral intubation first. Blind nasal intubation is a useful skill, when you can do it quickly and reliably. Listening to the patient's breath sounds is a useful guide as to where the end of the tube is, so don't try to intubate him while he is apnoeic from relaxants, unless you are expert.

INTUBATING THROUGH THE NOSE

INDICATIONS (1) Operations on a patient's mouth and oropharynx, such as dental operations and tonsillectomy.

CONTRAINDICATIONS (1) Purulent nasal discharge. It may infect his lungs. (2) Nasal obstruction; test for this by asking the patient to breathe through each nostril in turn.

EQUIPMENT You will need all the equipment described earlier for oral intubation, except a different kind of tube. For nasal intubation use a tube one size smaller than for oral intubation. Choose a tube which is two or two and a half times as long as the distance from the patient's nostrils to his ear, or use Fig. 13-6 as a guide to its length. Use a cuffed tube in adults and a plain one in children. Lubricate them well. Use a suitable oral tracheal connector and adaptor.

Instil ephedrine drops in the patient's nostril to shrink his mucosa.

METHOD FOR INTUBATING THROUGH THE NOSE

EITHER, bring the patient to the stage of surgical anaesthesia with ether. He must be well-relaxed, and breathing spontaneously.

OR, if you are more experienced, give him atropine, thiopentone, and suxamethonium. This saves time. He will be well relaxed and the tube will pass easily, but there will be no breath sounds to guide you.

Put a pillow behind his head. Bare his chest. Put your left hand under his head and tilt it backwards. This will leave your right hand free to control the tube.

Preoxygenate him (9.3).

Put the well-lubricated tube into his right nostril, and pass it vertically downwards along the floor of his nasal cavity towards the floor of the room. If you push it up towards his eyes, it will stick in his turbinates. Twist it from time to time to overcome any obstruction. Don't use force, or his mucosa will bleed.

If the tube sticks while it is still in his nose, this is probably because his septum is deflected, try a smaller tube, or his other (left) nostril.

CAUTION ! Fix the tracheal connector firmly on the tube, or the tube may disappear down a bronchus!

You now have a choice as to whether you will intubate him visually or blindly. Anaesthetists vary as to which they prefer to try first. Some always intubate visually and only do so blind if intubation under direct vision is impossible or fails. Others do the reverse. We advise you to try to intubate visually first.

INTUBATION UNDER DIRECT VISION

Look into the patient's pharynx with a laryngoscope. You may be able to see the end of the tube. Push the tube onwards until you can see it enter his larynx. If it is not far forward enough, lift up the distal end of the tube with Magill's forceps, while your assistant pushes the proximal end further down his nose. Intubation may be easier if you put the blade of the laryngoscope below the patient's epiglottis.

Push the tube between the patient's cords while they are maximally abducted in inspiration.

If the tube goes through his cords and then sticks, his head is too far extended, so flex it, and then push the tube onwards.

BLIND NASAL INTUBATION

This is only necessary if intubation under direct vision fails. If the patient is breathing spontaneously, listen at the proximal end of the tube, as you advance its tip into the pharynx. If breath sounds become louder, it means that the tip of tube is going in the right direction. The change from a high pitched sound to a low one shows that the tip of the tube is in his larynx. If the breath sounds disappear entirely, the tube may be in the oesophagus. Withdraw the tube a little and his breath sounds will return. If you now give it a gentle push during inspiration, it should slip through his vocal cords.

Gently push the tube along a line from the nostril through which you have passed the tube to his opposite sternoclavicular joint.

Watch the skin of the patient's neck. You may be able to detect the movement of the tube. You may feel it snap past his cords and see it distort the anterior wall of his trachea as it passes.

If the tube sticks in his pharynx, it may have stuck in his adenoids. Put a finger into his mouth and try to lift the tube past his adenoids.

If the tube sticks in the midline above his larygnx, it is either pushed up against the anterior wall of his larynx or it has stuck at the base of his tongue beside his epiglottis. So, first flex his head a little, and then push the tube gently onwards. If this fails, withdraw the tube, flex his head and again push gently.

If the tube pushes out the skin to one side of his larynx, withdraw it a little, rotate it towards the midline, and advance it again.

IS THE TUBE SAFELY IN HIS TRACHEA? It can be in his pharynx, his trachea, or perhaps in a bronchus. You can find out in the same way as with oral intubation—listen over both lungs. If you are not sure where the tube is, quickly compress his chest, and listen down the tube. The sound of air coming up the tube shows it is in the chest. Blow down the tube. If it is in the trachea, the chest will inflate, although air may

INTUBATING WITH MAGILL'S FORCEPS

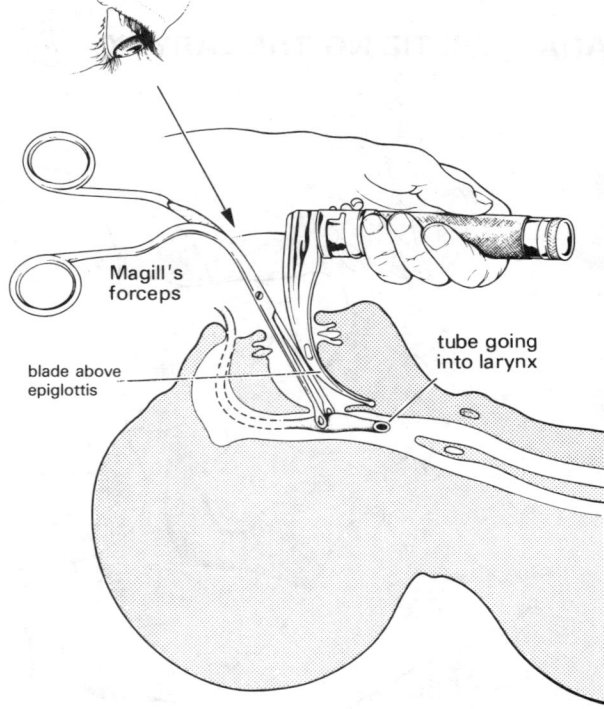

Fig. 13-13 INTUBATING VISUALLY WITH MAGILL'S FORCEPS. As you become skilled, you will be able to intubate a patient blind, so that you will need to do this only if blind intubation fails. *Kindly contributed by John Farman.*

103

leak out round the tube. If it is in the oesophagus, there will be a deep bubbly sound when you try to inflate, and no chest movement. If so, withdraw the tube, extend his head and try again.

CAUTION ! (1) Don't use force. (2) Don't persist with unsuccessful attempts for more than 30 seconds.

DIFFICULTIES WITH NASAL INTUBATION

If the patient's mucosa starts to bleed, you may be able to insert the tube before bleeding obscures your view. Suck out the blood and put a moist gauze pack in his pharynx. If you push too hard you can push the end of the tube into his pharyngeal mucosa and cause a large haematoma.

13.5 Local anaesthesia for intubation

There are two reasons for spraying lignocaine onto a patient's larynx before you pass a tracheal tube: (1) To make passing it easier when the patient is not having a general anaesthetic, or when he is only having a weak one, such as trichloroethylene. (2) To weaken the stimulus that a tube may cause during a long light anaesthetic. A tracheal tube moves up and down each time a patient breathes. Anaesthetizing his larynx will remove the stimulus that these movements cause, so that anaesthesia can be lighter. Local anaesthesia will also reduce his tendency to cough on the tube during the operation and immediately afterwards. This is useful if he needs an operation on his eye or his brain, when coughing can be disastrous. Also, an anaesthetized larynx will reduce the discomfort of a sore throat for the period immediately after any operation.

But an anaesthetized larynx can be dangerous—it will make the patient less likely to cough, and so more likely to inhale the contents of his stomach, if he vomits or regurgitates. So don't anaesthetize his larynx if: (1) He might have a full stomach. Or, (2) he needs an operation on his nose or mouth.

You can anaesthetize the larynx in several ways: (1) You can anaesthetize it with a spray can that delivers a calibrated dose at each puff. (2) You can spray the larnyx using a syringe and a stiff piece of catheter. (3) You can inject lignocaine solution through the patient's cricothyroid membrane. Whichever method you choose, he will find the whole procedure so uncomfortable that he will need constant encouragement.

ANAESTHETIZING THE LARYNX

INDICATIONS (1) To make intubation easier. (2) To make a lighter general anaesthetic possible. (3) Awake intubation (4) Intraocular and intracranial operations. Some additional indications for injecting lignocaine through the cricothyroid membrane are discussed below.

CONTRAINDICATIONS (1) Patients with a full stomach. (2) Operations on the nose or mouth.

DRUGS The maximum dose of lignocaine is 3 mg/kg.
CAUTION ! *Take care not to exceed the maximum dose in Fig. 5-1.* The maximum dose is 4 ml of 4% lignocaine for an adult. For a child of 15 kg, it is only 1 ml.

Either, use a pressurised spray can of lignocaine delivering 10 mg at each puff. Calculate how many puffs (or how much spray) you can safely use. One puff is the dose for a baby.

Or, use a syringe containing 2% or 4% lignocaine attached to a piece of stiff catheter tube. The 2% solution is safer.

SPRAYING LOCAL ANAESTHETIC FROM ABOVE

Wait until the patient is surgically anaesthetized with ether or thiopentone, along with atropine and a relaxant.

Get a clear view of his larynx with a laryngoscope.

Place the tip of the spray 2 cm away from each vocal cord, and give two puffs. Then pass the spray tip 2 cm through his vocal cords and give the rest of the dose. If he is breathing spontaneously, *spray during expiration*. This will help to prevent lignocaine reaching his alveoli where it will be quickly absorbed, and may cause toxic complications.

Then intubate him.

LOCAL ANAESTHESIA THROUGH THE CRICOTHYROID MEMBRANE WHILE THE PATIENT IS AWAKE

INDICATIONS (1) For laryngoscopy in abnormalities of the larynx. (2) Laryngeal oedema. (3) Ludwig's angina. (4) patients who are nearly dead from organic respiratory obstruction. All these conditions make intubation very difficult. Anaesthetizing a patient's larynx through his cricothyroid membrane may help.

METHOD If there is time, give the patient an anaesthetic lozenge to suck for half an hour. Give him diazepam 5 mg, intravenously.

Ask an assistant to stand by and prevent him clutching at the laryngoscope, or at your arms.

Spray his lips and tongue with 2% or 4% lignocaine.

Draw 2 ml of 4% lignocaine into a syringe, and attach a sharp 1 mm needle. Push the needle through the patient's cricothyroid membrane until you aspirate air. To find his cricothyroid membrane, find the prominence of his larynx (16-4). Follow this downwards. You will reach the depression occupied by his cricoid membrane just before you reach the much smaller prominences of his cricoid. Then, at the end of expiration, rapidly inject the whole contents of the syringe. If you inject it at the end of inspiration, he will cough it all out.

After a few minutes, gently put the laryngoscope into his mouth. Spray the rest of his tongue, and the posterior surface of his epiglottis.

Raise the base of his tongue until you can see his larynx, and then spray his larynx and trachea with more lignocaine, but don't exceed the maximum dose.

Now try to pass the tube.

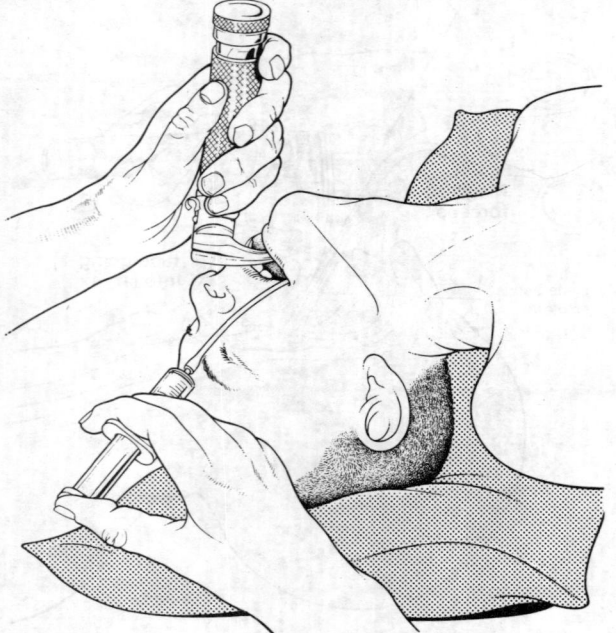

Fig. 13-14 ANAESTHETIZING THE LARYNX. This will make passing a tube easier if a patient is only lightly anaesthetized. It will also weaken the stimulus caused by the tube during a long light anaesthetic.
Kindly contributed by John Farman.

13.6 Intubating children

This is often necessary, and if you have the right equipment, particularly a suitable laryngoscope blade, it is not too difficult. A child does however have a small mouth, a large tongue, loose teeth, a floppy epiglottis, and delicate cords that you can easily injure.

An adult's larynx is the narrowest part of his respiratory tract, but in a child below the age of 10, the narrowest part is his cricoid ring, just below his larynx. This is round, so a round tube of exactly the right size will seal itself without the need for a cuff. Besides being unnecessary, a cuff increases the diameter of a tracheal tube (13.2), without increasing its lumen. So use a plain (uncuffed) tube, such as an Oxford tube. Oxford tubes have a preformed bend and are less likely to kink than Magill tubes, although they can do so.

In a small child, especially, be gentle. A tube that passes his larynx may stick at his cricoid ring, and if you push it through forcefully, inflammatory oedema may subsequenlty cause dangerous respiratory obstruction. A tube that is a little too small is safer than a tube that is too large. A little leak round the tube is unimportant. A tube about the diameter of the middle phalanx of his little finger will be about right for him. A neonate usually needs a 3 mm tube, a child of 6 months a 3.5 mm tube, and a 1 year old child a 4 mm tube, as shown in Fig. 13-6. The size at the larynx varies, so have tubes ready that are 0.5 mm larger and smaller than the one you think you will need.

If a baby is less than a month old, you can intubate him without an anaesthetic.

You can intubate a child over 3 months much the same way as an adult by any of the following methods: (1) You can induce him with an inhalation agent and then when anaesthesia is deep enough, you can intubate him. (2) You can induce him with an inhalation agent, give him suxamethonium and intubate him. (3) If you are good at it, you can give him thiopentone and suxamethonium, preoxygenate him, apply cricoid pressure and then intubate him. This is useful for emergencies and is the standard procedure for older children. It is progressively more difficult the younger he is.

In the method below, we describe the use of halothane and lignocaine. You can use ether, with or without lignocaine, in the same way as for an adult.

POSITIONS DURING INTUBATION

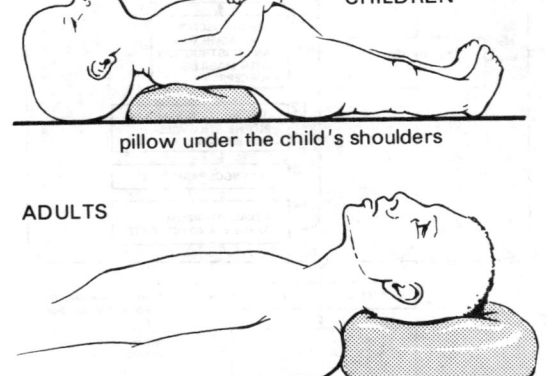

Fig. 13-15 THE POSITIONS OF PATIENTS OF DIFFERENT AGES DURING INTUBATION. Put the pillow under an adult's head and neck, but under a child's back. *Kindly contributed by Michael Wood.*

AWAKE INTUBATION FOR BABIES UNDER ONE MONTH OLD

INDICATIONS These include: (1) Abdominal and thoracic operations, such as pyloric stenosis and tracheo–oesophageal fistulae. (2) Repair of a meningocoele. (3) The respiratory distress syndrome in an infant being managed on an ICU.

EQUIPMENT A laryngoscope with a baby blade. If you don't have one, use the tip of an adult Macintosh blade.

INSERTING THE TUBE *Give the baby atropine. Intubate him while he is awake before you anaesthetize him. Wrap him in a towel, put a sandbag or a firm pillow under his shoulders, and ask a nurse to hold him with her hands each side of his face.*

Preoxygenate him for 2 minutes with 3 litres of oxygen a minute through a T-piece (18.2).

Take the laryngoscope in your left hand and open his lips with your right hand. Pass the blade behind his tongue. His epiglottis points directly backwards, so put the tip of the blade posterior to it. Lift the blade to expose his glottis. If you take care, this will not stop him breathing. There is no need to spray his cords.

Ask the nurse to press his larynx gently backwards while you pass the tube. Wait until his cords abduct and his glottis opens. Put the tube in gently. Don't screw it in.

Connect the tube to the system, and give him oxygen immediately.

If he coughs or breathes irregularly, control his respiration for a few breaths, until he breathes regularly again.

Listen to both his lungs with a stethoscope to make sure that air is entering them equally, and that the end of the tube has not gone into a bronchus.

Turn on the ether, and increase the concentration slowly up to 10% or 15% until he settles and stops moving his limbs.

When surgical anaesthesia is reached, as shown by relaxation of his hand grip, reduce the concentration of ether to about 5%.

If you are in doubt about his breathing, ventilate him gently.

REMOVING THE TUBE is a dangerous moment and severe laryngeal spasm is common.

If he is a neonate, leave the tube in until he is awake, coughing and turned on his side.

If he is an older baby, examine his pharynx with a laryngoscope while he is still moderately deeply anaesthetized. Suck out any secretions. Don't remove the tube until he is responding to stimuli. Insert an oral airway, turn him onto his side, and give him oxygen. Gently remove the tube, and substitute a face mask.

Alternatively, in order to avoid laryngospasm when you remove the tube, you can remove it when a baby is quite deeply anaesthetized, and then leave an airway in place.

INTUBATING A CHILD OVER ONE MONTH

Give the child atropine (2-4). Tape a stethoscope to his chest and listen to his heart sounds constantly (a slowing of his pulse and a reduction in their intensity indicates myocardial depression, and a need to reduce the ether or halothane).

Start by inducing him with halothane and follow this with ether. Or, use ether alone. This will not be easy because induction with ether alone is difficult in children. Use a face mask and a paediatric non-rebreathing valve and blow the agent over his face.

Don't try to pass the tube until anaesthesia is deep enough. Halothane will depress his respiration, and he may look deeply anaesthetized, and yet cough loudly when you try to intubate him.

If you are inducing him with halothane, give him some more 4% halothane for 4 minutes, spray his larynx, and then give him more 4% halothane for one more minute. Then pass the tube.

If you are inducing him with ether, give him 10–15% ether, until his abdominal muscles relax and his pupils are moderately dilated.

If there are no contraindications (13.5), insert the laryngoscope, and spray his larynx with 10 or 20 mg of lignocaine.

Reapply the facemask, and give him more ether for a few minutes while the lignocaine acts.

After you have intubated him by either method, remove the mask from the system and connect up the tracheal tube. You may need to assist his respiration for a few breaths until he starts to breathe spontaneously.

ALTERNATIVE EMERGENCY METHOD If he has a suitable vein, induce him intravenously with thiopentone or ketamine, as if he where an adult. Preoxygeneate him. Give him suxamethonium, apply cricoid pressure (16.5), and intubate him. Adjust the doses to his weight.

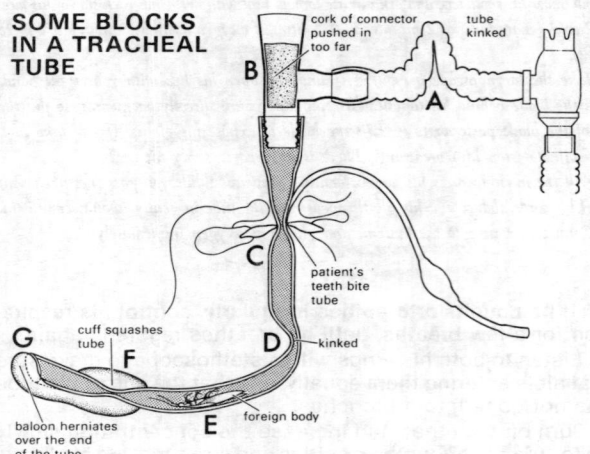

Fig. 13-16 SOME CAUSES OF BLOCKS IN A TRACHEAL TUBE. A, the catheter mount is kinked. B, the cork of the connector has been pushed in too far. C, the patient's teeth bite the tube. D, the tracheal tube is kinked. E, there is a foreign body inside it. F, the cuff squashes it. G, the cuff herniates over the end of it. *Kindly contributed by John Farman.*

13.7 Compliance, and the blocked tracheal tube

When you have paralysed a patient and are ventilating him, you can learn a lot from the feel of the bag. Is ventilating him easy or difficult? The feel of his lungs through the bag or bellows is called compliance. It can be abnormal in various ways, and depends partly on his lungs and partly on your anaesthetic equipment—compliance is easier to feel with a thin rubber bag, like that on an anaesthetic machine of the Boyle's type, than it is with a self[ninflating bag or a bellows.

If there is *high compliance,* the bag is easy to squeeze, and ventilation is good. This is usual in young paralysed patients.

If there is *low compliance* the bag feels stiff and ventilation is more difficult. You will find this in the elderly, in heavy smokers with chronic bronchitis, in obesity, in abdominal distension, and in pregnancy. Compliance is also low as muscle relaxants wear off, in acute bronchospasm, left ventricular failure, tension pneumothorax and when a tube is obstructed or when it is in one lung.

If you are using an anaesthetic machine of the Boyle's type, and the bag or bellows empty too easily, there is a leak in the system or the gas flow is diminished, or there is no gas flowing at all. Check the oxygen and nitrous oxide.

If the bellows or bag will not empty at all, the patient's airway is probably blocked completely, somewhere between the bag or bellows and his smaller bronchi, which may be in spasm.

Unfortunately, a tracheal tube does not absolutely guarantee a clear airway. It may become obstructed in several places: (1) There may be a foreign body in the tube, because you never looked to make sure it was patent before you passed it. (2) It may have kinked because it is old and worn. A soft tube may kink at the back of the patient's throat; a long one may kink as it comes out of his mouth. (3) The bevelled end of the tube may be blocked by the wall of his trachea, especially if his trachea is deviated to one side, for example, by a large thyroid. (4) The backward facing bevel of an Oxford tube can also be blocked by the posterior wall of his trachea when his head is flexed. So, when you use this tube in a small child, raise his shoulders slightly on a small folded towel as in Fig.13-15. (5) If the cuff is overinflated, it may compress the tube or herniate down beyond its tip and block the opening.

"THE PATIENT'S LUNGS WILL NOT INFLATE"

IF HE SHOWS MODERATE RESISTANCE TO INFLATION (1) The anaesthetic may not be deep enough—he may be waking up. (2) The relaxant may be wearing off. (3) He may have bronchospasm from bronchial or cardiac asthma, in which case expiration will be prolonged.

IF HIS LUNGS WON'T INFLATE AT ALL, consult Fig. 13-17. There must be (a) a block, or (b) a leak somewhere between the bellows (or bag) and his alveoli. The feel of the bag will help in diagnosis. Complete resistance to inflation is much more likely to be due to a kinked tube. First look at the non-rebreathing valve (1). Unscrew it gradually to ensure that it is working and allowing gas to escape. What you do next depends on whether he is intubated or not (2).

If a patient is intubated, first make sure there is no obvious kink in the tube, as in Fig. 13-16. Put your finger into his pharynx and feel for the kink. If you find a kink, replace

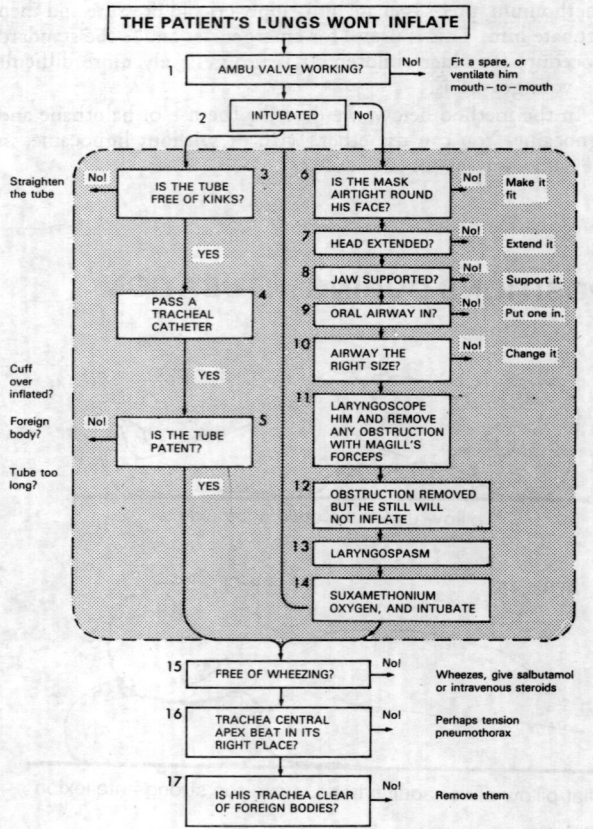

Fig. 13-17 THE PATIENT WHOSE LUNGS WILL NOT INFLATE. If you find you cannot inflate a patient when you squeeze the bag or pump the bellows, here are some of the reasons for it. *Kindly contributed by John Farman.*

the tube. If you can find no obvious kink (3), quickly disconnect the tube and pass a catheter down it (4). The cuff may have herniated over the end, or there may be a foreign body in the tube itself. It is hard to distinguish a complete block from bronchospasm, except by putting a catheter down the tube.

CAUTION ! When in doubt, take out the tube, and try again with a different tube.

If he is not intubated there may be a leak between the mask and his face (6). Or his tongue may have fallen back and blocked his airway, because you have not extended his head properly (7), or supported his jaw (8), or put in an oral airway (9), or because the oral airway is the wrong size (10). If none of these are the cause of the trouble, quickly laryngoscope him (11) and see if there is any obstruction, such as dislodged teeth or vomit in his pharynx or larynx (12). A common cause of trouble is laryngospasm—you will see his cords tightly together (13). For this he needs suxamethonium, oxygen and intubation (14).

You are now sure that his airway is clear right down to his trachea. The possibilities now are bronchial or cardiac asthma, (15) which will make him wheeze, or such rarities as a tension pneumothorax (16) or a foreign body in his trachea (17). Remember that cardiac and bronchial asthma are not the only causes of wheezing, and that both *a kinked tube and a foreign body can both cause wheezing*. Disconnect the tube and listen to the expiratory sound.

If you cannot diagnose the cause of the obstruction within a minute, remove the tube and give oxygen by mask. There may be a swab in the tube, or a blocked connection, and he cannot wait while you investigate.

Try lying him on his side, give him oxygen, and keep the sucker going.

14 Muscle Relaxants

14.1 Long and short–acting relaxants

Many operations, especially those in the abdomen, need well relaxed muscles. Until the introduction of relaxants, the only way to relax the muscles was to produce deep general anaesthesia with ether or to use nerve blocks, neither of which is completely satisfactory. After deep ether anaesthesia a patient takes 48 hours, or longer, to excrete the ether that has accumulated inside him and does not feel well until he has eliminated all of it. He has to recover both from the operation and from a heavy dose of ether. If he is already very ill, he may fail to do so.

If you give a patient a muscle relaxant, it will paralyse him, so that you need only give him just enough anaesthetic to keep him unconscious and free from pain. Two to 3% of ether may be enough, instead of the 10% to 15% that he will need if you don't use a relaxant. After the operation, he quickly excretes this small dose of ether and recovers rapidly. Relaxants also make intubation easier and induction quicker. If you paralyse him so that he cannot cough, and then intubate him, you can induce him with ether in 5 minutes instead of 20, so saving 15 minutes with each operation. For all these reasons, the combined use of general anaesthesia and relaxants has been one of the greatest advances in anaesthesia since ether was introduced in 1846.

Relaxants have some disadvantages: (1) You must control the patient's ventilation, so you will need the equipment for this. (2) Many of the classical signs of anaesthesia, particularly those caused by ether, depend on changes in the pattern of the patient's respiration, and are absent if he is paralysed. (3) Because the depth of anaesthesia is less easy to judge, you have to place much more reliance on the position of the control lever of the vapouriser. (4) Even more important, the most obvious sign of cardiac arrest—failure to breathe—is absent when you are controlling a patient's ventilation. The first sign that a patient's heart has stopped is an absent pulse, or heart beat, or an unrecordable blood pressure, so watch them both carefully, particularly his pulse. If the operation is being done under a tourniquet, even the sign that he no longer bleeds will be absent. This is why a precordial stethoscope with an earpiece is so essential.

ALWAYS MONITOR THE PULSE DURING CONTROLLED VENTILATION

There are two kinds of muscle relaxant: (1) Short–acting ones, which depolarise the motor end–plates (depolarising relaxants) and which don't need reversing. (2) Long–acting ones, which do not depolarise the motor end–plates and which do need reversing. Both types of relaxants are almost always given intravenously.

Depolarising (short–acting) relaxants include suxamethonium bromide and suxamethonium chloride ("Scoline")—'sux" to many anaesthetists. Chemically these drugs resemble acetyl choline, and like it, they combine with the motor end–plates. In doing so they make the muscle fibres contract, and cause a wave of fine twitching (fasciculation) to pass all over the body. This causes muscular pains after the operation, but these soon go. A depolarising relaxant is less rapidly

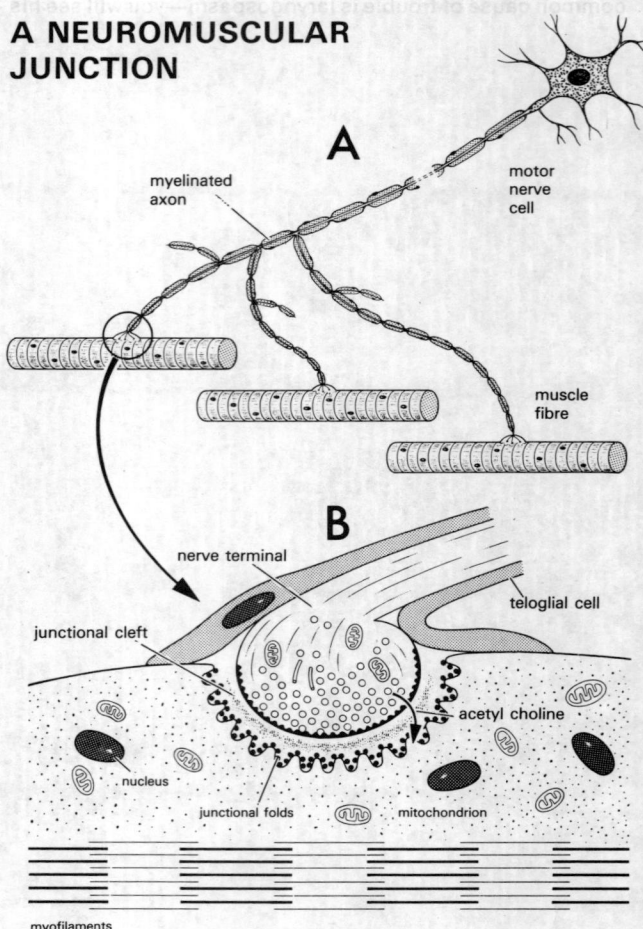

Fig. 14-1 A NEUROMUSCULAR JUNCTION. A, an electrical impulse comes down a patient's nerve fibre. B, at his neuromuscular junctions it releases the acetyl choline stored in the vesicles of his nerve terminals. This crosses his junctional folds, combines at special receptor sites, and causes his muscle fibres to contract. Cholinesterase (black dots) destroys acetyl choline and prevents it accumulating, until more is released by the next nerve impulse.

A depolarising relaxant (suxamethonium) combines at the same receptor sites as acetyl choline, but it stays attached to them much longer. Initially, it depolarises the muscles so that they contract (fasciculate). Then it prevents them repolarising ("recharging"), so that they remain paralysed, until the suxamethonium has been broken down after a few minutes by cholinesterase.

A non-depolarising relaxant (such as alcuronium) also combines at the same receptor sites as acetyl choline, but it does not depolarise the muscles. So they do not contract or fasciculate. It works by blocking the receptor sites and preventing acetyl choline acting, so that the patient is paralysed. Neostigmine reverses the paralysis by inhibiting cholinesterase and allowing acetyl choline to build up and stimulate the muscles to contract once more. *From Bowman and Rand's, Textbook of Pharmacology, with the kind permission of Blackwell's the publisher.*

removed from the motor end–plates than acetyl choline, so it remains on them for a few minutes. In doing so, it prevents them responding to acetyl choline, and so causes temporary paralysis.

Suxamethonium acts almost immediately and paralyses a patient for 3–5 minutes, after which he recovers spontaneously. No drug is needed to reverse the effects of suxamethonium. Neostigmine, which is necessary to reverse the effect of non–depolarising relaxants, *is contraindicated*. It inhibits the cholinesterase needed to destroy suxamethonium, and so prolongs the paralysis. Suxamethonium causes vagal side effects, particularly bradycardia, hypotension, and increased bronchial secretions, so always give atropine first.

Depolarising relaxants are easier to use than non–depolarising ones, and are safer in less skilled hands, so these are the ones to start with.

Solutions of suxamethonium chloride deteriorate in a hot climate, and so need to be refrigerated. For this reason, it is preferable to order suxamethonium bromide powder, which stores well. Dilute it as you need it.

Non–depolarising (long–acting) relaxants include alcuronium, tubocurarine, pancuronium and gallamine. Alcuronium is the most suitable one for routine use and usually the cheapest. Gallamine causes tachycardia and may increase bleeding. Pancuronium has to be refrigerated.

Non–depolarising relaxants combine with the motor end–plates, but they take longer to start paralysing a patient than the depolarising ones—1 to 3 minutes, instead of only 15 to 20 seconds. Paralysis lasts much longer—30 minutes or more. There is no fasciculation. You usually have to reverse a long acting relaxant with with neostigmine. This combines with the cholinesterase and inactivates it, so that the concentration of acetyl choline can increase and overcome the effect of the relaxant. Unfortunately, neostigmine also causes acetyl choline to build up at all the nerve terminals outside a patient's central nervous system. It slows his pulse, it dilates his blood vessels, and it lowers his blood pressure. It also constricts his bronchi, and it increases the flow of his bronchial secretions and saliva. It contracts the smooth muscle of his gut and urinary tract, and it constricts his pupils. Sometimes it stops his heart. You can counteract all these undesirable side effects by giving atropine, so always do this when you give neostigmine.

If you give a long–acting relaxant, you must control the patient's ventilation. This will be much easier after you have intubated him. So never use a long–acting relaxant without intubating.

Depolarising and non–depolarising relaxants have quite different actions, so never mix them! Give the depolarising relaxant (suxamethonium) first and then the non depolarising one (alcuronium) in a separate syringe.

DON'T GIVE A LONG–ACTING RELAXANT WITHOUT INTUBATING
DON'T MIX RELAXANTS

14.2 Suxamethonium

Use this: (1) To intubate a patient. (2) For procedures that require complete relaxation for a few minutes only, such as reducing a dislocated hip or shoulder. (3) To provide short periods of muscle relaxation during an operation, for patients you have already intubated. A long–acting relaxant is a much better way of doing this. But if you don't have long–acting relaxants, or cannot use them, you will find that using a little "intermittent suxamethonium" like this is sometimes very useful. It is *not* good anaesthetic practice, but it may be necessary. Follow the rules below, and don't give too much!

If possible, learn to give relaxants under the supervision of a trained anaesthetist. But, provided you can intubate a patient

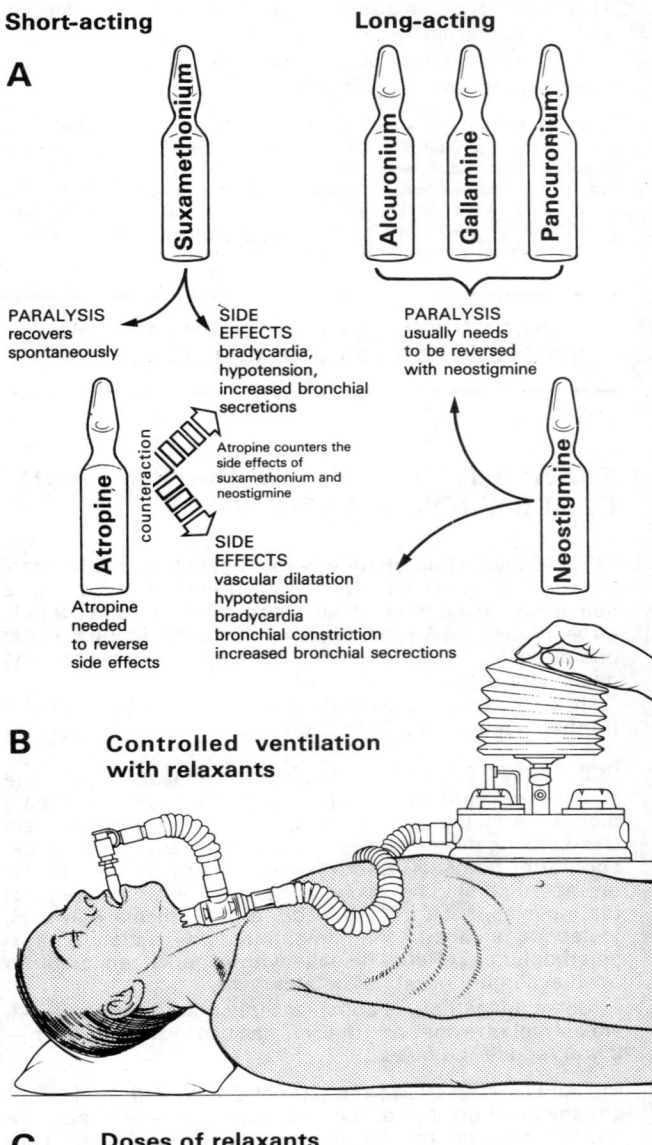

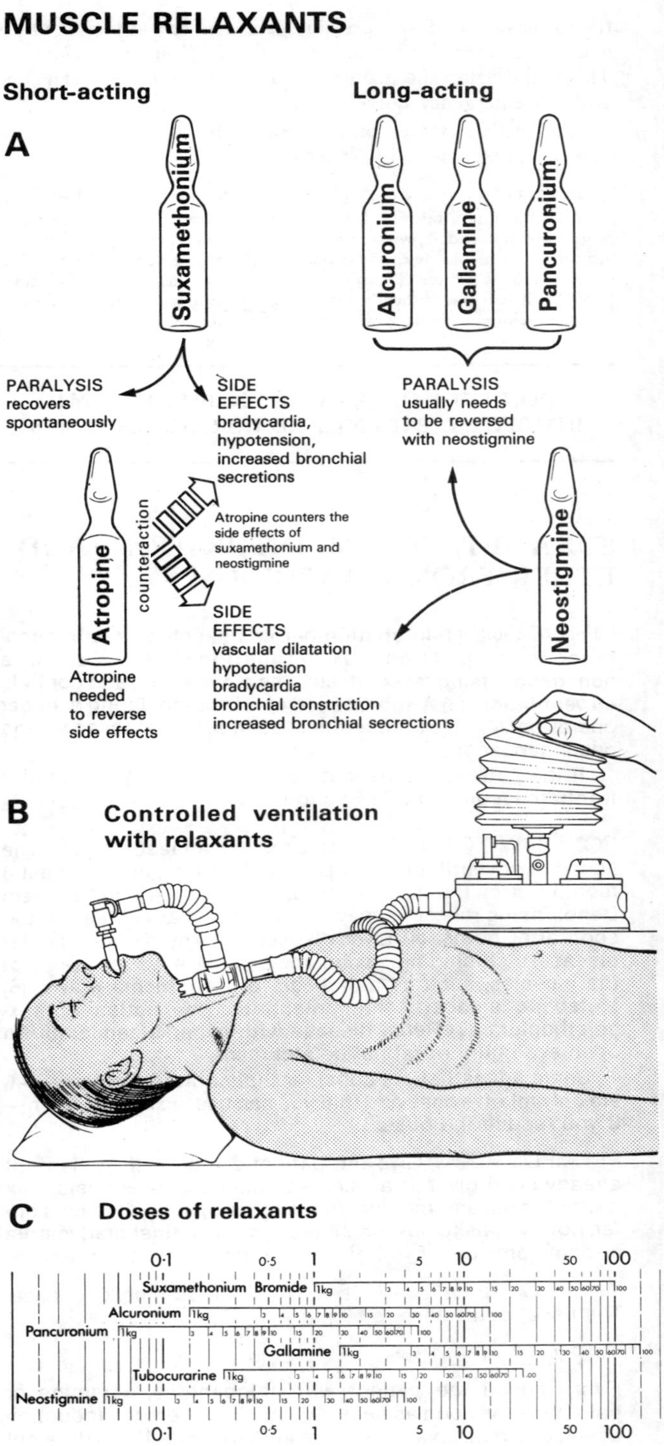

Fig. 14-2 RELAXANTS. A, the relaxants you can use. The paralysis caused by suxamethonium recovers spontaneously. That caused by long–acting relaxants needs reversing with neostigmine. Both suxamethonium and neostigmine cause side effects which you can minimise with atropine.

confidently and control his ventilation, you can use relaxants without formal training. Don't use them if intubation looks difficult, for example, when a patient cannot open his mouth or when his respiration is obstructed. You may find yourself in the desperate situation of having paralysed him and being unable to ventilate him!

The combination of thiopentone, suxamethonium and intubation is such a useful one in an emergency that you should try to master it, if you possibly can. *The best way to do this is to use the combination routinely on "cold cases" on an operating list.* This will develop and maintain your skills, so that you can cope with an emergency quickly and safely.

Very little suxamethonium crosses the placental barrier, so you can safely use it in obstetrics.

BERNADETTE (21) was to have a Caesarean section. The anaesthetic assistant had difficulty intubating her with the first dose of suxamethonium, so he gave her another dose, without first ventilating her with oxygen. After some difficulty he succeeded with the second dose. He then gave her gallamine, but she was dead. When the Caesarean section was done, her baby was still alive. LESSON If you have difficulty intubating a patient with your first dose of suxamethonium, ventilate with oxygen before you try again.

DON'T USE RELAXANTS UNLESS YOU CAN INTUBATE A PATIENT AND INFLATE HIS LUNGS

SUXAMETHONIUM, INTUBATION, AND ETHER FROM A VAPOURISER

INDICATIONS (1) Intubation before anaesthesia with spontaneous respiration. (2) Intubation before using a non-depolarising relaxant, such as alcuronium, and controlled ventilation. (3) A short period of relaxation during a longer operation. (4) Short procedures, such as bronchoscopy, and oesophagoscopy.

If the patient is a neonate or small infant, you can give it intramuscularly as in Section 18.2.

CONTRAINDICATIONS (1) An unskilled anaesthetist. (2) The absence of ventilating equipment. (3) Burns, until at least 3 months after the date of the burn, especially in children. Depolarising relaxants may cause cardiac arrest if given too soon after burns. (4) Liver disease. (5) Any neuromuscular disease, including those causing extensive disuse atropy of the muscles, such as paraplegia or myasthenia gravis. (6) Metabolic acidosis; this potentiates the action of suxamethonium. (7) Renal disease with hyperkalaemia. (8) An open eye injury or retinal detatchment.

Some anaesthetists consider that contraindications 4–6 are only relative ones and that you can use suxamethonium—if you reduce the dose.

PREMEDICATION Give the patient atropine. If he has not already been given it at the beginning of anaesthesia, mix it with the suxamethonium in the same syringe. Opinions differ, however, as to how much protection against bradycardia atropine provides if you give it mixed with suxamethonium.

INITIAL DOSE OF SUXAMETHONIUM Give 1 mg/kg of base. The usual adult dose is 50 mg.

THE METHOD FOR USING SUXAMETHONIUM
First, induce the patient with thiopentone, ketamine or halothane. As soon as he is unconscious from the induction agent, give him suxamethonium intravenously. Use a different syringe from the thiopentone, which is strongly alkaline and will hydrolyse the suxamethonium, if you put them in the same syringe.

CAUTION! Don't give suxamethonium while the patient is still conscious.

As soon as the fasciculations have stopped, ventilate the patient 3 or 4 times with oxygen and then intubate him. Don't try to intubate him while his tongue is still fasciculating. If intubation is difficult, don't allow him to become anoxic—ventilate him with oxygen again.

Suxamethonium causes paralysis for 3–5 minutes, and occasionally for 20 minutes or more.

When the tube is in, and you have checked the air entry to both his lungs, inflate the cuff, and use the apnoea time of the relaxant to quickly increase the ether concentration to 15%, or 10% if the patient is sick. He is paralysed, and cannot cough, so you can increase the ether concentration rapidly. Ventilate him adequately, but not excessively. Hypotension and cardiac arrhythmias can occur at this stage, so keep a finger on his pulse. Cardiac arrhythmias can also be caused by anoxia, so don't allow him to become anoxic.

Usually, by the time the relaxant has worn off, after about 5 minutes, there will be enough ether in his blood for him to continue breathing without coughing.

After 5 minutes, pause from time to time to see if he has started to breathe.

Give him enough ether to take him down to the level of surgical anaesthesia. Once the incision is made you can reduce the ether concentration to 6–8% and finally to about 6%.

CAUTION ! You can easily give a patient too much ether: (1) Don't over-ventilate him if he is paralysed, because this will increase his uptake of ether. (2) Be especially careful not to give him too much ether, if the return of spontaneous respiration is delayed.

FURTHER DOSES OF SUXAMETHONIUM

If you fail to intubate a patient the first time, and you need a further dose to intubate him, repeat the initial dose together with another dose of atropine in the same syringe, but make quite sure you give him a few breaths of oxygen first.

If you want to prolong the effect, give half of the original dose (0.5 mg/kg), and repeat it cautiously if necessary.

INTERMITTENT SUXAMETHONIUM You can use suxamethonium to produce short periods of relaxation during an operation. Mix 100 mg (two 50 mg ampoules) with atropine and dilute the mixture to 10 ml with water or saline. This will give you a solution of 10 mg/ml. Start with ¼ to ½ mg/kg. For example, a 60 kg adult would need 1.5 to 3 ml of this solution. Subsequently give him 1 to 2 ml (10 to 20 mg).

CAUTION ! (1) Intermittent suxamethonium is not good anaesthetic pratice. Don't give more than 6 mg/kg in any one operation. 300 mg at one operation is the maximum dose for an adult. The breakdown products from large doses cause another kind of paralysis accompanied by bradycardia, muscle weakness and persistently inadequate respiration. It is the second or third dose that causes the bradycardia. (2) *Don't prolong paralysis for more than 20 minutes, because there is no antidote.*

The effect of the atropine you gave with the first dose will have worn off, so some anaesthetists give another dose of 0.2 to 0.6 mg with each subseqent dose of suxamethonium mixed together in the same syringe.

DIFFICULTIES WITH SUXAMETHONIUM

If the patient does not become paralysed, or the paralysis lasts only a short time, the suxamethonium chloride solution may have deteriorated, because it was not stored in a refrigerator. Prevent this by buying suxamethonium bromide powder.

If the patient fails to breathe at the end of the operation, don't panic. Keep ventilating him. Don't give drugs to try to stimulate his respiration, because they don't work. He may be the one patient in 2,000 who lacks the enzyme that destroys suxamethonium. Or, he may have liver disease or chronic organophosphate poisoning. You may have to wait until the suxamethonium slowly hydrolyses in his plasma. So keep ventilating him, if necessary with relays of nurses working the bellows. They may need to go on for hours, or longer, but he will recover eventually. Remember that he is totally paralysed; and, although he may look peaceful, he will be terrified and can hear what you are saying. So don't talk about him, talk to him, and reassure him. If the operation is still proceeding, give him 4% ether, or 0.5% trichloroethylene, to prevent pain and keep him asleep.

14.3 Long-acting (non-depolarising) relaxants

This is the most complex procedure we describe. Long-acting relaxants, such as alcuronium, are very useful for major operations, especially those on old or high-risk patients. *But using long-acting relaxants needs skill, and you must be able to control a*

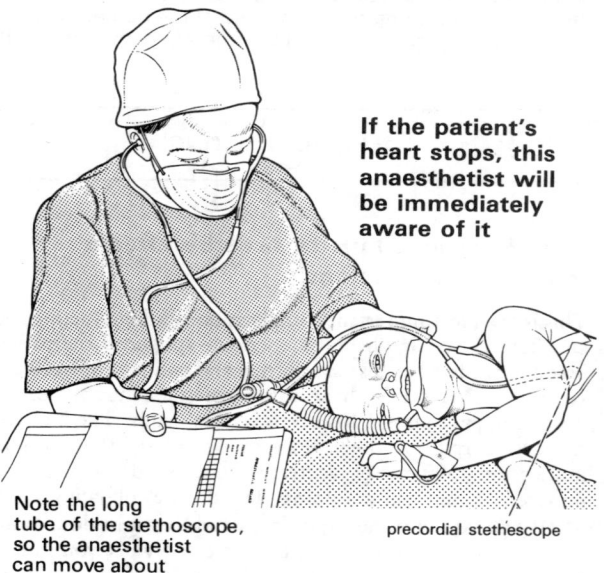

MONITOR THE HEART OF A PARALYSED PATIENT

If the patient's heart stops, this anaesthetist will be immediately aware of it

Note the long tube of the stethoscope, so the anaesthetist can move about

precordial stethescope

FIG. 14-3 MONITOR THE HEART AND PULSE OF A PARALYSED PATIENT. In a patient who is breathing spontaneously, one of the important signs of cardiac arrest is that he stops breathing. This sign is absent if you have paralysed him and are controlling his respiration. So you must always monitor his heart or pulse, or both of them. The first sign of cardiac arrest is an absent pulse. *Kindly contributed by Arthur Adeney*

patient's respiration during the entire operation. Even so, many trained anaesthetic assistants use them expertly. For relaxing a patient's muscles for major abdominal surgery, they are a useful alternative to deep ether anaesthesia (11.2) or intercostal blocks.

Alcuronium is one of the best general–purpose long–acting relaxants. Unlike gallamine, it does not cause tachycardia. And it is less dependent on good renal function than gallamine. It also lasts longer and is cheaper than gallamine. Often, alcuronium is not available, so if you are using some other relaxant, such as curare (d-tubocurarine) go on using it. Pancuronium is more expensive.

If you have paralysed a patient with a relaxant, you can keep him unconscious with a low concentration of ether, halothane or trichloroethylene. Because he will need only a little anaesthetic, he will recover rapidly with few side effects. You can use the combination of alcuronium, trichloroethylene and oxygen for almost any patient, however sick.

Induce the patient with thiopentone and intubate him under suxamethonium. As soon as he begins to breathe again, paralyse him with alcuronium. Its effects may have worn off spontaneously by the end of the operation, but you will probably have to reverse the paralysis with neostigmine and atropine. When the surgeon starts to close the skin, you can stop the ether or the trichloroethylene; they are eliminated only slowly. The patient will then wake up while you gently ventilate his lungs with air enriched with oxygen. As soon as the neostigmine has had time to act, he will start to breathe normally.

The timing of both the alcuronium (or any other long–acting relaxant) and the neostigmine are critically important: (1) Be careful not to give a patient alcuronium *until you are sure that the paralysis caused by the suxamethonium is wearing off.* If you wait until he starts to breathe before giving alcuronium and he does not breathe at the end of the operation, you will know that it, not suxamethonium, is responsible for his failure to breathe. (2) Don't give the neostigmine too early. It is only effective in reversing paralysis *if the patient has already started to recover spontaneously.* It will not work if he is still completely paralysed, or

it may partly reverse him, after which he may become paralysed again in the ward later. So wait to give the neostigmine until at least 20 minutes after you have given the alcuronium. It acts rapidly and its effect may have gone while the alcuronium is still present, so that he may become paralysed (recurarised) again later. If this happens back in the ward and nobody notices, he may die. Failure to observe this rule can be fatal as the story below of the patient Koo shows. Failure of the patient to breathe is one of the major complications of long–acting relaxants, especially if the patient has severe electrolyte imbalance. Even so, this may be the safest anaesthetic for him.

KOO (42) was having a laparotomy for a suspected carcinoma and was given a long–acting relaxant. She was quickly found to be inoperable, so she was given neostigmine only 5 minutes after her injection of gallamine. She was breathing weakly when she was sent back to a busy ward. An hour later she was found dead in bed. LESSON (1) Don't try to reverse a long–acting relaxant with neostigmine too early. (2) A busy ward is a dangerous place in which to to recover from an anaesthetic.

INHALATION ANAESTHESIA WITH RELAXANTS

This is the sequence of thiopentone, suxamethonium, intubation, controlled ventilation, ether and alcuronium.

INDICATIONS (1) Operations inside the abdomen which need a relaxed abdominal wall. (2) Major operations on shocked or old, poor–risk patients. (3) Operations inside the chest or skull, or in the face–down or lateral Trendelenberg position. (4) Operations on very fat patients, or on patients with large abdominal tumours or ascites.

CONTRAINDICATIONS (1) An unskilled anaesthetist. (2) The absence of ventilating equipment. (3) The previous administration of aminoglycoside antibiotics, such as streptomycin or gentamicin. (4) Electrolyte imbalance, particularly hypokalaemia and metabolic acidosis. Both (3) and (4) increase a patient's sensitivity to relaxants. So, if you have been unable to correct his acidosis adequately, or he has previously been taking an aminoglycoside, avoid long–acting relaxants or give them cautiously in low doses. (5) Renal failure, especially if a drug is predominantly excreted by the kidneys as is gallamine.

CAUTION ! If the patient has a ruptured spleen, sudden muscular relaxation may abolish the splinting effect of his abdominal muscles, so the operator should be prepared to be inside his abdomen tying off his spleen quickly.

METHOD OF USING NON–DEPOLARISING RELAXANTS

Induce the patient with thiopentone (12.1), give him suxamethonium (14.2), intubate him, and give him ether, or halothane, trichloroethylene or chloroform.

DOSES OF NON–DEPOLARISING (LONG–ACTING) RELAXANTS Wait until the patient tries to breathe again after the suxamethonium, or starts to swallow, or tries to use his abdominal muscles. This shows that the paralysing effect of the suxamethonium is wearing off. *Now, and not before* give him a long–acting relaxant.

The doses below and in Fig. 2-4 are for patients who have been given suxamethonium, and who are going to be maintained on ether. Under other circumstance you may need slightly larger doses. The repeat doses are suggestions only, and you may need to give less.

Alcuronium. Initial dose 0.15 mg/kg, average adult dose 7.5 to 15 mg. repeat dose 0.05 mg/kg. Adult repeat dose 2.5 to 5 mg. Duration 20 to 40 min. (Ampoules usually contain 5 mg/ml)

Gallamine. Initial dose 1.5 mg/kg, average adult dose 60 to 120 mg, repeat dose 0.75 mg/kg. Duration about 20 min. (Ampoules usually contain 40 mg/ml). Don't give this if tachycardia might be dangerous, as for example in mitral stenosis.

Pancuronium. Initial dose 0.05 mg/kg, average adult dose 2 to 5 mg, repeat dose 0.025 mg/kg. Duration 20 to 30 min. (Ampoules usually contain 2 mg/ml, 4 mg in 2 ml.)

Tubocurarine Initial dose 0.25 mg/kg, average adult dose 30 mg, repeat dose 0.125 mg/kg. Duration 30 to 40 min. (Ampoules usually 10 mg/ml, 1.5 ml containing 15 mg).

With all these drugs, paralysis will start in about a minute, and is quickest with pancuronium.

Control his respiration.

CAUTION ! Don't forget to monitor his pulse. An absent pulse is the first sign of cardiac arrest!

As soon as the patient is satisfactorily paralysed, reduce the concentration of the ether or halothane to the level required to keep him lightly asleep. You have no means of knowing that he is asleep, but 2 to 3% of ether is usually enough.

EXTRA DOSES The effect of the first dose of alcuronium will start to wear off very gradually in 20 to 30 minutes, and the effect of gallamine in 15 to 20 minutes. As the relaxant wears off, there will be less abdominal relaxation. You may see or feel from the bellows that the patient is starting to breathe.

If the patient becomes harder to ventilate, this is probably because the effect of the lon-acting relaxant is wearing off. Make sure it is not caused by bronchospasm (listen for wheezes over his lungs or at the non-rebreathing valve), a foreign body, a kinked tube (try passing a sterile suction catheter) or because sputum or secretions are accumulating (listen for rattling in the tube).

Don't give repeat doses any set time, but if they are necessary, give the repeat doses suggested above or less. If the operation is short, the patient will probably not need another dose.

AT THE END OF THE OPERATION AFTER USING RELAXANTS

REVERSING THE PARALYSIS (1) Always reverse the paralysis with neostigmine, even if the patient seems to be breathing normally. Although he may be breathing, he may be unable to cough. (2) Don't try to reverse the paralysis until at least 20 minutes after the initial dose of relaxant, or at least 10 minutes after the last extra dose. If you try to do so, the paralysis will not reverse, or will reverse only with difficulty, or reverse only temporarily.

Give atropine 0.02 mg/kg with neostigmine 0.04 mg/kg. For a 60 kg adult this is atropine 1.2, mg and neostigmine 2.5 mg (in round figures). For smaller patients calculate the doses carefully. You can mix these drugs in the same syringe, and you must give them slowly. If you make up this mixture early in the operation, keep it clearly labelled on a side table, where you will not confuse it with other drugs you are using during the operation.

The peak effect of neostigmine takes more than 5 minutes to develop.

If the patient's heart rate is still below 60 after reversal with neostigmine, repeat the dose of atropine.

REMOVING THE TRACHEAL TUBE Don't remove the tube until the patient is breathing adequately, showing that reversal is complete.

CAUTION ! Don't remove the tracheal tube if he shows any of these signs—

(1) Paradoxical movement of his chest, caused by poor intercostal movement. Observe or put your hand on his chest to make sure it moves outwards, not inwards, on inspiration.

(2) Chin or tracheal tug. His chin moves downwards on inspiration. If this sign is mild, only his larynx moves downwards.

(3) Muscular weakness. He cannot move his head off the pillow.

(4) Drooping eyelids.

(5) "Thrashing about" or fighting for breath.

If the patient shows any of these signs 5 minutes after you have given your first dose of atropine and neostigmine in the maximum dose for an adult, don't give more.

If he shows the above signs, and you have taken the tube out by mistake, reintubate him, and continue ventilating him until all signs of weakness have gone. Cyanosis and sweating are signs that he needs reintubating quickly.

If you run out of neostigmine, you can still use a long-acting relaxant if you use it with care. Use the smallest dose, and when this is starting to wear off, hyperventilate him. This will make him alkalotic and potentiate its action. When you stop hyperventilating him at the end of the operation, he will start breathing spontaneously. Some anaesthetists do this routinely.

KEEP VENTILATING!

14.4 A patient fails to breathe after a long-acting relaxant

This is the most important complication of a long-acting relaxant. The cause is probably not serious—provided the patient's blood pressure and pulse are normal and you are controlling his ventilation. Many anaesthetic disasters are the result of precipitate drug therapy, so don't rush to give him drugs. The best treatment is likely to be *careful* IPPV (not too fast), the infusion of more fluid (500 ml of dextrose saline), and waiting for 15 minutes. While you are doing this, do the following checks.

(1) Did you give the right drugs and the right dose of muscle relaxant? Check that you have injected what you intended to give . When did you give the last dose? If you have given too much, you can help the patient to get rid of the drug by giving him more fluid over the next 30 minutes. Have you adequately reversed the relaxant with neostigmine and atropine? For an adult the maximum dose of neostigmine is 5 mg. Don't give more. You should not normally give it within 10 minutes of the last dose of the relaxant.

(2) Have you been hyperventilating the patient? You may need to maintain ventilation to remove the volatile agents (ether or halothane) from his body. But hyperventilation will also remove too much of his CO_2 and reduce his respiratory drive. Give him one breath each time you breathe. Don't ventilate faster than your own respiratory rate—about 16 breaths a minute.

(3) Is he centrally depressed and not paralysed? Most analgesics depress the respiration if you give enough of them. Has he had too much of a volatile agent? Or, have you given him too much opioid, such as morphine or pethidine? Look at his pupils. If they are very small, give him naloxone, the adult dose is 0.2 mg.

Move the tube a little. If he tries to cough strongly or "buck", he is anaesthetised rather than paralysed. Ventilate him steadily with air and oxygen until you have blown away enough of the volatile anaesthetic for him to start breathing spontaneously.

(4) Is he hypovolaemic? If his peripheral veins are collapsed, his blood pressure low, and his pulse rapid and weak, he is probably hypovolaemic. Correct this using his urine output and if possible his central venous pressure as a guide. Give him 500 ml of 5% dextrose in saline or Ringer's lactate rapidly.

(5) Is his urine output adequate? Pass a urinary catheter. Gallamine is entirely excreted in the urine, and other long-acting relaxants are partly excreted. If his urinary output is low after correcting his hypovolaemia, increase it by giving him frusemide (20 to 40 mg for an adult). Remember that this is powerful and potentially dangerous, so don't give too much.

(6) Has he got a metabolic acidosis, because this prolongs the effect of non-depolarising relaxants? If he has been in prolonged shock and recieved a massive blood transfusion, this may well be the reason why he is not breathing. Only analysis of his blood gases will confirm it. If you suspect it, give him 1 to 2 mmol/kg of sodium bicarbonate (15.1). If you do not have bicarbonate, let his kidneys correct his acidosis. Give him alternate bottles of 0.9% saline and 5% dextrose. Give him frusemide as above.

If he has had a massive blood transfusion, give him 10 ml of intravenous 10% calcium gluconate very slowly and cautiously, with your finger on his pulse.

(7) Is he short of potassium? If he has lost fluid by diarrhoea, vomiting or an excessive diuresis for several days before the operation, he will have lost potassium with it and is probably short of it. If he is still able to produce urine, add 20 mmol of potassium chloride to every 500 ml bottle of intravenous fluid you give him.

(8) Is he hypothermic? This is an important cause of failure to breathe in children. Take his temperature, and warm him if necessary.

(9) Is he in renal failure? Has he passed urine? Consider passing a catheter. Is he in hepatic failure?

(10) Has he been given an aminoglycoside antibiotic, such as streptomycin or gentamicin? Give him 500 ml of dextrose saline containing 10 ml of 10% calcium gluconate or chloride, over 30 minutes.

MUSCLE RELAXANTS DON'T KILL PATIENTS, BUT RESPIRATORY INADEQUACY DOES

---

15 Fluid therapy

15.1 Intravenous infusions

Intravenous fluids are scarce and precious commodities in many hospitals. Methods of preparing them on a small scale are described in Appendix A. If your hospital can prepare any fluids, it can probably prepare all those in the following list. They all have their uses, so try to keep the complete range in stock. Here are the fluids you will need, and the main surgical indications for each of them.

Blood is the most useful and life–saving of all human spare parts. Methods of collecting it, storing it and cross–matching it are described elsewhere, so here we will only stress the great value of a district hospital blood bank and the importance of establishing the tradition that blood is not paid for, but is a gift from the well to the sick. The organisation of a local blood transfusion service is a responsibility in which local community organisations can play a major role. Blood transfusion has its risks, so don't give blood unnecessarily; and when you give it, give enough. An injured adult either needs at least 2 units (one litre) or he needs none.

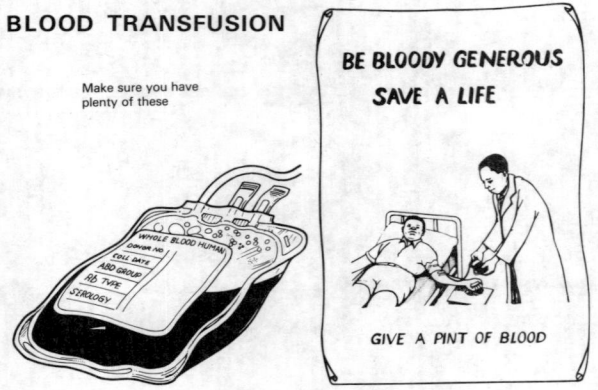

Fig. 15-1 THE MOST USEFUL HUMAN "SPARE PART". Do try to establish the tradition that blood is given free as a gift from the well to the sick. This poster was prepared by the Lions club of Nyeri, Kenya, and is an example of what a local community can do.

0.9% saline is physiological saline, and contains 154 mmol/1 of sodium, which is approximately the same concentration as in the extracellular fluid (135 mmol/1).

The main uses of saline are: (1) In quantities of 500 ml or less, to keep a drip open, so that drugs can be given without the need for repeated venipuncture. (2) As the first fluid given to a severely shocked patient, while waiting for blood. (3) To preload patients having spinal or epidural anaesthetics. (4) As a substitute for Ringer's lactate, when this is not available, to treat surgical dehydration (15.3).

One of the most common mistakes in fluid therapy is to give large volumes of "saline" when a patient has lost water out of all proportion to his losses of sodium and chloride, and so to overload him with these electrolytes.

0.18% saline in 4.3% dextrose is one fifth physiological saline and contains 31 mmol of sodium per litre. Its main use is to provide a balanced, basal water and electrolyte intake for a patient who is not taking fluids by mouth. When his water requirements are fulfilled by this fluid, he gets about 1 mmol/kg of sodium per day, which approximately balances his urinary sodium loss.

Ringer's lactate (Hartman's solution) contains 131 mmol/1 of sodium, which is slightly less than 0.9% saline, 5 mmol/1 of potassium, 112 mmol/1 of chloride and 29 mmol/1 of bicarbonate (as lactate). It is isotonic and is the best fluid for replacing the water and electrolyte losses of patients with surgical dehydration. However, most such patients have lost water out of proportion to their electrolyte loss, so part of their fluid requirements should be supplied as 5% dextrose in water, as described in Section 15.3.

Dextrose solutions, 5%, 10%, 25% and 50% provide a patient with intravenous water, without electrolytes, and with energy. A 5% solution is isotonic, but only provides 200 cal per litre. If you want to provide more energy than this without overloading the patient with fluid, you will have to use stronger solutions. You can give small quantities of stronger solutions as a bolus injection, to treat hypoglycaemic coma; but if you give the quantities necessary to provide a useful amount of energy through an ordinary drip, they will thrombose the veins. A 10% solution runs some risk of doing so, and a stronger solution certainly will. If you are going to use these solutions to provide energy, then you will have to give them through a cannula that you have inserted into a central vein. The main indication for 10% dextrose is for children undergoing surgery.

Half–strength Darrow's solution in 2.5% dextrose is the standard intravenous fluid for treating children with diarrhoea, and it may be the only fluid you have. It contains 65 mmol/1 of sodium and 18 mmol/1 of potassium. You can use it: (1) To replace fluid losses from diarrhoea or a colostomy. (2) To keep a drip running, so that you can inject drugs. (3) To preload a patient having a spinal or epidural anaesthetic (7.1). (4) You can also use it to rehydrate a surgical patient; however, the sodium and potassium content of half–strength Darrows in 2.5% dextrose is too low for it to be satisfactory as the sole fluid this purpose.

1 mmol/ml potassium chloride, and 1 mmol/ml sodium chloride in 50 ml bottles are the easiest way of giving a patient, particularly a child, calculated quantities of potassium or sodium. Tip the volume he needs into a bottle of 5 or 10% dextrose. At 1000 mmol per litre these are concentrated solutions, so he will only need *a small* volume in the range of 1 to 50 ml. *Never make these solutions up in 500 ml volumes,* because someone is sure to give a patient a whole bottle by mistake and kill him.

Some hospitals are so aware of the dangers of the ease with which imperfectly trained staff can give an overdose of potassium that they don't use these concentrated solutions. Instead, they use Darrow's solution for postoperative fluid replacement—the purpose for which it was designed. The full strength solution contains 36 mmol of potassium per litre and the half strength solution 18 mmol.

1 mmol/ml of sodium bicarbonate (8.4%) is the strongest

of the commonly used bicarbonate solutions. It contains 1 mmol/ml of sodium and the same quantity of bicarbonate. Use it to treat the low bicarbonate and high hydrogen ion concentration of metabolic acidosis (17.2). Provided a patient has enough fluid, and normally functioning kidneys, they will usually correct moderate degrees of metabolic acidosis satisfactorily, so you need only give sodium bicarbonate to more severe cases.

SODIUM BICARBONATE

Ideally, you should know the weight of the patient and the severity of his acidosis. If you don't know them, a first dose for an adult of 50 to 150 mmol is reasonable (or 1 mmol/kg for a child).

CAUTION ! (1) Give bicarbonate slowly. (2) Err on the safe side, give too little rather than too much. (3) If you use the more dilute solution (1.2% or 1 mmol in 7 ml) take care not to overload the patient with water. (4) If he is in cardiac failure the excess sodium you are giving him is undesirable. So try to balance the effect of this against the benefit of the bicarbonate.

If a patient is in cardiac arrest, or has been paralysed by relaxants, hyperventilating him will achieve much the same effect as giving him bicarbonate. It will blow off the CO_2 in his blood and temporarily correct his acidosis.

10% or 20% mannitol is a very effective diuretic. Use it for: (1) Reducing cerebral oedema following head injury or head surgery. (2) Protecting the kidney after trauma or in the presence of jaundice. If you are using it for its effect on the kidney be sure to give adequate fluids with it. Fluids are unnecessary if you are using it to treat cerebral oedema. Give 0.5 to 1 g/kg. If necessary, repeat the dose 4 hours later. It may make a patient with a head injury recover consciousness rapidly.

15.2 Intravenous lines

A reliable 'drip' or intravenous line will often save a patient's life and is no less important in anaesthesia than it is in surgery. To establish an intravenous line: (1) You can puncture one of the patient's peripheral veins directly, (2) you can cut down on a vein surgically, (3) you can cannulate one of his great veins. This is particularly necessary for measuring the central venous pressure, so it is described in Section 19.2. Here we describe the other two methods. Puncture is quicker, and there is less risk of infection, but a cut—down is easier for unskilled staff to look after. Auxiliaries soon become expert at managing drips, so do your best to teach them.

For direct puncture you can use: (1) An ordinary hypodermic needle, which is convenient for infusions that do not need to run fast. Its disadvantage is that the point of the needle easily punctures a vein so that fluid runs into the tissues. (2) A short wide (3×40 mm) intravenous needle. This is an inexpensive way of providing an intravenous line that needs to flow fast, as in a shocked patient. (3) A winged needle, which is merely a hypodermic needle with wings that you can fix with strapping. (4) A diaphragm needle, which is a useful way of maintaining an open vein for giving drugs, but is useless for intravenous fluids. (4) A needle and plastic cannula combination. This takes two forms. One is the needle—inside—cannula ('Medicut', 'Intracath', etc). (5) The less satisfactory form is the catheter—inside—needle. (6) If the patient is an infant, you can use a special set to put a needle into one of his scalp veins (Primary Child Care 9.27).

For a "cut—down" you can use: (1) A winged cannula. (2) The cannula part of a needle and cannula combination. (3) Any convenient length of fine plastic tube. (4) The plastic tube of a drip set, if you are cutting down on a patient's long saphenous or femoral vein in an emergency.

In hospitals where the nursing care is good, a cut—down is seldom done, because it is almost always possible to keep a drip going by puncture. But a cut—down can be life—saving, if your staff cannot care for a drip during the night, and cannot be relied upon to tell you when it has stopped. If a baby is to be operated on, a cut—down may be essential. One will probably be necessary somewhere in the hospital almost every day, and if you don't have a special cut—down set, the instruments are easily lost. One arrangement is to keep a cut—down set ready prepared under lock and key in the minor theatre, and for the ward staff who use it to sign for it. When it is returned its contents must be checked. Each time it has been used, the instruments must be washed and autoclaved, and the scissors put back in spirit.

ELIZABETH (19) had severe postpartum bleeding. The medical assistant set up an intravenous drip with saline, and summoned prisoners to donate blood. The doctor explored the birth canal and spent 45 minutes repairing a cervical tear and an episiotomy. The patient was so restless that the ordinary hypodermic needle that was being used came out of her vein and had to be replaced four times. She recovered uneventfully. LESSON At that time no needle—cannula combinations were obtainable in the country. They are almost indispensable.

• *GIVING SET, intravenous, plastic, to deliver 15 drops per ml, with soft rubber injection segment, disposable, but capable of being boiled for reuse, one hundred sets only.* A giving set, preferably a good one, with a standard size of drop, makes monitoring the rate of infusion much easier, and if it has a rubber segment, you can use a fine needle to inject drugs into it without leaks. You can also insert the needle of a second set into the rubber segment and so combine two sets. Most of these sets cannot be boiled for reuse, so be sure to order one which can.

• *NEEDLE—INSIDE—CANNULA venous, autoclavable, teflon, Luer fitting, (a) 0.5 mm, (b) 1 mm, (c) 1.5×150 mm needle, twenty of each size only.* Plastic cannulae and needles can be combined in two ways, the needle can be outside or inside the cannula, We have specified the needle inside variety, because there is less chance of the cannula being cut by the needle and embolising into the circulation. The needle has a plug to block it, while it is being inserted. Both the needle and cannula go together into the vein, the cannula is then advanced a little way, and the needle removed. Although both the cannulae and the needles are intended to be disposable, you can sterilise them and reuse them. They have been a great advance. The large size is for giving blood to adults, the middle size for solutions and the small ones for children, or for drug infusions.

• *NEEDLE, hypodermic, short bevel, 3×40 mm, one hundred.* This is a wide—short—bevel needle for resuscitation. Although these needles are less satisfactory than the cannulae—outside—needles described above, they are much cheaper. With one of these needles, you can pour fluid into a shocked patient fast. Try always to keep some in stock. A drip through one of these large needles is much better than trying to use two smaller ones.

• *NEEDLE, diaphragm, intravenous 0.9 mm, "Venflon" pattern, five only.* This provides the patient with an "open vein", and is highly economic because it saves fluids by removing the need to put up a drip merely to inject drugs. It is much more satisfactory than a syringe and needle strapped to a vein. You can stop blood clotting in the needle by filling it with ½ ml of 1:1000 heparin (500 units).

• *NEEDLE, winged, intravenous, assorted sizes, ten only.* This is a cheap and convenient way of maintaining an open vein; use it for slow—running infusions of crystalloids. If you insert it skillfully and don't leave it in too long, you can use the same vein repeatedly. But a winged needle does not run fast and easily penetrates the wall of a vein.

INTRAVENOUS LINES

Methods for cannulating a patient's subclavian and internal jugular veins are described in Section 19.2.

PUNCTURE

You can use much the same method with an ordinary hypodermic needle, a winged needle or a diaphragm needle. The method for a cannula is slightly different.

If possible, chose a vein in the patient's left arm (if he is right handed), unless you are inserting a cannula, or he is an infant. Choose a vein you can feel in one of the preferred sites in Fig. 15-3, preferably his cephalic vein, because it does not need a splint. Try to leave his arm free, and don't put the needle over a joint. Avoid his antecubital fossa and the veins of his leg if you can—they have thick walls, and they easily go into spasm, become infected or thrombosed.

Make the vein dilate by applying a rubber tube, or a

INSERTING AN INTRAVENOUS CANNULA

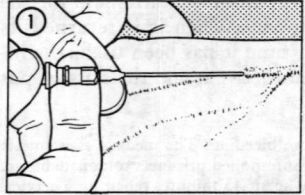
Push the needle through the skin at the side of the vein.

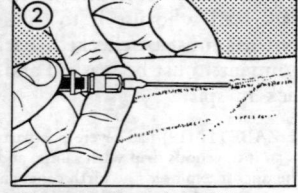
Depress the point of the needle so that it enters the vein.

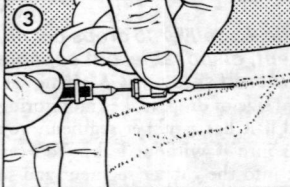
Hold the needle steady while you push the cannula further up the vein.

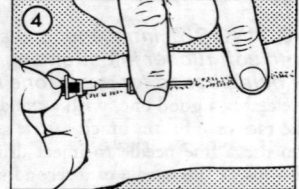
Press the skin over the cannula with your finger.

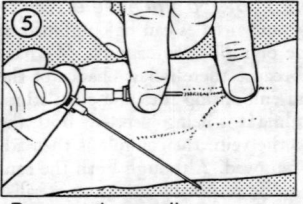
Remove the needle, and connect up the drip set

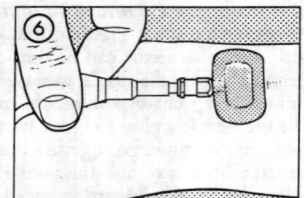
Apply a small sterile dressing.

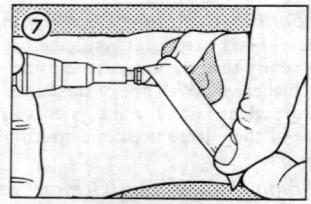
Fix the cannula with strapping.

Fig. 15-2 INSERTING AN INTRAVENOUS CANNULA
The tourniquet is not shown. Kindly contributed by John Farman

Push the cannula through the skin along the side of the vein, with the bevel upwards (1). Move the cannula so that its point lies over the vein.

Depress the point of the cannula so as to enter the vein, and push the needle a little way up it (2). Blood will flow back into the needle hub, confirming that the tip is in the vein.

Hold the needle steady, while you push the cannula a little further still up the vein (3). The point of the needle will now lie inside the cannula, where it cannot puncture the vein.

Remove the tourniquet.

Press the skin over the tip of the cannula with your finger (4), so as to prevent blood escaping. Remove the needle, connect the drip set, and lock it in place (5).

INTRAVENOUS LINES

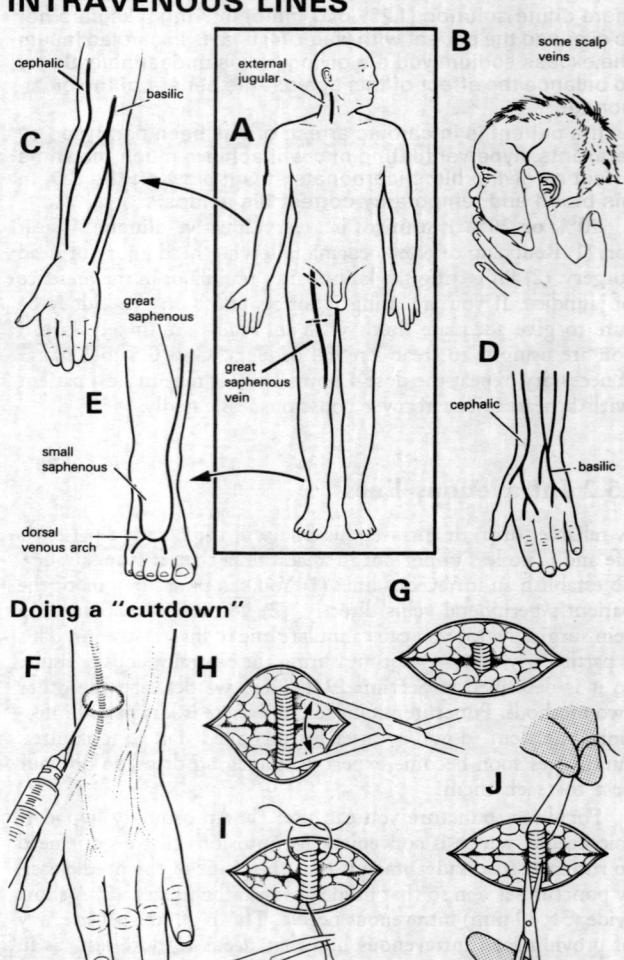

Fig. 15-3 INTRAVENOUS LINES. A, the main sites. B, in a very young child you may be able to use a scalp vein. C, the front of the arm. D, the back of the forearm and hand. E, the ankle. F, doing a cut–down on the hand. G, a transverse incision. H, exposing the vein. I, inserting the ligatures. J, opening the vein. K, the V–shaped nick. L, opening the nick. M, opening the flap of the 'V' to insert the cannula. N, the final cut–down. *Partly after Hamilton Bailey with kind permission.*

sphygmomanometer inflated to 30 mm of mercury to the arm, proximal to the puncture site. Look for a vein. If necessary, flick it to make it dilate. If you cannot find a vein, try warming the arm in warm water, with or without the tube on. Clean the patient's skin with iodine.

Using a fine (0.5 mm) needle, raise a small wheal with local anaesthetic solution intradermally beside the vein. If the local anaesthetic obscures the vein, press firmly on the skin to disperse the solution. The vein will then stand out again. Push the needle through the anaesthetized skin, then *with a separate movement* bring it over and into his vein.

If you use the external jugular vein, compress it just above the clavicle to make it distend. A needle here is uncomfortable and difficult to secure.

NEEDLE–INSIDE–CANNULA

Raise a wheal with anaesthetic solution, as above.

Try to prevent the vein from moving under the patient's skin when you puncture it. Do this by using the thumb of your free hand to pull his skin taught, so that it stretches longitudinally. Don't pull at right angles across the vein, because this will make it collapse.

Apply a small sterile dressing to the puncture site (6). Fix the cannula or needle firmly with strapping, making sure it lies along the line of the vein. Loop the tubing to prevent it being pulled out (7).

CAUTION! (1) If you are using a cannula–inside–needle, and leaving the needle in place, splint it with care to prevent the needle cutting the cannula. (2) With all methods, cover the skin puncture with gauze, and keep any adhesive strapping well away. It may promote infection. (3) Don't touch the sterilized puncture site or the cannula with your fingers.

"A CUT-DOWN"

INDICATIONS (1) When direct puncture has failed or looks impossible. (2) Hypovolaemic shock when the veins are tightly constricted and the patient requires a large intravenous line urgently. (3) Nurses who cannot be relied upon to look after drips through needles or cannulae.

CUT-DOWN SET (1) Dissecting forceps, Adsons, 120 mm, fairly fine with one into two teeth. (2) 2 skin hooks (Gillies). In infants skin hooks are the only appropriate retractors. (3) Sharp-pointed stitch scissors. (4) Scalpel handle No. 5, with No. 11 blade. (3) 2 fine curved haemostats (Halsteads). (4) 2 fine straight haemostats (Halsteads). (5) Small needle holder. (6) 2 straight, fine, cutting needles. (7) 2 lengths of fine polythene tube into which a suitably sized intramuscular Luer needle has been pushed. (8) Spool of 4/0 monofilament for the skin. (9) Spool of 3/0 chromic catgut for the vein. (10) 5 ml syringe. (11) 2 ml syringes for local anaesthesia. (12) If possible, also a pair of fine, curved pointed scissors, and fine non-toothed forceps.

METHOD Use any of the veins shown in Fig. 15-3 as being suitable for direct puncture, particularly the cephalic or basilic veins, or, if necessary, the long saphenous vein 2.5 to 3 cm in front of the medial malleolus.

Use: (1) The largest cannula you can easily insert; you can easily slow a fast flow, but it is more difficult to speed a slow one. (2) The cannula from a needle and cannula combination. Or, (3) any suitable piece of sterile plastic tube, including that of the drip set itself, as described below.

Apply a proximal tourniquet to make the patient's vein swell. Clean and drape the site. Make a 2.5 cm transverse wheal over the vein (F), and cut a 1.5 cm incision in this (G), spread the edges of the incision to expose the vein (H), pass two ligatures round it (I), tie the distal one, and leave the proximal one loose.

With fine scissors make a small V-shaped nick in the vein (J and K), using the proximal ligature to hold the vein while you do so. The main difficulty is to avoid cutting the whole vein. Enlarge each side of the V a little by passing one of the blades of the scissors into it (L). Pick up the tip of the V with forceps, and, holding the vein with the distal ligature, insert the catheter (M). Ideally, insert it through a small distal stab wound. Secure it with monofilament sutures (N).

To remove the tube, pull hard.

Alternatively, don't tie the vein distally and hope that it will recanalise.

USING THE TUBE OF A GIVING SET FOR A CUT-DOWN

The tube of a disposable giving set will be sterile inside its package. If you cut it obliquely, close to the distal adaptor, the pointed end makes an excellent large bore cannula for use in a large vein, especially if the patient is severely shocked. This is a very convenient method and is not used as often as it should be.

Cut down on your chosen vein, dilate the V-shaped slit with the beak of mosquito forceps, and push the tube of the giving set into it. The great saphenous vein, as it runs up the thigh, is particularly convenient for this method. Cut down on it 10 cm distal to the saphenous opening. If a patient is severely shocked and on the point of death after a severe injury, this is one of the most effective ways of getting fluid into him fast.

Alternatively, and less satisfactorily, make an incision in the crease just distal to the patient's inguinal ligament, deepen it to expose his saphenous vein, pick it up, cannulate it, and thread the cannula through into his femoral vein. This useful in severe burns, but it is a very easily infected site.

To attach a new giving set, cut the tube and plug in the cannula of the new set.

DIFFICULTIES WITH INTRAVENOUS LINES

If the cannulated vein becomes painful and you can feel a red cord running proximally from the site of the drip, thrombophlebitis has developed. For maintenance infusions minimise this risk by using fine needles, changing them regularly, and using them for short periods only.

CAUTION! Don't let a peripheral infusion run for more than 24 hours without changing it. Prolonged infusions are best done with a central cannula, or with needles and puncture sites that are changed regularly.

If the patient develops rigors immediately the drip starts, or soon after a fresh bottle has been put up, he is probably having a pyrogenic reaction to the intravenous fluid—change the bottle. This is rare with fluids made under ideal conditions, but is less rare with fluids made with the plant in Appendix A.

If the patient develops fever, rigors and sweating after the infusion has been running fo some hours or days, he may be septicaemic. One probable source of infection is the puncture site. Take a blood culture, remove the intravenous cannula, and then start antibiotics—the endemic hospital staphylococcus will probably be responsible. Minimise this risk by: (1) inserting intravenous lines aseptically, (2) anchoring needles and cannulae firmly so that they do not move, (3) keeping the puncture site clean and dry and not spilling fluids on it.

15.3 Replacing fluid before operating—surgical dehydration

If a patient's fluid and electrolyte state is disturbed, and you don't correct it before you operate, he is at greatly increased risk. Each kind of patient has his own particular needs. For example, fit adults for elective surgery need only water, but babies need milk. Bleeding, shocked, hypovolaemic patients have very special requirements (16.7).

This section tells you how to manage the common and important group of patients who arrive in hospital having lost much fluid, and whose electrolytes are severely depleted, as the result of diarrhoea or vomiting or the accumulation of fluid in their obstructed or atonic guts. They may have intestinal obstruction or peritonitis. They have substantial deficits of water, sodium and potassium, which you must replace quickly before you can operate on them safely.

Fortunately, you can correct a patient's electrolyte state very satisfactorily by following a few simple rules, without the need for a flame photometer to measure the serum electrolytes. The regime that follows is energetic and safe. First it restores his blood volume, then it promotes an osmotic diuresis that allows his kidneys to correct his acidosis, and so make the final correction to his electrolytes.

How much fluid does a surgically dehydrated patient need? The first step is to find out if the patient's dehydration is mild, moderate or severe, and to use this as a guide to the fluid he needs. The same clinical degree of dehydration produces a much greater percentage fluid loss in a child, so his age, and more particulary his weight, are important. His fluid needs are given in Chart A in Fig. 15-4, which shows the volume of fluid you must give to correct isotonic dehydration in mild, moderate, and severe dehydration. The fluid requirements shown in this figure are low rather than high, and a patient may need more fluid than this figure indicates. Give him half his fluid needs in the first hour and the other half in the next 4 hours.

ALPHONSE (18) was admitted severely dehydrated and moribund with a 4–day history of peritonitis. Looking at Fig. 15-4 and estimating his weight to be 50 kg, he was seen to need between four and five litres of fluid. He was given 2½ litres in the first hour and another 2½ litres during the next 4 hours after which he recovered rapidly.

Assess the severity of a patient's dehydration according to the following criteria:

Mild dehydration. These are the patients whose history indicates that they must be dehydrated, but who do not yet show any signs of it. For example, an adult who has had no fluid for 24 hours will be mildly dehydrated, but a child will be similarly dehydrated after only 12 hours. A patient in this state has lost about 5% of his body weight.

Moderate dehydration. In addition to having some reason for his dehydration, the patient with moderate dehydration also has a dry mouth, somewhat sunken eyes, and moderate reduction of his skin elasticity. A child may be restless or irritable, or abnormally quiet and drowsy. His systolic blood pressure may be low, or it may be normal. Vasoconstriction may enable the patient to compensate for a low blood volume, so that his blood pressure remains above 100 mm Hg until dehydration is severe. He has lost about 8% of his body weight.

Severe dehydration. A severely dehydrated patient has a very dry mouth, severely sunken eyes, and greatly reduced skin elasticity. An adult may be confused and a child delirious, comatose or shocked. Circulatory failure makes the patient's hands and feet cold and lowers his blood pressure. He has lost 10% or more of his body weight.

What fluid should you give a patient to correct his initial dehydration? A surgically dehydrated patient has lost water out of proportion to his losses of sodium and chloride. He will also have also lost potassium. As Fig. 15-4 shows, he needs about 100 mmol of sodium for every litre of water you replace. The easiest way to give him sodium and water in this proportion is to give him *the first half of his deficit as Ringer's lactate (or 0.9% saline), and the second half as alternate bottles of Ringer's lactate (or 0.9% saline) and 5% dextrose.* The most convenient way of giving him potassium is to add 10 mmol of

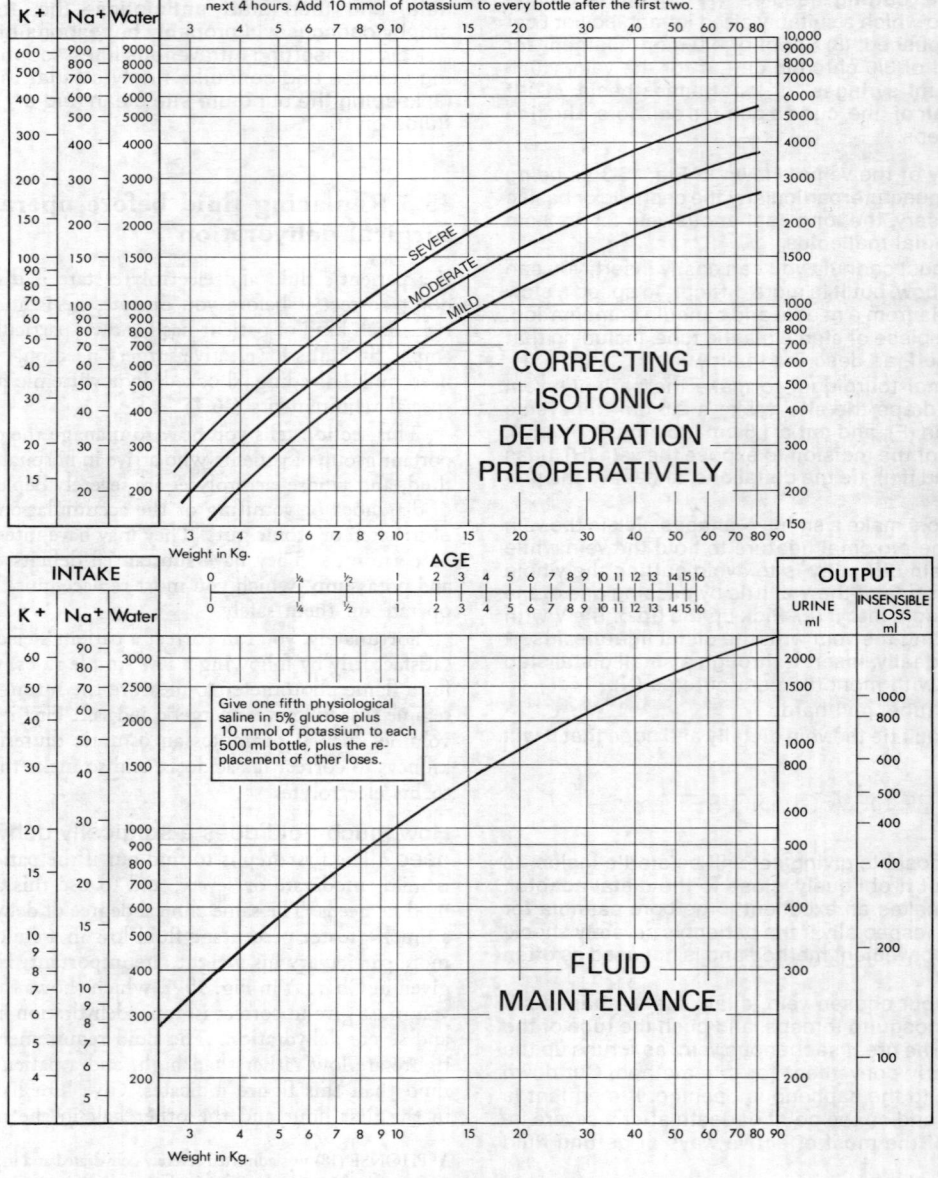

Fig. 15-4 TWO CHARTS FOR FLUID THERAPY. There is a second copy of this figure at the end of the book to tear out and paste up in the ward. *Kindly contributed by Peter Bewes*

potassium chloride to each 500 ml bottle of fluid after the first two, that is after about 15 ml/kg of fluid. The easiest way to give 10 mmol of potassium is to give him 10 ml of a solution of 1 mmol/ml.

This regime replenishes a patient's estimated sodium and water deficit satisfactorily, but only about a third of his potassium deficit. The immediate replacement of all the potassium he has lost would be dangerous without careful monitoring.

If a patient is severely dehydrated and also has panting respiration and an acid urine and, he is probably acidotic; so give him part, or, in very severe cases, all the fluid he needs as 1.2% sodium bicarbonate. Alternatively, give him part or all the fluid needs as 5% dextrose, and give him 1 mmol/kg of sodium bicarbonate. He will also need potassium as above.

Measuring a patient's serum electrolyte concentrations has its shortcomings, because they don't indicate the total electrolyte stores of his body, so that he can have a large deficit and yet his serum concentrations can be normal. In practice, knowing his electrolyte concentrations or blood urea would not be of great value, even if you could measure them. His blood urea will certainly be high if he is severely dehydrated, and it does not necessarily mean that he is in renal failure. His plasma sodium might be high, normal or low, so this would be of little help initially. It is a good working rule under these circumstances, that giving fluid with an approximately normal sodium value will keep a normal value normal, it will raise a low value, and it will lower a high one.

A patient's serum potassium is falsely high initially, due to potassium leaking out of his injured cells. But, as soon as he is rehydrated, this potassium will return to his cells and his plasma potassium will fall. But his body's total potassium stores will still be depleted, so you will have to replenish them.

If necessary, you can give Ringer's lactate only, but if so, the patient may need frusemide to promote a final diuresis and to correct his electrolyte imbalance.

If you can measure a patient's serum electrolytes, they will give you some measure of his electrolyte derangement, and later of your success in correcting it. *Don't delay operating because you cannot measure them, or because you have not got the results back.*

A COMMON ERROR IS TO GIVE ALL FLUID AS "SALINE"

How fast should you give the fluid? Severely dehydrated patients are often rehydrated too slowly. You must rehydrate them fast enough. *Give a patient half his total requirements intravenously during the first hour.* Give him the rest over the next 3 or 4 hours.

A patient's urinary output, as measured through an indwelling catheter, is a good indicator of how successful you are in rehydrating him. Observe his jugular venous pressure carefully. Or, observe his central venous pressure, as in Fig. 19.2. It should only rise 2 or 3 cm of water. If there is a sudden sustained rise of more than this, slow the drip.

If you rehydrate patients energetically like this, you should be able to operate on all of them within 4 hours of admission, and certainly within 6 hours. The only common exceptions are patients with pyloric stenosis. But these patients are not surgical emergencies, and they will not die during the 2 or 3 days that you need to prepare them for surgery.

DIFFICULTIES IN PREOPERATIVE FLUID REPLACEMENT

If a severely dehydrated patient has a haematocrit of less than 36% on admission, or his haemoglobin is less than 12 g/dl, he is certainly severely anaemic. His haemoglobin is falsely high, due to the great haemoconcentration that occurs in severe dehydration. So give him some of his initial fluid as whole blood.

If he has had peritonitis for two days or more, or he is malnourished or has liver disease, his plasma proteins will be low. If you give him an electrolyte infusion fast, he is at risk of pulmonary oedema, which can develop without a change in his central venous pressure. If possible, give him plasma or blood, or less satisfactorily 15 ml/kg of dextran 70.

If intravenous fluids are scarce or absent, use oral or rectal fluids where you can (15.5).

If a patient has intestinal obstruction and by mistake he has been given 0.18% saline in 4.3% dextrose, or 5% dextrose, he is likely to be seriously short of sodium and probably needs 0.9% saline given slowly to treat his sodium depletion. Hyponatraemia can cause fits, and both hyponatraemia and hypokalaemia can cause ileus.

CAUTION! Any drip of dextrose in water, when given on the wrong indications, can lead to water intoxication.

15.4 Replacing fluid during the operation

A patient who is not dehydrated needs no extra fluids if his operation is short and he will be eating later in the day. But if he is to have any kind of laparotomy, he needs a drip. If this is an emergency, a drip is an essential part of his pre–operative preparation. Not only will it enable you to give him fluid in a hurry, but you can also give him drugs more easily. It is one of the "Ten Golden Rules" described in Section 3.1 for all but the most minor anaesthetics.

Replacing insensible loss at open abdominal surgery. At least 2 square metres of warm moist surface line an adult's

FLUID-BALANCE CHART

Hosp. Reg. Number: 987461
Surname: JOAB MUTUMBI
Other Names: AGNES
Address: Mitobeka's village, Kilimanjaro district
Date of Birth: 5.1.81. Sex: M
Clinic/Ward: SICU

Date (as at 8.00 am): 6.3.82

PRESCRIPTION Fluid to be given: 13 kg. child

ORAL — Type of fluid: nil — Amount — Ml/hr
OTHER — Type of fluid: nil — Amount — Ml/hr

Time	INTAKE Intravenous Fluid type	Ml.	Intravenous Fluid type	Ml.	Oral Fluid	Ml.	Other Ml.	OUTPUT Urine Ml.	Gastr. Cont. Ml.	Faeces Ml.	Other Ml.	Time
8 am	Dext. 10%	300	Dext. 10%	300								8 am
9	NaCl mmol	9	NaCl mmol	9								9
10	KCl "	6	KCl "	6				20				10
11												11
noon								100				noon
1 pm												1 pm
2	Dext. 10%	300	Dext. 10%	300				20				2
3	NaCl mmol	9	NaCl mmol	9								3
4	KCl "	6	KCl "	6								4
5								100				5
6												6
7												7
8	Dext. 10%	300	Dext. 10%	300				60				8
9	NaCl mmol	9	NaCl mmol	9								9
10	KCl "	4	KCl "	4								10
11												11
mn								130				mn
1 am												1 am
2	Dext. 10%	300	Dext. 10%	300				20				2
3	NaCl mmol	9	NaCl mmol	9								3
4	KCl "	4	KCl "	4								4
5												5
6												6
7								210				7
8	Dext. 10%	300										

INTRAVENOUS: 1256   ORAL   OTHER   Urine: 540 Gastr. Cont.: 120 Faeces   Other

24hr. total intake = 1256 Ml.   24hr. total output = 660 Ml.

Fig. 15-5 A PRACTICAL FLUID BALANCE CHART

peritoneal cavity. All the time that his abdomen is open this surface is losing water. Each time his bowel is handled, however gently, it becomes slightly oedematous. To keep pace with this fluid loss, and in addition to replacing any blood the patient loses, *give him 15 ml/kg of fluid during the first hour of the operation, and 8 ml/kg/hour after that.* This is the minimum, if he is hypotensive, give more. If you give alternate bottles of Ringer's lactate and 5% dextrose, his electrolytes will look after themselves.

Replacing blood loss. A patient's normal blood volume is 80 ml/kg. Watch how much blood he is losing. If possible, weigh the blood soaked swabs on kitchen scales, and subtract the weight of an equal number of dry ones. Measure the volume of blood in the sucker bottle. A cold skin from vasoconstriction, a thready pulse, and hypotension are signs that the patient has lost more than 10% of his blood volume. An adult can compensate for a loss of up to about 1 litre (about 20% of his blood volume) without a blood transfusion, but only provided his haemoglobin before the operation was at least 10 g/dl.

Replace the blood you estimate has been lost with one and half times as much fluid. When more than one litre has been lost, replace further losses with blood. If a patient's blood pressure falls during the operation, go to Section 4.4.

15.5 Fluids after the operation

If a patient who has had an operation is not given adequate fluids and electrolytes, he will not live long. If he is about 60 kg, he will need sufficient fluid to replace the following volumes of water he loses: urine 1000 ml, water vapour from his lungs 400 ml, evaporation from his skin 900 ml (more if the weather is hot and he sweats much), stools 200 ml (more if he has diarrhoea). This adds up to about 2,500 ml in all. In a moderately hot climate, be safe and reckon that he needs 3 litres (for a very hot one, see below). This is the fluid for *maintenance* and is best replaced by mouth. But the patient may be nauseated and vomit as the result of the anaesthetic; he may be drowsy; and he may have ileus. So you may have to give him fluid intravenously.

If you have managed his fluids correctly before and during the operation, and he has no abnormal losses, he now needs only: (1) maintenance fluids (about 3 litres in a moderately hot climate) until he can drink. But: (2) If he had any *losses before the operation began* that you have not replaced, you will have to replace them now. (3) You will also have to to replace any *continuing losses* that he may have, for example, through nasogastric suction, or through fistulae.

If you don't give a patient enough fluid, his kidneys will be unable to excrete urine, so that he will become uraemic, and his skin and mucosae will become dry and more liable to infection. He will become dehydrated and will show the signs of dehydration described in Section 15.3. His circulating blood volume will fall, and he will go into peripheral circulatory failure and shock.

The fluid maintenance chart in Fig. 15-4 is calculated on the assumption that in a temperate climate, a patient needs to pass 1 ml/kg/hour or about 25 ml/kg/day of urine to eliminate waste products, which is about 1500 ml for a 60 kg man. *In practice, to allow for the water he loses through his lungs and in his sweat, he needs about 2500 ml and in a hot climate 3000 ml. This is the minimum daily intravenous fluid requirement for an adult surgical patient who is having no fluids by mouth.* It is about 4% of his weight. A child's needs are proportionately greater and are shown in the figure. The figures for insensible loss are for moderately hot climates. In very hot weather, or during fever, an adult may need 4 litres of fluid a day or more.

A patient also needs about 1 mmol/kg/day of sodium. Water and sodium in about this proportion are most easily provided in the form of 0.18% saline in 4.3% dextrose.

To know if you are giving a patient enough fluid, be guided by: (1) His urine output. If an adult's kidneys are producing 30 to 60 ml (preferably 60 ml) an hour, they are being adequately perfused. For a 60 kg adult, 60 ml/hour is 1 ml/kg/hour, or about 1500 ml/day. 20 ml/hour is the *absolute* minimum. (2) His urine specific gravity. If this is 1.030, and he is pasing little urine, he is probably hypovolaemic. (3) Signs of dehydration, such as sunken eyes. A dry mouth is less reliable.

---
1 ml/kg/hour IS THE MINIMUM URINE OUTPUT

A patient will also be short of potassium if: (1) He is passing urine, and has been on intravenous fluids for 3 days or longer. He will lose potassium in his urine after trauma and major surgery, and you should replace it. (2) He is vomiting or has diarrhoea or a fistula. The signs of hypokalaemia include weakness, confusion, and ileus. Give potassium as described below. But if he is not passing urine, giving him potassium is likely to be unnecessary and dangerous.

The regime described below will provide a patient with enough water, sodium and potassium. It will also give him enough glucose to reduce his catabolism significantly.

A fluid balance chart will be necessary if you are going to maintain a patient's fluid and electrolyte state adequately after an operation. This must be a chart that is practical under district hospital conditions. Many hospitals find keeping even the simplest chart difficult or impossible. Even some teaching hospitals find that only the intensive care unit can maintain a fluid balance chart accurately. The chart in Fig. 15.5 has been developed over many years. There is a blank version of it at the end of the book, which you can photocopy. Use a new sheet each day, and start it at 8 a.m. Prescribe intravenous fluids in the column down the left hand side, and oral and other fluids along the top. Ask the ward staff to enter a bottle as having been given, only when it is empty. At 8 a. m. work out the input and output for the previous day. Use Fig. 15.4 to calculate the patient's insensible loss and his fluid requirements. The ward staff are more likely to fill charts in carefully if you don't use them unnecessarily and if they feel the charts are important; *so make sure you use their charts and tell them how important their charting is.* Ask ward staff to record only the volumes of fluids. They are concerned only with "ml", not "mmol". These, and any interpretations, are your concern. Make sure that they stick a strip of paper down the side of the bottle and mark where the level of the fluid should be each hour.

Measuring the patient's urine output may be difficult. When the patient is catheterized try to use a closed system and see that the bag is changed before it is full. A good method is to connect the catheter to a used fluid giving bag.

POSTOPERATIVE FLUIDS

MAINTENANCE NEEDS To replace water, sodium and some energy, give an adult 2,000 to 2,500 ml of intravenous fluid daily in a moderately hot climate. In a very hot climate give him 3000 ml or even more. Give it as: (1) 0.18% saline in 4.3% dextrose. Or, (2) one bottle of Ringer's lactate (or 0.9% saline) to 2 bottles of 5% dextrose (some surgeons give one bottle of saline to 3 or 4 bottles of 5% dextrose). Or, (3) Darrow's solution; in a very hot climate give this half strength.

If the patient has had a big operation and has been well hydrated, give him only 2000 ml in the first 24 hours; start giving him 3000 ml when his postoperative diuresis starts.

POTASSIUM If the patient is passing urine, add 10 mmol of potassium to each bottle of 4.3% dextrose in saline. Add it as 10 ml of a solution of 1 mmol/ml. Or, if you are worried about the safety of more concentrated potassium solutions, use Darrow's solution, half or full strength, depending on the climate.

CAUTION ! (1) Balance the saline or Ringer's lactate, and

the 5% dextrose you give. If you give too much sodium, the patient's kidneys may not be able to excrete it. So don't give him too much 0.9% saline or Ringer's lactate at this stage. (2) If you only give 5% dextrose, he will get water intoxication. (3) Don't give potassium if he is not passing urine. (4) The maximum maintenance dose of potassium for an adult is 80 mmol/day. (5) Don't give bolus intravenous injections of potassium—it may all reach his heart suddenly and cause cardiac arrest! (6) If the weather is very hot, he may need 4 litres of fluid or more. Give the extra fluid as 5% dextrose.

REPLACING OTHER LOSSES Replace any gastric fluid that is aspirated with an equal quantity 0.9% saline. For each 500 ml bottle of aspirate add 20 mmol of potassium to the patient's intravenous fluids. Replace any loss from diarrhoea or from an ileostomy or colostomy with half-strength Darrow's solution in 2.5% dextrose. Alternatively, calculate his losses from Fig. 15-6 and replace them with suitable volumes of solutions of sodium and potassium chloride of 1 mmol/litre.

REPLACING FLUID RECTALLY Provided that that the patient does not have diarrhoea, you can replace his post-operative fluid losses through his rectum with a solution made up in tap water. This saves sterile fluids and is particularly useful in gastric surgery. Give the fluid through a Malecot catheter into his rectum. Give him the volume shown in Fig. 15-4, as tap water containing half a teaspoonful of sodium chloride, and quarter of a teaspoonful of potassium citrate to each litre. Replace gastric losses with an equal quantity of saline (a level teaspoonful of salt in a litre of tap water), containing 20 mmol of potassium per litre.

SPECIAL TESTS If you did not adequately replace the blood a patient lost at the operation, he will have diluted his remaining blood by the first day, so measure his haemoglobin or his haematocrit. Give him blood as necessary.

STARTING ORAL FLUIDS If a patient has no nasogastric tube, try to start oral fluids on the first postoperative day, starting with small volumes and slowly increasing them.

If he does have a tube down, start oral fluids as soon as his stomach is empty, his bowel sounds have returned, and he has passed flatus. Don't change abruptly from intravenous

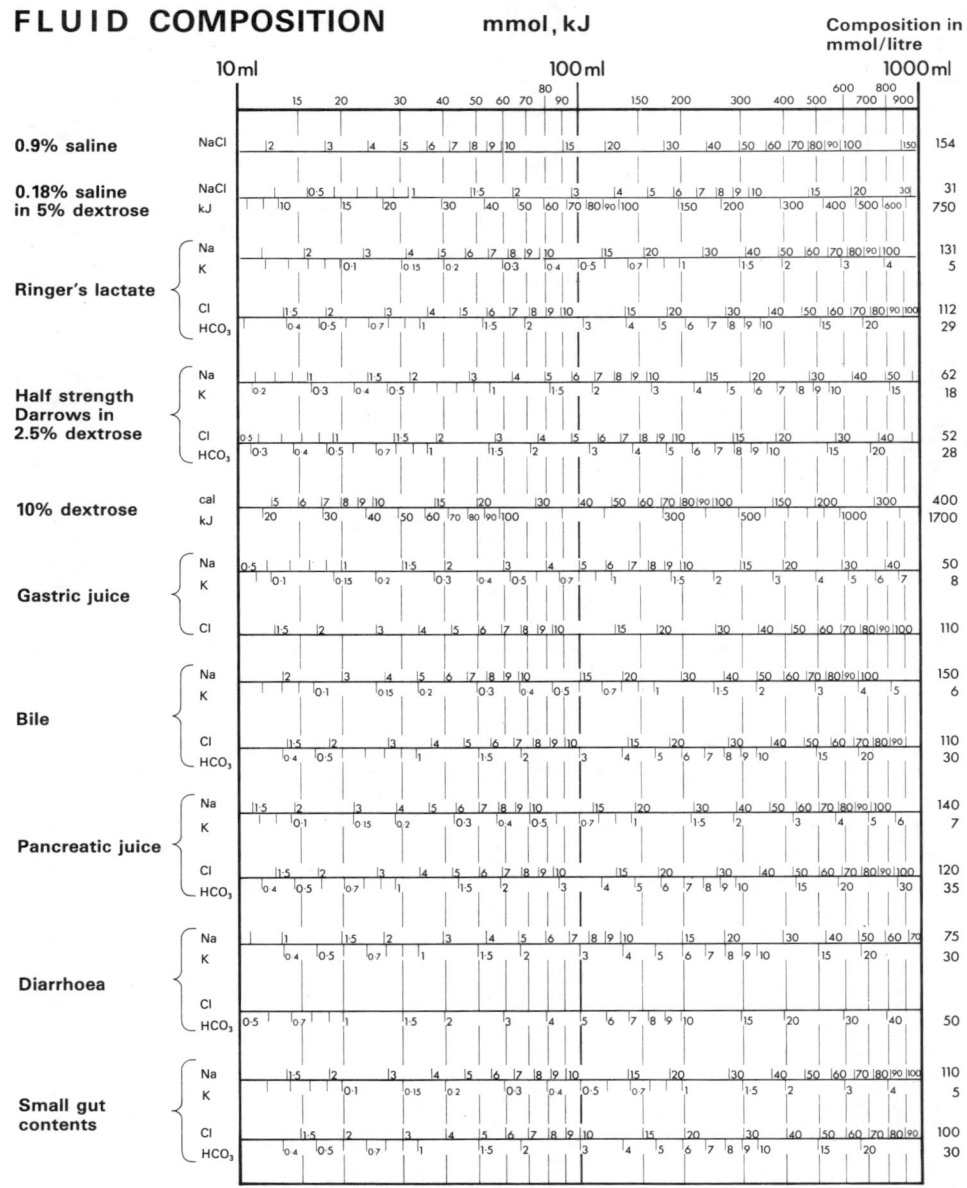

Fig. 15-6 THE COMPOSITION OF SOME IMPORTANT FLUIDS. This figure will tell you how much sodium, potassium, and bicarbonate there is in any volume of fluid between 10 ml and a litre. It will also give you the energy content of some of them. The column of figures on the right gives you their composition in mmol/litre. Use it if you want to balance a patient's intake and output somewhat more accurately than with the rule-of-thumb methods we have given here.

to oral rehydration. Reduce his intravenous fluids as you give him fluids by mouth.

Keep his drip up until the third day.

DIFFICULTIES WITH POSTOPERATIVE FLUIDS

If the patient has sacral oedema, you have probably given him too much saline.

If he has tachycardia, prominent neck veins and crepitations at his lung bases, you have overloaded him with fluid.

If his haematocrit is raised, he is haemoconcentrated.

If he has fever, there may be bacteria or pyrogens in the infusion fluid or the bottle.

If he bled severely before or during the operation be prepared to give him plenty of fluid. He may have lost far more blood than you think. Examine the filling of his peripheral veins. Cold or anxiety can also constrict them, but if they are full, he is not hypovolaemic. Watch his jugular venous pressure, or use a central venous catheter (19.2). Changes in its level are more important than its absolute value. If you watch his central venous pressure carefully, you are unlikely to overtransfuse him. A rise of jugular venous pressure of more than 12 cm above his sternal angle, with an acceptable systolic arterial pressure, shows that you have given him too much fluid. The jugular pressure of an old patient with a poor myocardium may rise above 12 cm while his arterial pressure remains low. If it does, treat him for cardiac failure and give him digitalis.

If he is not passing urine, when should you switch from active fluid replacement for hypovolaemia to fluid restriction for acute renal failure? This is a common problem and a difficult one. His blood urea is no help, and his urine output is the best guide. He should pass 1 ml/kg/hour. If he does not, he is likely to be in renal failure. Be suspicious of flows much greater than 1 ml per minute. They may show that you are over-transfusing him. The specific gravity of the urine is useful also.

16 Anaesthesia for special circumstances

16.1 The patient with the full stomach

The normal reflexes of the body keep the contents of a patient's stomach out of his lungs most effectively. One of the major risks of general anaesthesia is that it weakens or abolishes these protective reflexes, so that the food in his stomach reaches his lungs, either because he vomits actively or because he regurgitates passively. Several anaesthetic procedures, particularly intubation, are designed to prevent this disaster, and there is also some immediate treatment should vomiting or regurgitation occur.

16.2 Vomiting

Vomiting is an active process which requires that the patient uses his muscles. The danger is that he may inhale his vomit, or lumps of food may stick in his larynx. Because he has to use his muscles to vomit, he cannot vomit actively if they have been relaxed by deep anaesthesia or a relaxant. He is most likely to vomit during induction or while he is recovering from anaesthesia. If you treat him correctly, and he is lucky, he lives. If you are less skillful and he is not so lucky, he dies immediately, on the table, from asphyxia or bronchospasm, or later from the acid aspiration syndrome (16.3).

Sometimes a patient rejects his oral airway, closes his jaw tightly and vomits. If he is in the correct position with his head down, vomit drains out of his nose, or between his teeth, and away from his larynx. But if there is much vomit, he can still inhale it.

A patient with intestinal obstruction is at particular risk from inhalation of vomit, because he is already vomiting. All that is said here about preventing the inhalation of vomit applies with particular urgency to him. Above all, you must pass a nasogastric tube and leave it in place when you operate.

ADSONI (18 months) was about to have a herniorrhaphy. The operation was postponed until 11 am because of an emergency in the delivery room, and then tea time. The assistant induced him with open ether, while the doctor scrubbed up. Just as the incision was being made Adsoni retched, whereupon the doctor immediately picked him up by the ankles, and a large quantity of milk flooded onto the floor. His skin was closed and the operation postponed. His chest was clear on auscultation, he was given ampicillin prophylactically, and he recovered uneventfully. LESSONS (1) Always do elective surgery on a child early in the morning. Adsoni's mother had fed him in an unobserved moment because he was crying. (2) A child's stomach is seldom empty. (3) Picking a child up by his feet can be lifesaving. It would be useful if adults could be picked up in the same way.

If a patient shows any sign of vomiting or regurgitating, treat him like this.

IMMEDIATE TREATMENT OF VOMITING OR REGURGITATION

ADULT If an adult vomits or regurgitates, quickly lower the head of the table while you keep his chin up. To make this possible, *always* anaesthetize a patient on a table or trolley that has a head you can lower—one of the "Ten Golden Rules" in Section 3.1.

Turn the patient's head to one side. Ask as assistant to help you turn his body to one side. Suck out his throat. This is life-saving, so ALWAYS have a sucker ready AND WORKING, whenever you give an anaesthetic.

If necessary, intubate the patient, and suck through the tube. Inflate him with oxygen, a high pressure may be needed.

CAUTION ! The patient is most likely to vomit during induction, and while you are intubating him. You must always be able to turn him quickly while you are doing this. So don't restrain him in any way, or put him into stirrups, until induction and intubation are completed.

USING FERGUSSON'S GAG

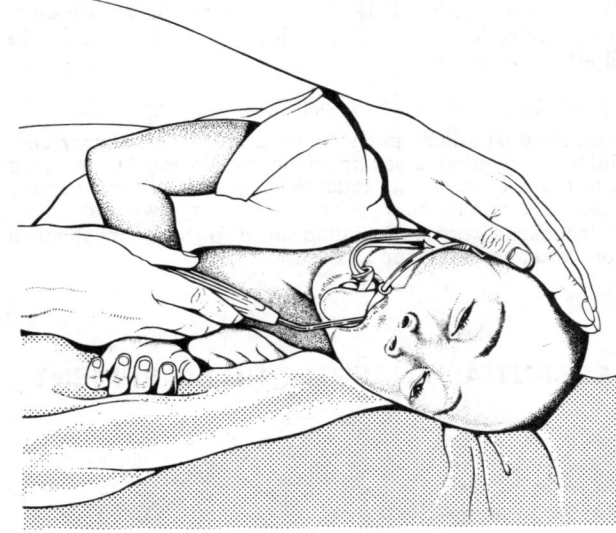

Fig. 16-1 USING FERGUSSON'S GAG ON A PATIENT WHO HAS VOMITED. **This should seldom be necessary; you can usually open his jaws by pressing behind his back teeth.** *After Brenda Vaughan, permission requested.*

CHILD If the patient is a child, pick him up by his feet, and let the vomit fall out of his mouth. Then treat him as above.

IF A PATIENT VOMITS BEHIND CLENCHED TEETH suck him out, but first you will have to open his mouth. There are several ways you can do this: (1) Put your finger behind his back teeth and force his jaws open. (2) Open his jaw by inserting the blades of a Fergusson's gag between his back teeth or behind them. Or, (3) use an anaesthetic wedge or a tongue depressor. Twist it to open his teeth enough to insert the jaws of the gag.

As soon as you have opened his mouth far enough under direct vision, suck out his pharynx.

16.3 Regurgitation

The second way in which the food and drink in a patient's stomach can get into his lungs is less dramatic, but even more dangerous. *Fluid can flow passively out of his stomach into his lungs without there being any muscular activity.* Because this fluid flows by gravity only, the patient is in particular danger when he is lying on his back in the horizontal position. The stomach is never completely empty and always contains some fluid, so *regurgitation can happen at any time, even in a paralysed patient with an "empty" stomach.* Active vomiting is always obvious, but with passive regurgitation there may be no signs, or the first sign may be a mouth and pharynx full of fluid, by which time the damage is already done. Regurgitation is more dangerous than vomiting, because it is more often overlooked.

The acid aspiration (Mendelson's) syndrome is the result of aspirated stomach contents. A patient with this syndrome develops bronchospasm, hypotension, and pulmonary oedema, either during an operation or some hours later. The contents of the stomach are always acid, so that even a small quantity of fluid can cause this syndrome and kill him. It is most common in obstetric anaesthesia, but it can happen whenever the pharyngeal and laryngeal reflexes have been lost. The only certain way to prevent it is to intubate the patient.

A way to minimise the effects of the acid aspiration syndrome is to give antacids preoperatively to all patients who are particularly likely to regurgitate. They include obstetric patients, patients with large abdominal tumours, those who give a history of regurgitation when lying down, and anyone who may have a hiatus hernia. Give an antacid such as 30 ml of magnesium trisilicate mixture, not more than 15 minutes before the operation. Lay the patient first on one side then on the other to mix his stomach contents. If he does regurgitate, his gastric secretions will be less acid, and he will be less likely to suffer the ill effects of aspiration.

TREATING THE ACID ASPIRATION SYNDROME
Intubate the patient, and give him oxygen. If necessary, control his respiration. Give him aminophylline. He will also need a broad spectrum antibiotic. Strictly limit his intravenous fluids to a minimum, or pulmonary oedema will get worse.
If necessary go on ventilating him. If you have a mechanical ventilator, you may need to use it.

ESSENTIAL ANAESTHETIC EQUIPMENT

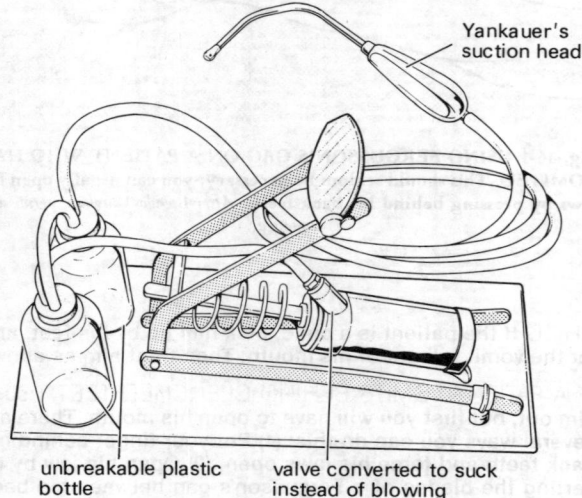

Fig. 16-2 ESSENTIAL EQUIPMENT FOR ANY ANAESTHETIC, INCLUDING KETAMINE AND "COCKTAILS". An effective sucker is one of the "Ten Golden Rules" (3.1) before any anaesthetic.

16.4 Preventing vomiting and regurgitation

There are several other ways of preventing this disaster, besides: (1) always anaesthetizing a patient on a trolley that you can tilt, and (2) always having suction ready. (3) You can starve him. (4) You can empty his stomach before operation. (5) You can anaesthetize him head down. And (6), most importantly, your assistant can apply cricoid pressure during induction.

Starve the patient If a patient is going to have a "cold" operation, you can starve him. Unfortunately, you cannot do this if he needs an urgent operation after an injury. Anxiety and pain both delay the emptying of his stomach. Trauma can also delay the emptying of of the stomach, even though the patient last ate 12 hours ago and his injury is small. Find out when he had his last meal, and assume that whatever was in his stomach at the time of the accident is still there now.

If the patient is going to have an anaesthetic, he should have had no food during the previous 6 hours, and no fluid during the previous 2 hours. Unfortunately, when nursing skills are scarce, you can seldom be sure about this. So, be wise and assume that *any patient you anaesthetize might have a full stomach.* If he has had an accident and needs an operation, there will not be time to starve him. This is where the local anaesthetic methods in Chapter six are so useful. Ideally, you should starve a patient even for these, because there is always the possibility that the local anaesthetic might fail so that he needs a general anaesthetic, or he might have a convulsion and aspirate his vomit. Starvation before local anaesthesia is however much less necessary before a general anaesthetic (3.1).

INDUCTION HEAD DOWNWARDS

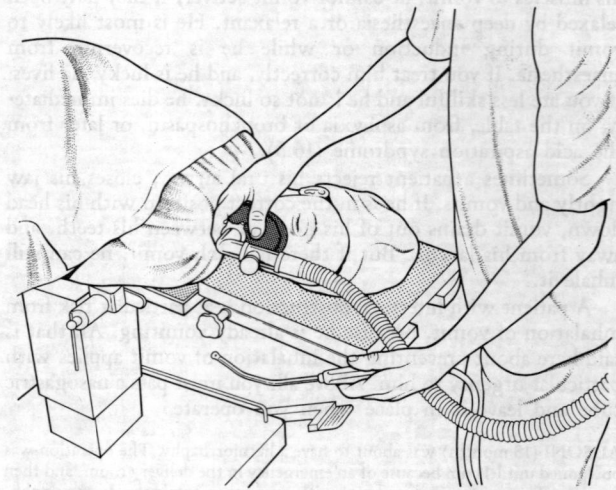

Fig. 16-3 INDUCTION HEAD DOWNWARDS. Use this method if you cannot intubate a patient. If you can intubate him, always do so, using cricoid pressure. The table is tilted, the patient's head is on his side, and the sucker is instantly ready. He is being induced with ether and has not been given thiopentone.

Empty the patient's stomach if it *might be full.* Try to empty it before you induce him. Fluid is easier to remove than food. If the patient has had an accident soon after a large meal, his stomach is sure to still be full of food. If he has intestinal obstruction or peritonitis, he will have mostly fluid in his stomach. If his gut is obstructed, the only way he can empty his stomach is to vomit. Unless you empty it for him with a tube, he is sure to come to the operation with it full. A small tube, such as a Ryle's tube, is useless for removing food from the stomach, so use a large one.

EMPTYING A PATIENT'S STOMACH

REMOVING FLUID Pass a nasogastric tube immediately before you induce a patient. Aspirate it, leave it in, and let it drain without a spigot into a bag or receiver.

REMOVING FOOD Use a large tube about 1 cm in diameter in an adult. Lubricate it and don't let the patient see it.

Tilt the table and lay him head downwards on his side, to minimise the risk of him inhaling his vomit. This is wise even if he is conscious.

Stand behind his head. Pass the tube through this mouth down into his stomach in one swift movement. If he vomits while you do this, he will vomit through and around the tube. If he does not vomit, move the tube about until he does.

CAUTION ! A stomach tube can be misleading because it may not empty his stomach completely. So leave a nasogastric tube in. But even this may leave fluid in his stomach so learn to insert a tracheal tube using cricoid pressure, as described in the next section.

ASSUME THAT EVERY EMERGENCY PATIENT HAS A FULL STOMACH

16.5 Anaesthesia with a full stomach, "crash induction"

Some patients are at special risk from vomiting or regurgitation. They include: (1) A mother having a Caesarean section, especially if her labour has been prolonged. (2) A patient with an acute abdomen, especially if his gut is obstructed. (3) *Any injured patient.*

The most dangerous method of anaesthetizing a patient with a full stomach is to give him thiopentone followed by ether, or some other inhalational anaesthetic, without cricoid pressure or intubation. If you are giving him ether only, he may vomit, but he will usually do so early on, at a stage when he still has his protective laryngeal reflexes. But if you have given him thiopentone or halothane, they will depress his protective reflexes, so that if he vomits, he will probably inhale his vomit.

The acceptable methods, if you cannot wait for a patient's stomach to empty naturally, are these.

(1) The local blocks in Chapter 6 are the safest.

(2) Subarachnoid (7.4) and epidural anaesthesia (7.2) are reasonably safe. They would be completely safe, were it not for the fact that an occasional patient does have complications, and it is during these, particularly unconciousness from a high subarachnoid in which the drug ascends to his brain stem, that he may regurgitate.

If you are going to give a patient a general anaesthetic, you can empty his stomach with a tube. Unfortunately, even this may not empty it completely, or remove the danger of aspiration entirely. So he will be safer if you combine the use of a nasogastric tube with one of these methods.

(3) *If, for any reason you cannot intubate him under suxamethonium,* you can induce him with ether head downwards. This is the easiest method.

(4) *If you can intubate a patient under thiopentone and suxamethonium,* you can ask your assistant to press on his cricoid while you do so. This will prevent him regurigitating, but not actively vomiting. It will press the patient's oesophagus against his spine, and keep it shut, so that any fluid in his oesophgus cannot escape up into his pharynx and then down into his lungs. But if this is to work, *your assistant must press firmly and continously from just before induction starts until you have inflated and clamped the cuff of the patient's tracheal tube.* If an older patient vomits actively while you do this, before you have paralysed him with suxamethonium, he can rupture his oesophagus. Fortunately, this is rare in younger patients, such as mothers having Caesearean sections.

If you are going to apply cricoid pressure and intubate a patient, the steps are to preoxygenate him, to give him atropine, to induce him with ketamine or thiopentone, and then to apply cricoid pressure, followed by suxamethonium and intubation. Finally, you can give a ketamine drip or ether or some other suitable anaesthetic. This is described below, and is probably the best method—if you can do it.

Preoxygenation is an important step. If the patient subsequently regurgitates, you have more time to suck him out before he goes blue. Preoxygenation also removes the need to ventilate him with oxygen before inserting the tracheal tube. This is important because, in ventilating him, you may blow oxygen into his stomach and displace the contents of his stomach up into his oesophagus. By itself, a stomach full of oxygen does not matter, but he will be more likely to regurgitate. When he does so, the oxygen in his stomach may bring back fluid with it.

BJORN (35) had appendicitis, and was quite certain that he had taken nothing by mouth for 12 hours. He was induced with thiopentone and then given ether, while the doctor scrubbed up. When the incision was made the blood was very dark. Strange noises were coming from the head of the table. The mask was full of vomit, and the patient's lungs too. He died from cardiac arrest. LESSONS (1) In many hospitals patients are seldom intubated, because it is thought to be too much bother, it is said to take too long, and nobody has learnt how to do it. (2) Every patient who is being operated on for an acute abdomen should be intubated.

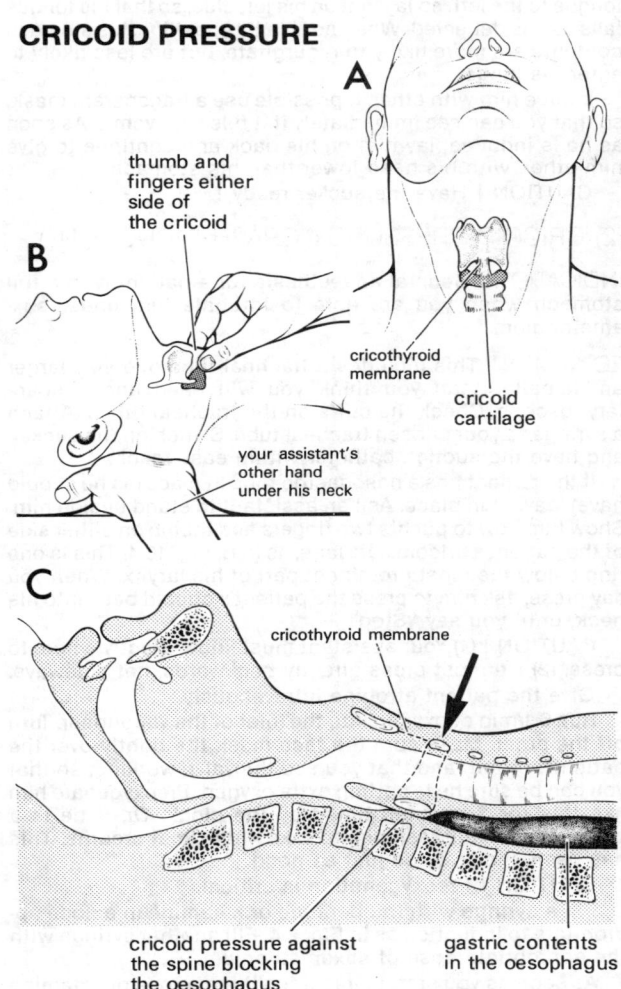

Fig. 16-4 CRICOID PRESSURE. This is one of the most life–saving methods in anaesthesia. Your assistant must know where the cricoid cartilage is, and press it from the moment induction starts, until the cuff is inflated. *Kindly contributed by Michael Wood.*

ANAESTHESIA WITH A FULL STOMACH

If you cannot wait until the patient's stomach is empty, and methods of local anaesthesia are impractical or unsuitable, anaesthetize a patient like this:—

CAUTION ! Avoid thiopentone, unless you are going to apply cricoid pressure and intubate him.

EMPTY THE PATIENT'S STOMACH Do this as described above. Many anaesthetists who are skilled at intubating under cricoid pressure don't do this routinely.

After you have emptied the patient's stomach with a large stomach tube, pass a nasogastric tube. Aspirate it and leave it in place.

CAUTION ! Make sure you aspirate the nasogastric tube just before you induce the patient, and leave the tube without a spigot during the operation. This will keep his stomach free of air and make him less likely to regurgitate.

EQUIPMENT Have a good drip running. Have suction tested and ready. Assemble all the necessary equipment.

(1) INDUCTION HEAD DOWNWARDS

INDICATIONS General anaesthesia for anyone with a full stomach, when you cannot intubate under suxamethonium.

METHOD Tilt the table 15° head downwards, so that when the patient lies on his side, the lower angle of his mouth is lower than his larynx. Don't tip the table too steeply, or he will fall onto the floor!

Most laryngoscopes are arranged to deflect a patient's tongue to the left, so lay him on his left side, so that his tongue falls as it is deflected. When he is in this position, his stomach contents are more likely to regurgitate, but are less likely to enter his lungs.

Induce him with ether. If possible use a transparent mask, so that you can see immediately if it fills with vomit. As soon as he is induced, lay him on his back and continue to give him ether, with his head lower than his stomach.

CAUTION ! Have the sucker ready !

(2) CRICOID PRESSURE ("CRASH INDUCTION")

INDICATIONS General anaesthesia for a patient with a full stomach when you are able to intubate him under suxamethonium.

EQUIPMENT This includes a tracheal tube one size larger and smaller than you think you will need and a spare laryngoscope. Check the cuffs on the tracheal tubes. Attach a syringe to your chosen tracheal tube. Switch on the sucker, and have the suction catheter within easy reach.

If the patient has a nasogastric tube in place (as he should have) leave it in place. Ask an assistant to stand beside him. Show him how to put his two fingers and thumb on either side of the patient's cricoid cartilage, as in B, Fig. 16-4. This is one ring below the most prominent part of his larynx. When you say press, ask him to press the patient's cricoid back into his neck, until you say "Stop".

CAUTION ! (1) Your assistant must know exactly where to press. (2) He must press directly backwards, not sideways.

Give the patient atropine intravenously.

Run 6 1/min of oxygen into the inlet of the vapouriser. Turn off the ether. Make sure the face mask fits tightly over the patient's mouth and that you see the valve working, so that you can be sure he is getting extra oxygen. Preoxygenate him like this for 3 minutes timed by the clock. Or, if he is a cooperative adult, ask him to take 4 maximal breaths. This has been shown to be just as good.

CAUTION ! Preoxygenation is critical.

Fill a syringe with thiopentone or ketamine in a dose appropriate to induction as in Fig. 2-4. Fill another syringe with the appropriate dose of suxamethonium.

As soon as you start to inject the thiopentone or ketamine say "Press". Give the rest of the thiopentone, and then the suxamethonium quickly.

Don't wait until the eyelash reflex has gone or waste time testing for it. Don't try to ventilate the patient manually. When he stops breathing, remove the mask. Open his mouth, but do not try to insert the laryngoscope or try to intubate him until his tongue has stopped fasciculating, showing that he is completely relaxed. If you intubate him too early, he will cough and vomit.

As soon as his tongue has stopped fasciculating, intubate him, and blow up the cuff. Check the air entry into both sides of his chest. Only now, say to your assistant "Stop pressing".

Give him ether (11.3).

If at any time he looks as if he is going to vomit, turn him onto his side, relax cricoid pressure and let him vomit.

COUGH EXTUBATION At the end of the operation, suck out the patient's pharynx, using a laryngoscope to enable you to see what you are removing.

Turn him onto his left side, with the table still tipped 15° head downwards. Inflate his chest. Quickly let down the cuff of the tracheal tube. Pull out the tracheal tube while his chest is still full of air. He will cough and in doing so remove any secretions that may be around the lower end of the tube.

ALL INJURED PATIENTS HAVE FULL STOMACHS!

16.6 Obstetric anaesthesia

Until a mother has been delivered, you have two people to anaesthetize—her and her baby. Both have their anaesthetic problems. Besides having a large mass in her abdomen, she also has a high gastrin level, which makes her stomach contents more acid than normal. This, and fact that her stomach is likely to be full, means that she is at particular risk from the acid aspiration syndrome. She may also be dehydrated and anaemic. Her baby will soon need to breathe, so you have to be careful about giving her drugs that might depress his respirations. But once she is delivered, you can give her what she needs, including pethidine (2.9) or gallamine, without any fear that it will endanger him. Although Caesarean section is the most common obstetric occasion for anaesthesia, any difficult delivery may require one.

Pregnant women are also at risk from another important syndrome.

The supine hypotensive syndrome A mother at term who is conscious automatically adjusts her position, if she is allowed to, so that the weight of her uterus does not press on her aorta or her inferior vena cava. But if she is anaesthetized and put flat on her back, her uterus will press on these vessels and obstruct the flow in them. The blood that pools in the lower part of her body reduces the flow to her heart, so that her cardiac output falls. She tries to compensate by constricting her peripheral blood vessels. But she is unable to do this adequately, so her blood pressure falls. Her uterine blood flow also falls, and her baby becomes anoxic, particularly if there is also placental insufficiency. Occasionally, she dies suddenly from cardiac arrest. This syndrome is also the most important cause of difficulty in resuscitating a depressed baby after Caesaran section. If you tilt your mothers to the side, you will notice a marked improvement in the condition of their babies after delivery.

So, prevent the supine hypotensive syndrome by always tilting a pregnant mother 15° to the left, either by tilting the table or by putting a pillow or wedge under her right buttock, as in Fig. 16-5.

If a mother is hypotensive, and is not bleeding, don't start to anaesthetize her until her blood pressure is normal. If tilting her to the left does not restore the blood pressure, try tilting her to the right.

Beware of the mother with a pulse of 140 to 160, who is a little sweaty and who feels nauseated or is vomiting. Although her blood pressure may be normal, she has signs of a reduced cardiac output, and is trying to compensate for it. If you induce her without trying to correct the syndrome, she may suffer from severe hypotension, and perhaps cardiac arrest.

If the mother's blood pressure falls during the operation, ask an assistant to lift her uterus or move it to one side. You will notice the improvement. The final danger period is when the surgeon is applying fundal pressure. If the uterine incision is too small, and he presses hard for longer than is necessary, the sydrome can arise again.

THE SUPINE HYPOTENSIVE SYNDROME

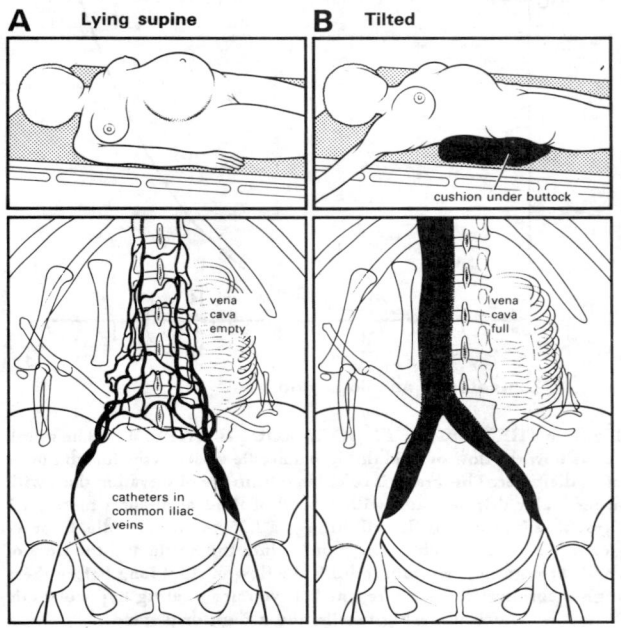

Fig. 16-5 THE SUPINE HYPOTENSIVE SYNDROME. These are both venograms. A, the mother is lying on her back, her uterus is occluding her vena cava, and all the blood from the lower part of her body is flowing through her paravertebral veins. B, a pillow has now been put under her right buttock tilting her to the left. Blood is now flowing normally in her vena cava. *Kindly contributed by Murray Carmichael.*

Methods of local and regional anaesthesia have been discussed in Section 6.9 (local anaesthesia), and Section 7.2 (lumbar epidural anaesthesia). You can use an epidural block for an assisted vaginal delivery or for Caesarean section. An epidural block removes the pain of labour completely; it is a useful aid in correcting abnormal uterine action; it is excellent in a high–risk labour needing manipulation in the second stage and it will allow you to do a symphysiotomy painlessly. But an epidural block increases the need for instrumental delivery in the second stage; it needs monitoring by a highly trained midwife; and it increases the risk of the supine hypotensive syndrome. One of the disadvantages of epidural anaesthesia is that it takes at least 15 minutes longer than general anaesthesia, so it is contraindicated if the mother needs caesarean section in a hurry.

The standard type of subarchnoid anaesthesia for a lower abdominal operation is dangerous for Caesarean section because it aggravates the supine hypotensive syndrome, so that an occasional mother "dies on the table". This typically happens when the operator, having given the patient a subarachnoid anaesthetic, and without having tilted her, or preloaded her with saline, goes to scrub up. When he looks round again, she is dead. The best method of subarachnoid anaesthesia for Caesarean section is the "augmented saddle block" (7.7). One of its advantages is that it is very safe for the baby.

The important measures for preventing the complications of epidural or subarachnoid anaesthesia are: (1) to use the saddle block method of subarachnoid anaesthesia, (2) to prevent supine hypotension with a left lateral tilt, as in Fig. 16-5, (3) to preload a mother with a litre of fluid intravenously, and (4) to be able to intubate and ventilate her when necessary. With these precautions both subarachnoid and epidural anaesthesia are much safer.

Ketamine anaesthesia is discussed in Section 8.1. You can, if absolutely necessary, do a Caesarean section under ketamine alone. This is not ideal, because by itself ketamine produces no muscular relaxation. Ketamine raises the blood pressure, so a ketamine drip with relaxants (8.4) is suitable for most pregnant mothers, except those suffering from severe hypertension, and its complications, and those in cardiac failure. It is also contraindicated in eclamptics and psychotics.

General anaesthesia is our main concern here. If you use ether alone, the baby will be very sleepy; but this is not a major disadvantage if you can resuscitate him actively and intubate him. Stimulating him to make him breathe is useless, because he is already receiving more than enough stimulation from a hostile world. He needs intubating and ventilating soon!

There are several acceptable alternatives for general anaesthesia in obstetrics, depending on your skill.

(1) If you cannot intubate the mother, induce and maintain her with ether using a mask. Induce her while she is lying on her side, with the table tilted, as shown in Fig. 16-3.

(2) If you can intubate her and have the necessary equipment, the best anaesthetic is described below. It is similar to that already described for a full stomach (16.5), and consists of atropine, preoxygenation, cricoid pressure, thiopentone or ketamine, suxamethonium, intubation and the minimum amount of ether. Relaxation is obtained, either with more suxamethonium in successive small doses or with a long–acting relaxant. Remember that oxytocin potentiates the action of suxamethonium, so that paralysis may last 20 minutes. The use of suxamethonium in these circumstances therefore needs skill.

CORRECT DEHYDRATION BEFORE YOU OPERATE

GENERAL ANAESTHESIA

Empty the mother's stomach with a large bore tube.

PREMEDICATION give her 20 ml of magnesium trisilicate as soon as possible before the operation, and have her roll over a few times to distribute this in her stomach.

Give her atropine 0.6 mg at the operation. Don't give her any other premedication except perhaps 10 mg of diazepam intravenously. Even this is likely to make her baby "floppy"
Put up a drip.

METHOD Tilt the table 15° to the mother's left, or place a wedge or pillows under her right hip. Check your instruments carefully. Place an introducer in the tracheal tube.

When the surgeon is ready, preoxygenate the mother and induce her with thiopentone 4 mg/kg or ketamine 1 mg/kg; then immediately give her suxamethonium 1.5 mg/kg (14.2). Intubate her while applying cricoid pressure (16-4). Thiopentone is better if she is hypertensive; ketamine is better if she is hypovolaemic or has bronchospasm.

EITHER, give her *small* increments of suxamethonium to relax her, and control her ventilation. The easiest way of doing this is to mix two (50 mg) ampoules of suxamethonium (100 mg) with 10 ml of water, and to inject 1 ml at a time.

OR, give her alcuronium, or tubocurarine or pancuronium bromide, as in Section 14.3, and reverse them with neostigmine at the end of the operation.

CAUTION ! Don't give gallamine; it crosses the placental barrier.

Keep the mother anaesthetized with an inhalation anaesthetic until delivery. If she is unpremedicated, and you are using ether, she will need 3% to 4 %. If you have premedicated her, she will only need 2% to 3%. As soon as she has been delivered, increase the ether to 10% as necessary and allow her to breathe spontaneously as the paralysis wears off.

Give her a litre a minute of extra oxygen. Don't hyperventilate her.

When the cord is clamped, give her an oxytocin drip of 5 units in 500 ml at 30 drops a minute. Avoid bolus injections of oxytocic drugs.

Extubate her while she is awake lying on her side, and when she can lift her head from her pillow, showing that she is sufficiently awake.

When she wakes from the anaesthetic, make sure she finds the baby at her breast. This will help greatly to establish the bond between them.

CAUTION! Breast feeding must start within 3 to 6 hours of birth. Its failure will be a particular disaster for him.

DIFFICULTIES WITH OBSTETRIC ANAESTHESIA

If you have tried to intubate a mother and failed, proceed as follows. We presume that you have preoxygenated her, given her thiopentone, and suxamethonium, and have applied cricoid pressure, but have been unable to pass the tube.

Check that your assistant is applying cricoid pressure correctly, and is not pushing her larynx to one side.

Don't panic.

Has the suxamethonium worked? If there have been no fasciculations, give her another 50 mg.

Carefully do another laryngoscopy.

Try blind intubation carefully, with the end of a plastic intoducer protruding 4 cm from the tracheal tube. The larynx and epiglottis are often oedematous in pregnant mothers.

If you fail and can ventilate her with a mask, *maintain cricoid pressure* while surgery proceeds. As the suxamethonium wears off, change to spontaneous ventilation with 1% hlothane, and trichloroethylene.

If you cannot ventilate with a mask, maintain cricoid pressure, get her onto her side, pass a nasogastric tube with suction ready, and let the suxamethonium wear off. Her life is more important than that of her baby. Operate under local anaesthesia (6.9).

If a mother has PIH (pregnancy induced hypertension, or pre-eclampsia) or eclampsia, control her convulsions and her hypertension properly before anaesthesia starts. Monitor her CVP (19.2), and adjust it to 6 to 8 cm of water. Intubation may cause dangerously high blood pressures if you don't first control her hypertension.

If she has been sedated with diazepam or barbiturates, reduce the dose of the induction agent. If she has been given magnesium sulphate, she will need only a small dose of suxamethonium.

If a mother has eclampsia or any evidence of a coagulopathy, avoid regional anaesthesia and ketamine.

If a mother has an antepartum haemorrhage, use general anaesthesia or local infiltration.

If a mother is diabetic, control her blood sugar preoperatively. If she is well controlled, fast her overnight, and set up a 5% dextrose drip early next morning. At the same time give her a dose of insulin equal to half her daily requirement.

In the theatre check her blood sugar. If it is high, delay lest it cause a rebound hypoglycaemia in the baby. For the same reason avoid giving her too much dextrose during anaesthesia.

General and regional anaesthesia are suitable, but avoid the latter if she has a neuropathy.

If a mother is in cardiac failure, and you cannot refer her, use local infiltration without added adrenaline.

If her baby baby does not breathe immediately, control his ventilation. If she has been given opioids, give him naloxone 0.01 mg/kg into his umbilical vein or intramuscularly. Less satisfactorily, give him 0.25 to 1 mg of nalorphine by the same route. These drugs will not help him to breathe, if his respiratory depression is not caused by opioids.

DON'T FORGET THE LEFT LATERAL TILT IN CAESAREAN SECTION

THE FLOW THROUGH A NEEDLE

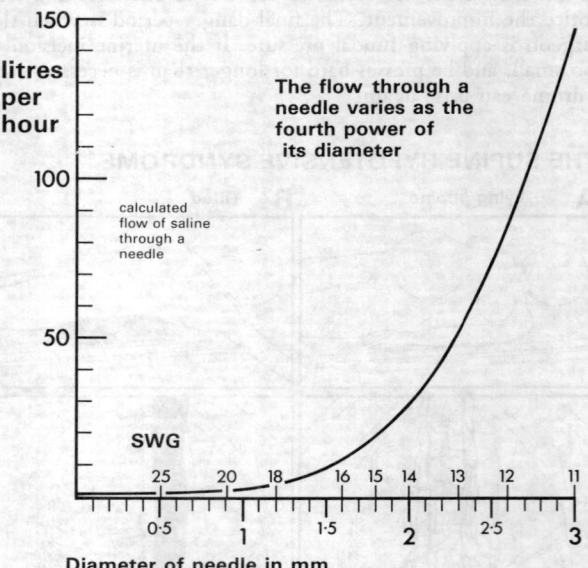

Fig. 16-6 THE FLOW OF FLUID THROUGH A NEEDLE. The graph shows how the flow of fluid through a needle varies as the fourth power of its diameter. This graph is calculated from the observation that, with a particular drip set, and with a head of fluid of about a metre, 4.5 litres of saline an hour flowed through a 1.25×40 mm needle. In practice other factors, such as entry of air into the bottle and the flow of fluid through the drip tubing limit the flow of fluid long before these high theoretical flows are reached. If you are treating hypovolaemic shock use a big needle and a high drip stand!

16.7 Anaesthesia for hypovolaemic shock

The resuscitation of patients in hypovolaemic shock is described in Section S 51.2 of Primary Surgery. We assume that you have resuscitated such a patient by the methods in that section, and now have to anaesthetize him. If he has been severely shocked, he should have been given sodium bicarbonate 1 mg/kg to correct metabolic acidosis as well as fluids to correct hypovolaemia.

General anaesthesia abolishes the compensatory vasoconstriction of hypovolaemic shock, so give a shocked patient only the smallest possible dose of anaesthetic. Avoid any drug that will dilate his blood vessels and make his hypotension worse. Subarachnoid and extradural anaesthesia are particularly dangerous for a hypovolaemic patient. For induction, ketamine is a much better agent than thiopentone. Although it raises the blood pressure of a normal patient, it is a myocardial depressant and may cause a fall in the blood pressure of a severely shocked one who is already maximally vasoconstricted, so it is not entirely safe. Ether is better than trichloroethylene. Avoid halothane. If possible, give the patient a relaxant and intubate him. Opinions differ about which long-acting relaxant is best, so use your usual one.

When you treat a patient's hypovolaemia try to: (1) Maintain his blood volume by giving him enough fluid, such as Ringer's lactate, fast enough. He is unlikely to die from anaemia, but he may die from hypovolaemia. (2) If he is bleeding into his abdominal cavity, don't wait until his blood pressure is normal, if necessary operate quickly and tie off the bleeding vessels. (3) As soon as he has stopped bleeding, give him what little blood you may have, because it will now stay in his circulation. If you have to give large volumes of fluid, the optimum ratio is one bottle of blood to two bottles of Ringer's lactate. Blood is unnecessary unless 1,000 ml, or in emergency 2,000 ml have been lost. Even if you have plenty of blood, start by giving him 500 to 1000 ml of Ringer's lactate.

The first essential is to be able to give intravenous fluids fast over a short period—to be able to pour fluid in. This is possible only if you use a short wide needle or cannula. If the pressure of fluid going through a needle is constant, the flow through it is inversely proportional to its length, but it is proportional to *the fourth power of its diameter,* as shown in Fig. 16-6. For example, halving the length of a needle enables a given volume of fluid to be given twice as fast, but doubling its diameter enables you to give the same volume of fluid 16 times as fast. So, use a short needle, and, even more important, use a wide one. Using a wide needle is more effective than raising the height of the bottle and is safer than trying to pump blood in under pressure, For all drips on adults try to use at least a 1.5×40 mm needle or a cannula; if you are treating shock, use a 3 mm needle. You never know when you may need to give fluid in a hurry.

If the patient has bled into his peritoneal cavity less than 24 hours previously, you may be able to collect this blood and transfuse it back into him.

If you treat hypovolaemia properly, it is very rewarding, because the prognosis is so good—if you operate quickly. *The patients who "die on the table" are often those with unreplaced loss of blood, in whom the unavoidable vasodilation of anaesthesia was the last straw that caused their cardiovascular collapse.*

The steps that follow are nearly the same as for the patient with a full stomach, but there are some important extra measures.

ANAESTHESIA FOR HYPOVOLAEMIC SHOCK

Follow the steps in Section 16.5, but alter them in the following way. If the patient is bleeding severely into his abdomen (or chest) don't wait to correct his blood pressure before operating.

If the patient has been injured, pass a nasogastric tube, and empty his stomach before he comes to the theatre, especially if you suspect a ruptured spleen or upper abdominal bleeding. If you pass a nasogastric tube, his stomach will then be empty and out of the way during the operation.

Because he is hypotensive, he will already be hypoxic, so allow a longer period of preoxygenation, and give him oxygen throughout the operation.

Make sure the drip really will "pour in".

Give him 100% oxygen from a mask. Induce him with ketamine 75 mg (1 mg/kg), suxamethonium and atropine.

Then give him gallamine or pancuronium (14.3) and 2% to 4% ether, or 0.5% trichloroethylene or a ketamine drip (8.3).

If a relaxant is not available, either use more ether, or combine the ketamine drip with local anaesthesia or, if necessary, intermittent suxamethonium (14.2).

CAUTION ! Patients with a ruptured abdominal viscus, such as a liver or spleen, rely on the tone of their abdominal muscles to limit their blood loss, so don't give any long–acting relaxant until the surgeon in absolutely ready to start operating.

Operate quickly!

Keep pouring fluid in until the bleeding vessel has been clamped. When the bleeding has stopped, give the patient donor blood, or give him his own blood from his peritoneal cavity.

POSTOPERATIVE CARE In severe cases, where the patient has lost more than 7 ml/kg of blood, his plasma osmotic pressure will be low, and he is in danger from postoperative pulmonary oedema. Also, give him frusemide 40 mg intravenously. For children, give proportionately smaller doses.

16.8 Anaesthesia for head injuries

Always anaesthetize a patient with a head injury, even if he is comatose. If you don't, he may wake up during the operation, as his intracranial pressure is reduced. Aim to: (1) Keep him unconscious. (2) Safeguard his neck, because he may also have a neck injury (S 64.5). If you have not x-rayed his neck, keep it still. Intubation can be very dangerous if his neck is broken. Even so, intubation is mandatory, so try to do a "crash induction" (16.5) using thiopentone and cricoid pressure, while keeping the patient's neck as still as possible. Try to use an armoured non–kinking tube, and good connections because they will be hidden by the drapes.

The ideal anaesthetic for head injuries includes relaxants and intubation followed by maintenance with trichloroethylene. You can also use halothane if you can control a patient's ventilation. If you can paralyse and intubate him, you can hyperventilate him, which will reduce his intracranial pressure and make evacuating an extradural or subdural haematoma easier. Put the non–rebreathing valve under the drapes and lead the exhaust gases through a tube to the floor. If you cannot intubate him, avoid thiopentone, because it may depress his respiration so that he needs ventilating urgently, perhaps for some time. Whether you intubate him or not, give him oxygen.

Although you can make burr holes and raise depressed fractures under local anaesthesia as described in Section S 65.3, doing so is likely to be a horrible experience for everyone, especially the patient. Make sure you have several strong men ready to hold him down. Even so, a good local anaesthetic may be better than poor general anaesthesia in which he bucks, coughs, strains or vomits, and in doing so raises his intracranial pressure. All too often he does all these things. This kind of struggling encourages venous bleeding, and may make his brain ooze like toothpaste from the hole in his skull.

A combination of pethidine and diazepam with muscle relaxants is another possibility for anaesthetizing a patient with a head injury.

16.9 Anaesthesia for eye surgery.

Nobody can do a neat tidy operation on an eye that is moving about, so the first essential for a success is that the eye must be still—both during the operation and afterwards. If the patient coughs or vomits, his eye may bleed, or his vitreous may herniate, so you must prevent this. Although you can use ketamine for eye surgery, it is far from satisfactory. It raises the intraocular pressure, and in small doses it does not stop the eye moving about, although it will do if you increase the dose. You will probably be holding the patient's eye with a superior rectus suture, so this will also help to prevent it moving about. In practice you will probably find ketamine a convenient anaesthetic for eye injuries. If he has an eye injury, remember that his stomach may be full. If you are going to give him a general anaesthetic, you must intubate him.

EYE ANAESTHESIA

THE INTRA–OCULAR PRESSURE

RAISING the intra-ocular pressure is raised by—(1)Hypercarbia. (2) Coughing and vomiting. (3) Light anaesthesia. (3) Struggling or excitation, at any time. (4) Ketamine. (5) Suxamethonium.

CAUTION ! Be particularly careful to avoid suxamethonium if the patient has glaucoma.

LOWERING The intra–ocular pressure is lowered by—(1) Hyperventilation. (2) All inhalational anaesthetics except nitrous oxide. (3) Long–acting relaxants. (4) Dehydration. (5) Deep anaesthesia.

PREMEDICATION is critical, both for local and general anaesthesia.

ATROPINE Unless glaucoma contraindicates it, give atropine. Stimulation of the eye is apt to cause bradycardia (oculocardiac reflex), and atropine will help to prevent it.

LOCAL ANAESTHESIA If possible use retrobulbar and facial nerve blocks (6.5). You can use a combination of ketamine and local anaesthesia if the patient is restless or bronchitic, and so liable to cough.

GENERAL ANAESTHESIA Induce the patient with thiopentone and suxamethonium, intubate him and continue with any general anaesthetic. Suxamethonium is not ideal for eye surgery; the alternative, which is to intubate him under a long-acting relaxant, is not a method for an inexperienced anaesthetist.

If you want to reduce his intra-ocular pressure, hyperventilate him.

Remove the tube while he is still quite deeply anaesthetized, so that he does not cough.

16.10 Anaesthesia for oral and facial surgery.

A patient with a maxillofacial injury will present you with some serious anaesthetic problems, because you will probably be unable to intubate him with an orotracheal tube. Nasotracheal intubation may be difficult and can be dangerous because it can carry bits of bone and foreign bodies into his lungs. If you need to intubate him for several days or more, it will probably be best done at the end of the operation after his wound has been cleaned up. You can usually wire a patient's jaws as a 'cold' operation when you have cleaned up his wound, and when nasal intubation will be safer. If you cannot secure his airway in any other way, do a tracheostomy (5.7). If he has a major injury, this will probably be necessary. If possible, use local anaesthesia. You can manage most maxillary fractures with sphenopalatine blocks, bilaterally if necessary, and wire his jaws under ketamine (8.1).

ANAESTHETIZING A PATIENT ON HER SIDE

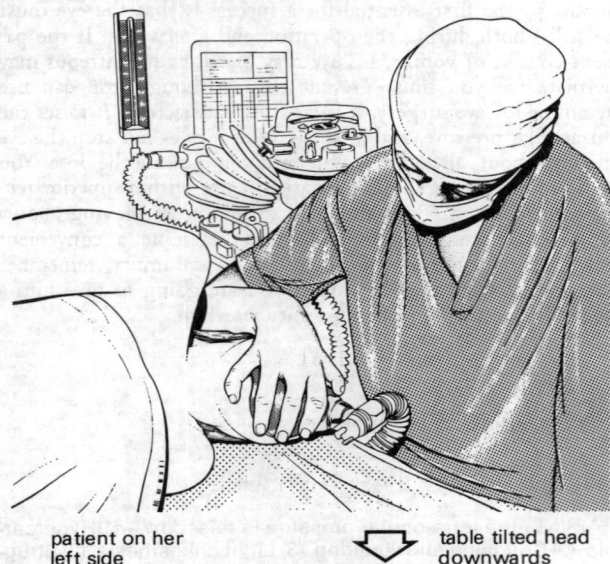

patient on her left side   table tilted head downwards

Fig. 16-7 ANAESTHETIZING A PATIENT ON HER SIDE. *Kindly contributed by Clive Cory.*

16.11 Anaesthesia for outpatients

The ideal anaesthetic for an outpatient allows you to operate on him safely, and then lets him walk or drive home shortly afterwards, fully alert. Local infiltration anaesthesia and regional blocks are best, particularly an intravenous forearm block. If a caudal epidural block does not go too high, he may be able to walk out of the operating theatre.

General anaesthesia is unsatisfactory for an outpatient because: (1) You can never be sure that he really has starved. (2) Recovery is slow, and may not be complete for 24 hours. You can use ketamine (8.1), thiopentone, or a pethidine—diazepam cocktail (8.8), for all of which he should be starved. Ketamine allows you the longest operating time (an hour or more if necessary), the cocktail is intermediate (3 to 20 minutes), and thiopentone the shortest (less than 3 minutes). He will be able to go home sooner with thiopentone or the cocktail, than with ketamine, which will make him sleepy all day, but even these make him sleepy for several hours; so try to operate on outpatients early in the day, so that they have longer to recover. The danger with thiopentone and the cocktail is that, although, a patient's final recovery is quicker, he is in more danger immediately after the operation from airway obstruction or aspiration of his stomach contents, especially if he is is not carefully watched (4.5). This can happen without anyone noticing it while you are busy with the next case, especially if you are treating a long line of outpatients in a busy hospital. Although a patient is sleepy for longer, these disasters are less likely with ketamine.

Admit a patient if he has any general medical condition, such as sickle cell anaemia or a cardiac mumur. You can only be sure about this if you examine him first.

After the operation someone must accompany the patient home, and he must not go back to work, drive a car, or operate machinery for 24 hours. As a test of his fitness to go home, ask him to walk along a straight line or stand still with his feet together and his eyes shut (Romberg's test).

AFTER INTUBATION THE PATIENT CAN BE IN ANY POSITION

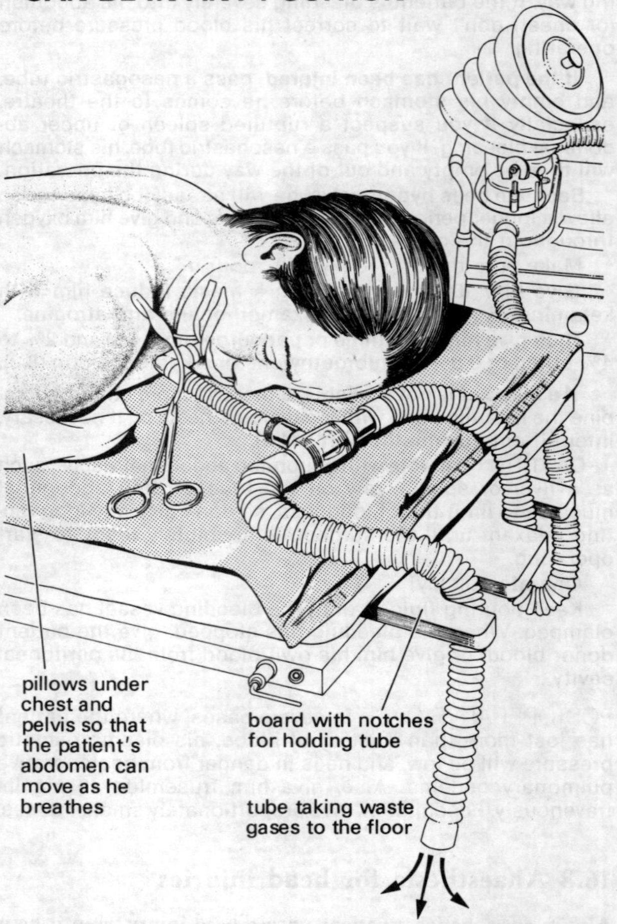

pillows under chest and pelvis so that the patient's abdomen can move as he breathes

board with notches for holding tube

tube taking waste gases to the floor

Fig. 16-8 AFTER YOU HAVE INTUBATED A PATIENT YOU CAN TURN HIM INTO ANY POSITION. *Kindly contributed by Arthur Adeney.*

16.12 Anaesthesia with the patient in unusual positions

Most operations are done with a patient flat of his back. If you need to anaesthetize him in other position, do it as described below. Unusual positions are some of the many occasions in which intubation is so useful. Both a steep Trendelenberg and the prone position make ventilation difficult, they cause an early increase in carbon dioxide tension, and a later decrease in oxygen tension.

POSITIONS DURING ANAESTHESIA

If possible, intubate the patient. Ideally, use a reinforced non-kink tube. Before you move him make sure that: (1) The tube is tied in place. (2) Its connections are firm. (3) It is supported and not kinked. (4) The patient's pressure points are protected.

If you operate on him face down, with his arms by his side, make sure you put pillows under his chest and pelvis, so that his abdomen is raised clear of the table. His abdomen can then expand as he breathes. If you don't do this properly, you cannot ventilate him adequately.

If his arms are above his head, bent at the elbows along either side of his head and supported on padded boards, they take away some of the pressure on his chest; but he still needs a pillow under his chest and his buttocks.

If you have to operate on him while he is on his side, as for a kidney operation, put his upper arm on a support, so that his chest is not compressed.

If you have to do some procedure on the floor, such as reducing his dislocated hip, remember that you cannot tip him head down if he vomits or regurgitates. Subarachnoid anaesthesia, epidural anaesthesia or a regional block are the safest methods. Or, you can intubate him on the table and move him to the floor.

If an operation has to be done with the patient's neck in extreme flexion, use a Portex or armoured tube. Check the airway repeatedly as the flexed position is reached.

If it is necessary to keep a woman's gut out of her abdomen during a hysterectomy or other pelvic operation, avoid a steep head-down tilt. Relax her well, and use only a slight head-down tilt.

If she has to be put into stirrups, don't anaesthetize her in this position, because you will not be able to turn her quickly if she vomits. So intubate her first, and then put her into stirrups. Intubate her even if she has to go into stirrups for a few minutes, as when applying forceps.

17 Some medical constraints on anaesthesia

17.1 Anaemia

Anaemia increases the risks of surgery, especially major surgery. It is so commom in some communities that it is almost normal. You must answer two questions before you can anaesthetize an anaemic patient safely.

"Is the figure for the patient's haemoglobin on the report slip correct?" (1) Laboratories can make mistakes. (2) His haemoglobin may not be a correct measure of his anaemia because severe dehydration or severe burns can raise a low haemoglobin to an apparently normal level, and only after you have rehydrated him will you see how anaemic he really is.

"Is his haemoglobin level acceptable?" You will have to answer this in relation to what is practicable. The blood of a patient with a haemoglobing of 15 g/dl, has an ample reserve of oxygen—carrying power. As the haemoglobin falls, so does this reserve; but there is usually no need to treat a patient's anaemia preoperatively unless it is below 10 g/dl at sea level. This is the figure at which "anaemia" can conveniently be said to start.

ANAEMIA

If a patient's haemoglobin is only 5 g/dl, operate only in emergency, or when he refuses to wait.

If his haemoglobin is only 2 or 3 g/dl, he is a medical emergency. He has a high cardiac output and almost no functional reserve. Operate only in the gravest emergency, and then only if his relatives understand that he will probably die.

If the operation is not urgent, try to raise a patient's haemoglobin first with iron or folic acid, when this is indicated. If he has a severe iron deficiency, oral iron will raise his haemoglobin about 1 g/dl a month, intramuscular iron will raise it the same amount in a week. The need to raise it depends on how much blood he is likely to lose during surgery. A man of 60 can safely have a cataract operation with only 9 g/dl, but if he needs a sequestrectomy, it should be 11 g/dl, or more.

If you have to operate without oxygen or blood, a high preoperative haemoglobin is even more important.

If a patient needs a transfusion before surgery, try to give him packed cells and to finish the transfusion 24 hours before the operation. This will give his circulation time to adjust to the increased volume.

If his haemoglobin is very low when you transfuse him, watch his jugular venous pressure carefully, because he will have a normal blood volume, but his heart will not be working normally because of oxygen lack. If possible give him packed cells and frusemide.

Anaesthesia for anaemia Remember—a severly anaemic patient has no reserve oxygen—carrying capacity, and hypotension and hypoxia will rapidly cause cardiac arrest. So, don't let his blood pressure fall; take great care of his airway; give him oxygen, and induce him with ketamine rather than thiopentone. Keep anaesthesia light so as not to depress his heart, which may be infiltrated with fat as the result of chronic anaemia. He needs a high cardiac output, so give him atropine. If you are in doubt, digitalise him before the operation, rather than as an emergency during it. Finally, replace all the blood he loses during surgery with blood, not with saline.

Sickle cell anaemia An operation may provoke a crisis; so use local anaesthesia if you can, but avoid an intravenous forearm block, because the tourniquet that you have to apply will make the patient's arm temporarily ischaemic. If he must have a general anaesthetic, give it with the greatest care, as described above. Correct his anaemia preoperatively, by exchange transfusion if you can. If possible, give him 7 ml/kg of a large molecular weight dextran (Dextran 70, or 110) intravenously an hour before operating. Afterwards, get him out of bed and walking about as soon as you can.

17.2 Metabolic acidosis

The hydrogen ion content of a patient's plasma can rise, and its bicarbonate fall, as the result of: (1) Loss of bicarbonate from his gut in acute diarrhoea, or into it in acute obstruction. (2) Shock causing hypoxia, which causes organic acids to accumulate. (3) Diabetic ketosis. (4) The inability of his kidneys to conserve bicarbonate in renal failure.

The most characteristic sign of severe metabolic acidosis is deep, sighing hyperventilation (Kussmaul's breathing). Another useful sign is an acid urine. Less distinctive are cold clammy extremities, hypotension, generalised muscle weakness, and cardiac dysrhythmias

If you anaesthetize a patient who is in metabolic acidosis: (1) He may stop breathing when you give him oxygen, because his oxygen deficiency drive has been keeping him breathing. This is not a reason for not giving him oxygen, but merely an additional indication for ventilating him when necessary. (2) He may not start breathing again after a long acting relaxant, or he may die postoperatively. If you learn to recognise metabolic acidosis, you will save many deaths on the operating table.

The regime described in Section 15.3 will treat moderate cases of metabolic acidosis satisfactorily. Only if hyperventilation is marked, need you give isotonic sodium bicarbonate. Then, give 1 mmol/kg (about 6 ml/kg of the 1.2% solution).

If a patient is severely acidotic, give him all the fluid he needs as 1.2% bicarbonate, rather than as Ringer's lactate or saline. If you are using a 1 mol/ml solution of sodium bicarbonate (8.4%) you can give him 5% dextrose as the fluid and 1 mmol/kg of this solution.

Give him oxygen, treat the cause of his acidosis, and avoid long—acting relaxants, or give them in reduced doses. Suxamethonium is probably safe if you give it cautiously.

IF A PATIENT IS HYPERVENTILATING, SUSPECT ACIDOSIS

17.3 Hypertension

During an operation a hypertensive patient is in danger from a sudden rise, or a sudden fall, in his blood pressure.

Intubating any patient raises his blood pressure. If he is already hypertensive, this rise may be so severe that it causes a cerebral haemorrhage or precipitates cardiac failure. So minimise the stimulus of intubation by premedicating him with an opioid (2.9). Anaesthetize his larynx before you intubate him (13.3), and do so very gently. If his blood pressure rises after the operation, this may be because of pain; if so, give him an analgesic.

When a hypertensive patient reaches the stage of surgical anaesthesia, his blood pressure may fall severely. He will probably have a low blood volume to begin with, and he will be unable to constrict his blood vessels normally to compensate for even mild bleeding. So don't give him any anaesthetic that will lower his blood pressure. A high subarachnoid block is particularly dangerous, but a low one is quite suitable. During the operation, give him fluids readily, and if necessary raise his feet. Vasopressors are not usually necessary and are dangerous.

When is a hypertensive patient fit for operation? This depends on several factors, and especially on whether or not he is being treated.

HYPERTENSION

If a hypertensive patient is not being treated, he is usually fit for operation without significantly increased risk, if: (1) His diastolic blood pressure does not rise above 120 mm when recorded over 24 hours. (2) He is not in cardiac failure and never has been. (3) He has no previous myocardial infarct or present angina. (4) He is not obese or anaemic. If he has any of these things, you will have to balance the added risks of operating against the risks of not doing so.

If he is being treated, and his hypertension is controlled, (diastolic blood pressure below 120 mm), keep him on his full medication and give him his last dose on the night before the operation.

If he is being treated, and his hypertension is not controlled (diastolic blood pressure above 120 mm), try to control his blood pressure before you operate.

17.4 Congestive cardiac failure

This is the patient who is breathless on exertion, whose jugular venous pressure is raised, and who has basal crepitations, ankle oedema, low blood pressure, cyanosis, or ascites. Any general anaesthetic is likely to cause serious hypotension; so, try to delay an elective operation until you have treated the cause of his heart failure, and improved his general condition with digoxin and diuretics. In an emergency, use local anaesthesia or a low subarachnoid or epidural anaesthetic.

If a patient who is in cardiac failure must have a general anaesthetic, try to refer him, because the risks are high. If you have to anaesthetize him yourself, use the minimum of sedatives and induction agents; induce him with 1% trichloroethylene or up to 6% ether, until his eyelash reflex is lost; then give him a long—acting relaxant in the full dose (pancuronium is better than alcuronium, and alcuronium is better than gallamine). Or, induce him with halothane and follow this with ether. Assist his respiration until he is well relaxed; intubate him; and then ventilate him with 0.5% trichhloroethylene or 3% ether, while giving him a litre of oxygen at the same time. Reverse his paralysis with atropine and neostigmine in divided doses, and avoid loading him with sodium. Give him oxygen from a mask until he is fully conscious.

Another approach is to preoxygenate a patient with 100% oxygen, to give him thiopentone in half the usual dose, to follow this with suxamethonium and a lignocaine spray; and then to wait for one minute and intubate him.

17.5 Hepatic failure

Some or all of the following signs should alert you to the possibility that a patient is in liver failure—jaundice, ascites, a large liver, a characteristic smell in his breath, altered consciousness, a bleeding tendency, oedema, and anastomotic vessels. If possible, treat such a patient symptomatically before you operate on him. He may need diuretics, a low—protein diet, vitamin K and fresh blood or plasma.

Both surgery and anaesthesia are dangerous for a patient in hepatic failure because: (1) His failure to metabolise drugs normally may greatly prolong his 'recovery from anaesthesia. (2) He may bleed severely. (3) He may go into circulatory failure. (4) If he has hepatitis, he may be a risk to the hospital staff.

Anaesthetize such a patient in the same way that you would if had cardiac failure—use the minimum of of sedatives and induction agents. Avoid suxamethonium, because his plasma cholinesterase is likely to be low. If he needs an analgesic after an operation, give it intravenously in low doses until you get just the effect you want, but no more. A patient with hepatic failure may develop renal failure postoperatively, especially if he has obstructive jaundice, so maintain a high urine flow and give him 10% mannitol (15.1).

17.6 Renal failure

Suspect that a patient is in renal failure if he is drowsy, if he has a low urine output (less than 0.5 ml/kg/hour), and is anaemic. Confirm your suspicion by measuring his blood urea. It may be high as the result of chronic kidney disease, urinary obstruction, or hypovolaemic shock.

If the patient is shocked, restore his blood pressure. If necessary relieve his urinary obstruction, and treat his renal failure symptomatically as far as you can. Minimise his sodium and potassium intake, and, in particular, avoid Ringer's lactate. Instead, use 0.18% saline in 4.3% dextrose.

If possible use local, regional, low subarachnoid or epidural anaesthesia. If he needs a general anaesthetic, avoid drugs that are excreted in the urine, especially gallamine. Induce him cautiously with thiopentone, give him oxygen, and anaesthetize him in the same way you would if he was anaemic (17.1). Give him only enough fluid to balance his urine output, plus his insensible loss plus any other loss.

17.7 Diabetes

The main dangers for a diabetic patient undergoing surgery are ketosis, especially if it is undiagnosed, and hypoglycaemia. Hyperglycaemia may also occur, but by itself is much less dangerous. He may never recover from the anaesthetic if you operate on him while he is ketotic. So don't anaesthetize him while he is in this state, especially if his diabetes is of the juvenile type. Try to control his ketosis first. You can do this most easily by stopping any long—acting insulins he might be having and controlling his diabetes with soluble insulin.

Sometimes, you may not be able to control his diabetes until you have treated some infection, such as a carbuncle. If his diabetes is of the milder adult type, you may be able to operate, even though it is not fully controlled.

Diabetic neuropathy can affect a patient's autonomic nerve fibres, even before he shows any loss of sensation. Because he is unable to constrict his blood vessels to compensate for hypovolaemia, he is in particular danger from hypotension. So, beware of this, avoid high subarachnoid anaesthesia, and correct hypotension energetically if it occurs. Unilateral spinal blocks are safe (7.6); so are other local blocks.

A diabetic patient is in particular danger from hypoglycaemia if you give him too high a dose of soluble insulin just before an operation. If you cannot measure his blood sugar, operate when you expect him to be mildly hyperglycaemic.

The main principle in managing any crisis that occurs while a diabetic patient cannot eat or drink is to *continue to give insulin*, using a drip bag, a paediatric drip set, or an infusion pump. The following method assumes you don't have the latter.

Some anaesthetic agents are more dangerous than others for a diabetic patient. Avoid thiopentone, curare, and to a lesser extent ether.

DIABETES

Check the patient's blood sugar the day before surgery. If possible, refer him, especially if his blood glucose is more than 15 mmol/l.

CAUTION ! (1) "Dextrostix" and similar tests for blood sugar may not work properly, especially if they have been stored in the theatre for a long time. (2) If you are giving an insulin drip, give it at a steady rate through a separate needle from that used for fluid replacement. (3) The first 24 hours after surgery will be a dangerous time for the patient. If his blood sugar is not high, don't give him insulin without food, or he will become hypoglycaemic.

INSULIN–DEPENDENT JUVENILE TYPE DIABETES

If a patient is receiving insulin, and is having a minor operation and will not need a post-operative drip, omit long-acting insulins the night before, and all insulin on the morning of operation. Operate on him early in the morning. Measure his blood sugar on the morning of the operation. If it is below 4.5 mmol/l, set up a 5% dextrose drip and give him an injection of 25 g of dextrose as a 50% solution into the drip.

On his return from the theatre before mid-day, give him half to ¾ of his normal morning insulin requirement. Give him some carbohydrate with it.

Measure his blood glucose after the operation, and four hours later.

Give him his normal evening insulin. If his postoperative blood glucose is more than 15 mmol/l, give him soluble insulin and repeat it 6 hourly. Or, test his urine and dose him as follows: 2% glycosuria (32 units of soluble insulin), 1% (20 units), ½% (12 units) 0% (8 units).

If the patient is receiving insulin and is having a major operation, give him his normal dose of short-acting insulin the night before. Start the following regime in the morning before breakfast. Begin an infusion of 5% dextrose containing 16 units of soluble insulin per litre. Run it at the rate appropriate to his fluid requirements. Adjust his insulin dose as follows.

If his blood glucose is less than 4 mmol/l, give him no insulin/l.

If his blood glucose is 4 to 15 mmol/l, give him 16 units of soluble insulin/l.

If his blood glucose is 16 to 20 mmol/l give him 32 units of soluble insulin/l.

If his blood glucose is more than 20 mmol/l review him carefully.

Measure his blood glucose 2 hourly until he is stable, and then 6 hourly. Test his urine as a check against erroneous blood glucose readings.

As soon as he starts to eat, and the intravenous drips have been removed, give him soluble insulin twice daily. If his blood glucose is high (more than 15 mmol/l), give him additional doses at noon or bedtime, or both. If necessary, adjust the regime daily.

If you have to operate in the afternoon, give him a drip of 10% glucose in water. Give him his morning dose of insulin as soluble insulin. Measure his blood glucose every 3 hours and give him soluble insulin if it is more than 10 mmol/l.

NON–INSULIN–DEPENDENT ADULT TYPE DIABETES

This is the patient who is well controlled (random blood glucose value less than 12 mmol/l) on diet or oral hypoglycaemic agents.

If he is well controlled, omit the tablet on the day of the operation, and fast him for the operation as usual.

If he has been on a long-acting sulphonylurea, check his blood glucose before the anaesthetic. If it is less than 4.5 mmol/l he may become dangerously hypoglycaemic. Give him a 5% dextrose drip, and into it inject 25 g of glucose as a 50% bolus injection. Check his blood sugar soon after the operation. If it is over 15 mmol/l start soluble insulin subcutaneously. Give him his usual tablets on the following day.

CAUTION! If he is on chlorpropramide, be careful, it has a half life of about 36 hours. So omit it on the day of operation, and beware of hypoglycaemia.

If he is poorly controlled (random blood glucose more than 15 mmol/l), start him on soluble insulin, using one of the regimes above.

DIFFICULTIES ANAESTHETIZING DIABETICS

If you anaesthetize a controlled juvenile type of diabetic, do so 3 to 4 hours after his last meal, and his last dose of soluble insulin. If the operation is delayed, give him a 5% dextrose drip.

If you cannot monitor his blood glucose, don't give him insulin, either just before or during the operation. Hyperglycaemia will cause much less harm during the operation than hypoglycaemia.

SOME MEDICAL CONDITIONS

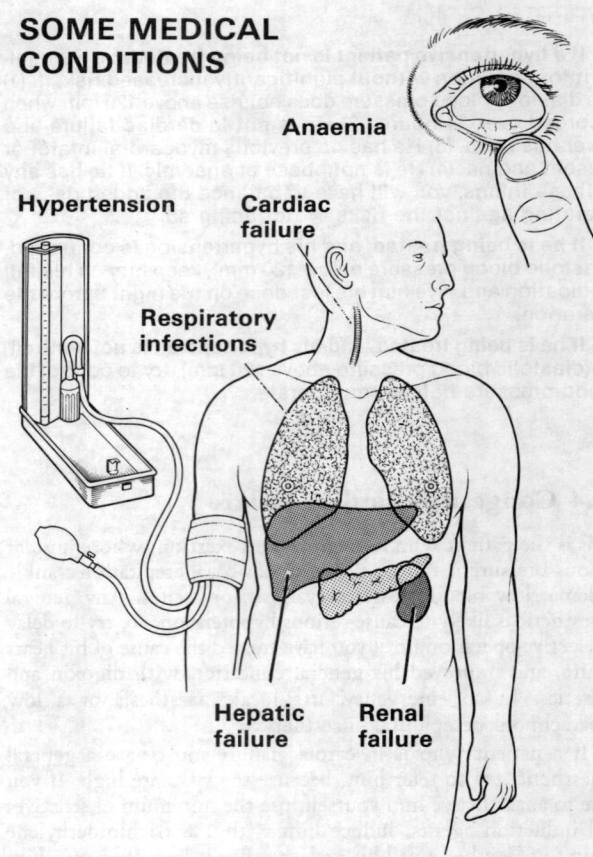

Fig. 17-1 SOME MEDICAL CONDITIONS THAT INFLUENCE ANAESTHESIA

17.8 Respiratory infections

If you anaesthetize a patient who has a respiratory infection, you run the risk of making his infection worse and precipitating bronchospasm.

An acute respiratory infection, including the common cold, contraindicates general anaesthesia and especially intubation. Even a local anaesthetic is unwise during respiratory infection because, if it fails, a general anaesthetic may be needed.

A chronic respiratory infection, producing sputum should be assumed to be tuberculous until proved otherwise. The patient may infect the equipment and the other patients. If possible treat him first; two weeks treatment will probably make him non–infectious. If you have to operate on him when he is infectious, and you have any disposable equipment, use it. Autoclave any metal instruments you have used. An expiratory spill valve is less likely to be destroyed by autoclaving than a non–rebreathing valve.

If a patient has not got tuberculosis, and his sputum is yellow, give him antibiotics until his sputum is white or greatly reduced in volume. Explain to him how important it is to remove pus from his lungs by postural drainage. Continue this for several days before you anaesthetize him. Do it intermittently for at least four hours each day, with the foot of his bed raised. Measure the sputum he coughs out each day.

If possible, use local or regional anaesthesia. If you have to give a general anaesthetic, intubate the patient, and keep large suction catheters ready. Ether will increase his respiratory secretions, but it will also make them easier to suck out. Listen beside his tracheal tube for the rattle of accumulated sputum, and suck it out. If it gathers dangerously, tip the table 20° head down, and then suck the sputum out. Emphysema may have destroyed much of his lung tissue, so that a volatile anaesthetic will take longer than normal to be absorbed. Induction will therefore be slow.

Asthma can cause serious difficulties during anaesthesia. Ask carefully if a patient is allergic to any drugs. Operate when he is at his best and is not infected. Continue his usual drugs, and premedicate him well to minimise his anxiety. If possible, give him a local, subarachnoid or extradural anaesthetic. If you hear any wheezing when he comes to the theatre, give him prophylactic aminophylline, and anaesthetize his trachea before you intubate him. Avoid thiopentone, tubocurarine, and gallamine; induce him with diazepam, ketamine or halothane. Ether is a good bronchodilator, so use it for maintenance; but don't try to induce him with it. Beware of bronchospasm. If it occurs, give him more intravenous aminophylline, and have hydrocortisone ready. If you paralyse a patient with relaxants, make sure he is breathing normally before you send him back to the ward. When he gets there, have oxygen available, and observe him carefully for at least 30 minutes. Asthmatics need very careful postoperative care.

18 Anaesthesia for children

18.1 Children are different

A child differs from an adult physiologically. The smaller he is, the greater these differences are, and the greater the risks of both anaesthesia and surgery. When you operate on a child, especially if he is very small, remember that:—

He has a high metabolic rate At rest in a warm room he needs twice as much oxygen per kilogram as an adult, and if he is febrile he needs even more. If he becomes apnoeic at any time, during intubation for example, he goes blue in half the time that an adult does, so act quickly.

His glycogen store is small It is quickly exhausted, and when it is, he becomes hypoglycaemic. If you don't prevent hypoglycaemia he may become confused postoperatively and may even die. So don't interrupt a child's feeds more than you must. Stop giving him milk 4 hours before surgery, but give him 3% dextrose water freely until 2 hours before. During the operation any intravenous fluids you give him should contain 5% dextrose. Give 15 ml/kg during the first hour, and 8 ml/kg/hour after that. He will probably feed immediately he wakes.

His circulation compensates badly for any blood he loses during an operation, because his vasomotor tone is poor. You will find that his blood pressure will be difficult to measure if you don't have the necessary sizes of children's and infant's cuffs. The best way to monitor anaesthesia is to strap a monaural stethoscope to his left chest and to observe the following signs.

(1) *The intensity of his heart beat.* If it is becoming fainter and if he is losing blood or fluid, this is a sign that his blood volume is falling; so speed up the drip, and his heart sounds may become dramatically louder.

(2) *The intensity of his breath sounds.* Monitor his ventilation both by the pressure you apply to the bellows, and by the air you hear going in and out of his lungs.

(3) *The slowing of his heart rate.* In a baby, particularly a neonate, this is an important sign of oxygen lack.

(4) *The blood he loses.* Measure it; weigh the swabs. Give a baby blood if he loses more than 5 to 10% of his blood volume (estimate this at 80 ml/kg or from Fig. S 53-1). His blood volume is small, he can easily bleed to death from what might seem to be only minor blood loss.

He has a large surface area for his weight This means that a child can gain or lose heat very quickly, so monitor his temperature with a thermometer in his rectum. Correct abnormal swings up or down as soon as possible. In most climates cold is a greater danger than heat, so keep the theatre warm— warm enough for you to feel mildly uncomfortable. A small baby can easily become hypothermic, even in a hot climate, especially if the theatre is air–conditioned and he is paralysed and ventilated. If there is an air–conditioner, turn if off. Wrap him well before you move him anywhere. Avoid draughts, wrap his limbs in cotton wool, and warm any infusions or fluid used for washing his peritoneum. If his temperature falls, correct it with hot towels, not hot water bottles, which may burn him.

If a child's rectal temperature has fallen at the end of the operation, raise his body temperature actively. While he is paralysed, he produces little heat; and if he is below 30°C when you reverse him, he may fail to start breathing until he warms up. So, let him struggle a little on his tube. The exertion of doing so will warm him. If necessary, warm him in a warm bath, or under a lamp.

He has poor vagal tone This is one reason why a baby's heart beats faster. However, anything that increases vagal tone slows a child's heart much more than it does an adult's. So, always premedicate a child with atropine to reduce the effects of sudden fluctuations in his vagal tone.

The anatomy of his airway is different The best way to secure a child's airway depends on his age, which in turn, is related to his weight:

If he is below 10 kg, place a folded towel under his neck and shoulders (13-15). Lifting his chin may obstruct his respiration, so put your fingers under the angle of his mandible to lift his jaw.

If he is between 10 and 20 kg, start to induce him in whatever position he is lying, and try to disturb him as little as possible. When he is unconscious, support his head or shoulders on a 5 cm pillow.

Atropine is dangerous if the ambient temperature is over 30°C. Atropine may raise a child's temperature, and if it rises high enough, he is in danger from hyperpyrexia and may have convulsions.

Finally, remember that he is small. You can very easily overdose a child with drugs, especially if he is a neonate. An overdose of a local anaesthetic is a particular risk.

HOLDING A CHILD—for "tie and cry anaesthesia"

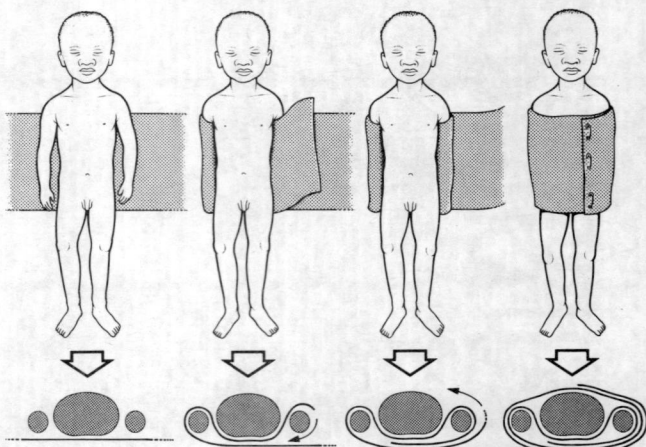

Fig. 18-1 HOLDING A CHILD FOR "TIE–AND–CRY" ANAESTHESIA. If you have no special anaesthetic skills or no ketamine, the less anaesthetic a child has the better. The safest method may be to give him the minimum of anaesthesia and restrain him.

18.2 Which methods are appropriate for children?

For all the reasons listed above and others, a child is at greater risk than an adult when he is anaesthetized. He also needs to be anaesthetized differently. Hence the reason why too many

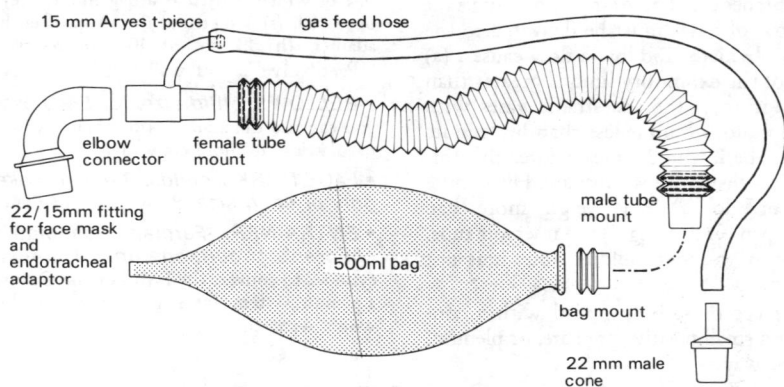

Fig. 18-2 FITTINGS FOR AYRE'S T-PIECE. You will usually need the bag only for older children.

children in district hospitals die under anaesthesia, particularly where care is poor. Some anaesthetic methods are much worse for children than others. Firstly, some of the less suitable methods.

Extradural and regional anaesthesia both need the patient's co-operation, they are unsuitable for anyone less than 15 years old.

Ether from a draw-over vapouriser has disadvantages unless you use it as described later:(1) Although vapourisers for ether and halothane are flow compensated, the range of their compensation is limited. Children do not draw enough air through these vapourisers to receive an accurate concentration of vapour. At low flow rates, they are highly inaccurate, and may deliver only half the concentration they say they do. Fortunately, the error is on the safe side. (2) An infant breathes faster than an adult, so he has more work to do in moving the column of air in a vapouriser. (3) An adult's non-rebreathing valve offers too much resistance and has too much dead space for a small child to work it in the way an adult can. For all these reasons, you have to use special methods, and special equipment, for children, particularly those weighing less than 15 kg. The standard adult equipment can kill them!

Standard machines of the Boyle's type can be equally dangerous, unless they are fitted with paediatric equipment. There may be such a large dead space between a small child's alveoli and the bag that a long anaesthetic is fatal. So don't use adult equipment on anyone weighing less then 15 kg, and don't try to improvise paediatric equipment if you are not sure of what you are doing!

Relaxants can be used if you have the right equipment, such as a paediatric self-inflating bag and the right tracheal tubes. Calculate the dose carefully, and don't let the child get cold. Remember that a relaxed child loses heat very rapidly. Relaxants are especially dangerous in newborn babies under the age of 1 month. Unless you have been carefully trained, don't use them for children under the age of one year. They are seldom necessary. A small baby has weak abdominal muscles, and a surgeon can usually return his gut to his abdomen without the help of relaxant drugs. If you need to, you can give suxamethonium intramuscularly in babies. Dilute it to make it easier to measure and give a neonate or small infant 2 mg/kg intramuscularly. It will give 10 to 15 minutes of relaxation, and will start to work in about a minute. If necessary, repeat it. If you want to, you can intubate a neonate while he is awake, as in Section 13.6.

Open ether is described in Section 11.4 and is particularly suitable for children unless they are very small. Don't use it for neonates because of the large dead space under the mask.

Ketamine is often the most suitable anaesthetic for a child (8.1). You can safely use it for children of any age, even a newborn baby—provided you adjust the dose carefully to his weight. It is much the safest way for the inexpert to anaesthetize children. You can usefully combine ketamine with lignocaine or chloral hydrate.

"Tie-and-cry anaesthesia" may be the safest way of anaesthetizing a child if you have no special paediatric equipment, or no ketamine. If your skills are limited, the less anaesthesia a child has the better. Under such circumstances, the safest anaesthesia for an abdominal operation in a child under 15 kg is diazepam 0.25 mg/kg intramuscularly, combined with the local infiltration of lignocaine, being careful not to exceed the safe dose. Tie the child's arms and legs to splints. He remains at least partly conscious and cries, hence the name given to this method of anaesthesia. Because his abdominal muscles are not relaxed, returning his intestines to his peritoneal cavity may be difficult, but it can be done. Such anaesthesia is far from ideal, but when anaesthetic skills really are minimal, it probably gives the child the best chance of living. It really is a procedure for desperate emergencies only.

DON'T USE RELAXANTS FOR CHILDREN UNDER THE AGE OF ONE YEAR, UNLESS YOU ARE EXPERT

18.3 Anaesthetic systems for children

For the reasons you have just read in the last section, you will have to use special methods to give a general anaesthetic to a child under 15 kg. If you are using the Dräger Afya" vapouriser, you can attach an AMBU "Paedivalve" directly to it. If you are using the the EMO system, there are two things you can do:—

(1) You can use a paediatric non-rebreathing valve, such as the "Paedivalve" (10.3), for for both spontaneous and controlled ventilation, by connecting it directly to the corrugated tubing of the EMO, as in Fig.10-7. A minor disadvantage of using this valve is that the EMO may give less than the indicated concentration of ether.

(2) You can use a vapouriser and Ayre's T-piece, which consists piece consists of two tubes joined to make a 'T'. The top of the T is made of 1 cm diameter tube. The child breathes through a mask or tracheal tube attached to one end of the top of 'T'; a 1 cm diameter corrugated rubber reservoir tube is attached to the other end. A thin tube forms the stem of the 'T' and delivers the anaesthetic gases. As he breathes in and out, his expired gases are carried away by the flow of fresh gas passing up the stem and out through reservoir tube. The T-piece has no valves, so it offers very little resistance to breathing, which can be controlled or spontaneous. There are two important points: (1) A continous flow of gases must be delivered to the T-piece, or the child will asphyxiate. Too low a flow causes: (a) rebreathing if the volume of the expiratory limb is greater than his minute volume; (b) dilution of the anaesthetic gases with air if the volume of the expiratory limb is less than his minute volume. The flow rate must be 2½ to 3 times greater than his minute volume, and never less than 4 litres a minute. His minute volume is about 200 ml per kilo. (2) If he weighs more than 10 kg, you must attach an open−ended bag to the reservoir tube. You can also use a bag with younger children, but it is not necessary.

The stem of Ayre's T-piece must be supplied with a continuous flow of gases under a small positive pressure, or plenum. You can supply it in three ways—

(a) You can use the paediatric bellows, or if necessary the Oxford Bellows. This is the simplest method, but it does mean that the bellows have to be pumped continously.

(b) You can use a flow of pure oxygen from a cylinder. Lead 6 to 8 litres a minutes of pure oxygen into the inlet port of the EMO, either through a special fitting, or through a makeshift one described below. With this method there is the theoretical danger that, by using pure oxygen, the splinting effect of nitrogen on his alveoli will be lost, causing them to collapse.

(c) You can use Farman's entrainer. This simple device also fits into the inlet port of the EMO. Oxygen under pressure from a cylinder goes through a fine jet inside it. As it does so, it sucks in (entrains) some of the surrounding air, so that a mixture containing 33% oxygen goes into the vapouriser. A total flow of about 10 litres a minute is delivered. This flow rate is reached when oxygen is supplied to it at a pressure of about 100 mm of mercury. The easiest way of measuring this is to fix a sphygmomanometer to the side tube of the entrainer. It only needs 2 litres a minute of oxygen, so it is cheaper to run than when pure oxygen is used.

If you have a Boyle's machine, you can use Ayre's T-piece, oxygen, and nitrous oxide in the same way as with an EMO vapouriser. The nitrous oxide and oxygen from the machine will form the plenum. You can add ether, halothane, or trichloroethylene to the mixture, just as you would with an adult. As always with Ayres T-piece, you must maintain an adequate flow. You cannot use a ''Paedivalve'' with a Boyle's machine, because a non−rebreathing valve has no way of discharging the excess gases of the plenum.

Which method is best? Ayres T-piece is standard practice with Boyle's machines, and with the plenum systems it is well tried with the EMO. You can also use it for operations close to the mouth.

The use of the ''Paedivalve'' with draw−over vapourisers in children is comparatively new. Its place in district hospitals in the hands of anaesthetic assistants is therefore still uncertain, but it may be the method of choice. It is simple, you can use it in exactly the same way as an adult AMBU E valve. One minor disadvantage is that it is bulky, and because it has to be close to the child's mouth, it gets in the way when operations are done on his face. But for operations on his eyes it is far enough away to cause no trouble. It is certainly safe with children down to 10 kg.

Here is the equipment you will need for use with a vapouriser—

• VALVE, paediatric, (''Paedivalve'') non−rebreathing anaesthesia type, for controlled or spontaneous respiration, with 15 mm male inlet cone, 22/15 mm patient cone, and 15 mm outlet cone, complete with 4 spare leaflets, and 15 mm male to 22 mm female plastic adapter, as (AMB) 1-101-100, two only. These are the complete specifications for the ''Paedivalve''. You can also use some other non−return valves.

• AYRE'S T-PIECE CHILD CIRCUIT KIT, complete, one only. This consists of: (a) 15 mm to 15/22 mm elbow connector, (b) 15 mm Ayre's T-piece, (c) 15 mm male tube mount, (d) 15 mm female tube mount, one of which is used as a bag mount, (e) 500 ml reservoir bag with open tail, (f) 1 metre of 6 mm gas feed hose, (g) 22/6 mm gas feed adapter, (h) 21 cm of 10 mm reservoir hose. If you use the ''Paedivalve'', you will not need this.

• BELLOWS, child size, for EMO system, one only. Although you can use the adult Oxford bellows for children, you will find the paediatric size more convenient.

• FACE MASKS, childs, Rendell−Baker, sizes 0, 1 and 2, three only of each size. Between them these fit all sizes of child.

• ENTRAINER, Farman's paediatric, for use with EMO children's circuit, one only. This uses the pressure of oxygen in cylinder to convert the EMO or the Oxford Miniature vapouriser into a plenum system. Here again, if you use the AMBU ''Paedivalve'', you won't want this.

THE PRINCIPLE OF AYRE'S T-PIECE

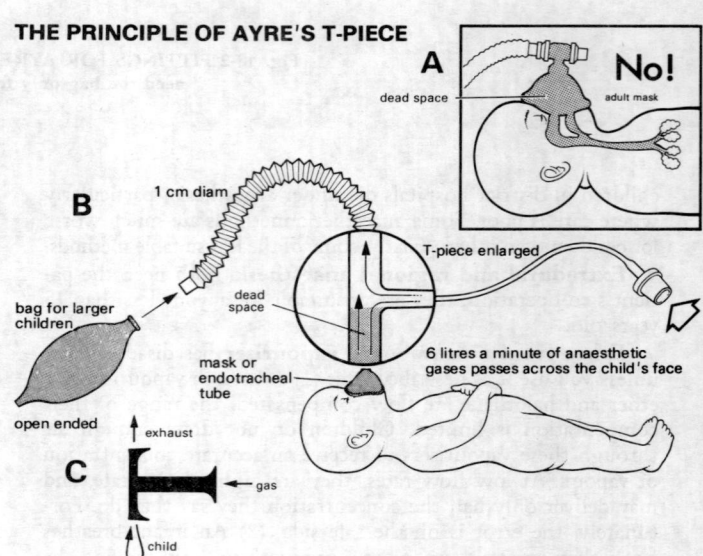

Fig. 18-3 THE PRINCIPLE OF ARYES T-PIECE. A, shows what a large dead space there can be under an adult mask if you use this for a child. B, the various parts of the T-piece, with the T much enlarged. C, the arrangement of the various limbs of the T.

The dead space lies between the point of inflow of fresh gases and the patient, and must be small, so the length of the tubing between the T-piece and the child must be short. The length of tube between the T-piece and the bag is unimportant. Select the smallest face piece.

A, kindly contributed by Georg Kamm.

CHILDREN'S ANAESTHETIC SYSTEMS

THE PAEDIVALVE

THE SYSTEM FOR THE PAEDIVALVE Use an EMO, or OMV, and an Oxford Bellows, preferably the paediatric version. Don't use a catheter mount, because it has too large a dead space. Instead, plug the adaptor of the tracheal tube straight into the ''Paedivalve'', as in Fig. 10-3. This will connect the tube to the valve with the minimum of dead space.

CAUTION ! The ''Paedivalve'' is a non−rebreathing valve, so inactivate the non−return valve (M, in Fig. 10-8) of the Oxford Bellows with a magnet.

Give oxygen through the oxygen attachment. Join this to the inlet of the EMO, or the OMV.

SPONTANEOUS RESPIRATION WITH THE ''PAEDIVALVE'' Raise the bellows sharply 6 to 8 times a minute, and allow them to empty slowly by themselves. They will draw anaesthetic mixture through the vapouriser, and deliver it to the child under a small pressure, so that he can breathe as he wants to. Because, by this method, he inflates his own lungs, and the bellows do not do it for him, his ventilation is not being controlled.

FARMANS ENTRAINER AND AYRES T-PIECE

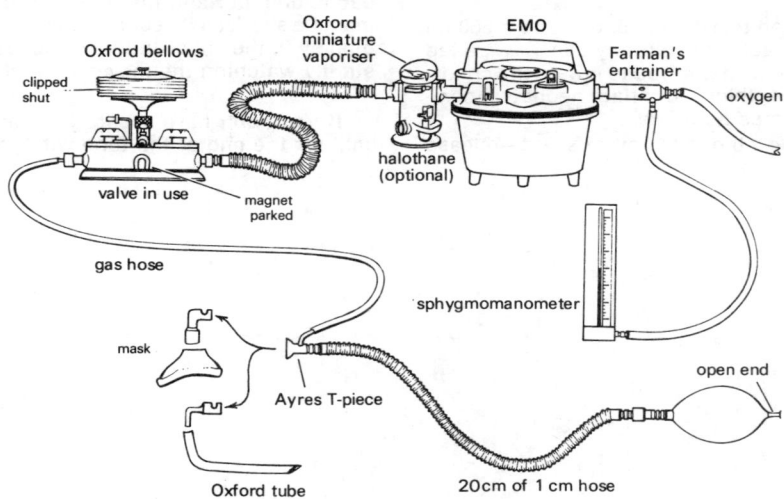

Fig. 18-4 FARMAN'S ENTRAINER PROVIDING A PLENUM FOR AYRE'S T-PIECE. In this circuit Farman's is providing the plenum. The Oxford bellows is clipped shut and is being used only for its valves.
Kindly contributed by Michael Wood.

CONTROLLED VENTILATION WITH THE PAEDIVALVE Do this exactly as in an adult.

AYRE'S T-PIECE WITH A VAPOURISER

PROVIDING A PLENUM FOR AYRE'S T-PIECE. There are three ways of doing this

(1) The Oxford bellows. Park the magnet out of use. Lift the bellows sharply and then compress them very gently, about 6 times a minute. Try to maintain a constant flow of air.

(2) Pure oxygen from a cylinder. Find some way of running 6 litres a minute of pure oxygen through the vapouriser. If you have the oxygen attachment for the EMO (9-5), remove its corrugated tube, and replace it by a cork (a special fitting is also made).

(3) Farman's entrainer. Fit the entrainer onto the inlet port of the vapouriser, and connect it to the oxygen supply. Attach a sphygmomanometer to the side arm of the entrainer. Adjust the oxygen flow, so that the sphygmomanometer reads 100 mm. You will need about 2 litres of oxygen a minute. To avoid waste, turn on the entrainer only when you are using it.

THE T-PIECE ITSELF Fit a Rendell-Baker face mask, or a tracheal tube with its adapter, to an angled connector. Join this to the T-piece. To the other end of the T-piece fit 20 cm of 1 cm corrugated tubing to act as a reservoir. The diameter and length of this tube are important. If it is too short, the child will breathe ordinary air. For children over 10 kg, fit a 500 ml open ended bag to the end of the reservoir tube.

CAUTION ! (1) If the oxygen cylinder empties unoticed and the flow of gas stops, the child may die; so watch the pressure in the oxygen cylinder carefully. If the oxygen runs out, disconnect the T-piece, and let him breathe the air of the theatre. This is such a serious hazard that some anaesthetists fit a bag between the entrainer and the EMO. If it deflates it is a sign that the pressure in the system is inadequate and the oxygen has run out. (2) 500 ml bags sometimes come from the makers with a closed end, the bung must be removed or the end cut off; otherwise there is no way for the child to breathe out.

SPONTANEOUS RESPIRATION WITH AYRE'S T-PIECE Let the child breathe from the T-piece spontaneously.

CONTROLLED VENTILATION WITH AYRE'S T-PIECE The method depends on the child's weight.

A child less than 10 kg, including a neonate. Block the end of the corrugated tube intermitenlty with your thumb. This will divert the flow of gases entering the T-piece into his lungs. When you remove your thumb from the tube, he will exhale spontaneously.

If the Oxford bellows are providing the plenum, **they have the necessary valves, but be careful not to overinflate the child.**

If an oxygen cylinder is providing the plenum, **no valves are needed, but be careful not to overinflate him. Adjust the flow of oxygen to 6 litres a minute.**

If the entrainer is providing the plenum, **no valves are needed.** When the end of the corrugated tube is blocked, the gas is under just enough pressure to inflate the lungs of a small baby, without being able to overinflate him.

A child over 10 kg. The lungs of a larger child take too long to inflate by closing the end of the corrugated tube with your finger. So if you will need an open ended 500 ml bag fixed onto it, a 1000 ml bag is less satisfactory. Pinch the end of the bag shut, while you squeeze it gently to inflate him.

The circuit needs some method of preventing the gases going back up the tube while you do this.

If the Oxford bellows is providing the plenum, you will need its non-return valve (B), so park the magnet out of use. You will need an assistant to work the bellows.

If an oxygen cylinder or entrainer is providing the gas mixture, valves are needed with a child of this size, so put the Oxford bellows or the Penlon bellows in the circuit; but clip them shut, park the magnet, and use them for their valves only.

CAUTION ! With all three methods, take care not to overinflate the child.

ETHER AND HALOTHANE WITH A VAPOURISER

The method is similar with the "Paedivalve" and Ayre's T-piece.

Set the control indicator of the vapouriser to 4 or 5% ether. Lower the mask gently over the child's face.

Increase the concentration slowly until you are giving 15 to 20% ether. Don't give a fixed concentration for a fixed time.

CAUTION ! (1) Be careful not to give too much ether. (2) Keep the airway clear.

HALOTHANE In children under a year of age either give ether alone or halothane alone. Unless you are expert, don't try halothane induction and ether maintenance in young children. Always give oxygen with halothane (1 litre a minute).

Halothane induction. Set the OMV to 0.5% halothane only. Then introduce ether as usual and turn off the halothane when the child is taking a sufficiently high concentration of ether.

Halothane only maintenance. Use 1-2% halothane only.

AYRES T-PIECE WITH A BOYLE'S MACHINE

Connect the hose of Ayres T-piece to the top circuit of an

anaesthetic machine of the Boyles type in place of the Magill attachment.

Use a 25 ml thin-walled bag for neonates, and a 600 ml bag for older children. Attach an expiratory bag *without* a tap valve in its tail. This bag will enable you to inflate the child's lungs and observe his breathing. To inflate neonates, compress the bag 40 to 60 times a minute.

CAUTION ! (1) Never allow the bag to overdistend—release it. (2) The length of the tubing between the T-piece and the bag is unimportant, that between the T-piece and the child must be short. (3) Select the smallest face piece that will adequately fit the child. Judge the adequacy of inflation by constantly watching the movements of his chest.

If you don't have a bag, you can alternately block and unblock the end of the tube with your finger.

19 Primary Intensive Care

19.1 Special care for those in special need

As intensive care has evolved, it has largely fallen to the anaesthetists to develop and manage, so it is appropriate that this chapter should be devoted to it. Intensive care is a way of concentrating skills and facilities round a few critically ill patients. Also, there are a few procedures, such as monitoring the central venous pressure and the use of a ventilator, that are particularly important in intensive care, and are best discussed as part of it. Because we are primarily concerned with surgery, we do not discuss its more medical aspects, such as coronary care and management of poisoning.

Some of the procedures in this chapter are beyond many, perhaps most of the hospitals for which we write. They will however give some of our readers in more fortunate hospitals something to aim for, particularly those who have already attained the level of anaesthetic care described earlier, and want to progress to the use of a ventilator, to measure the central venous pressure, and to monitor the ECG. The main constraint on these methods is less the equipment than the nursing care.

About two patients in a hundred need continuous care of a very high level, usually for a few hours or days only, after which you can move them to an ordinary ward. They may have severe injuries, acute illness such as tetanus, metabolic disturbances or circulatory or respiratory failure. Trained staff must watch them constantly. They may also need oxygen, suction, intubation, intravenous therapy, or an accurate fluid balance chart.

How can the critically ill and injured get this care under the exacting circumstances of a district hospital? Are they best left scattered through the wards, or should you gather them into an intensive care unit (ICU)? If your hospital is minimally equipped and staffed, you may find it best to concentrate a proportion of your limited facilities round a few critically ill patients, in what will probably have to be a very simply equipped ICU. Trying to care for them adequately wherever they are in the hospital is much less practical. You may find it useful to set aside two or three beds in a special room, or part of a ward, for such intensive care facilities as you may be able to provide, or perhaps combine the ICU with a recovery room. *The more poorly developed your hospital and the more rudimentary its facilities, the more impor-*

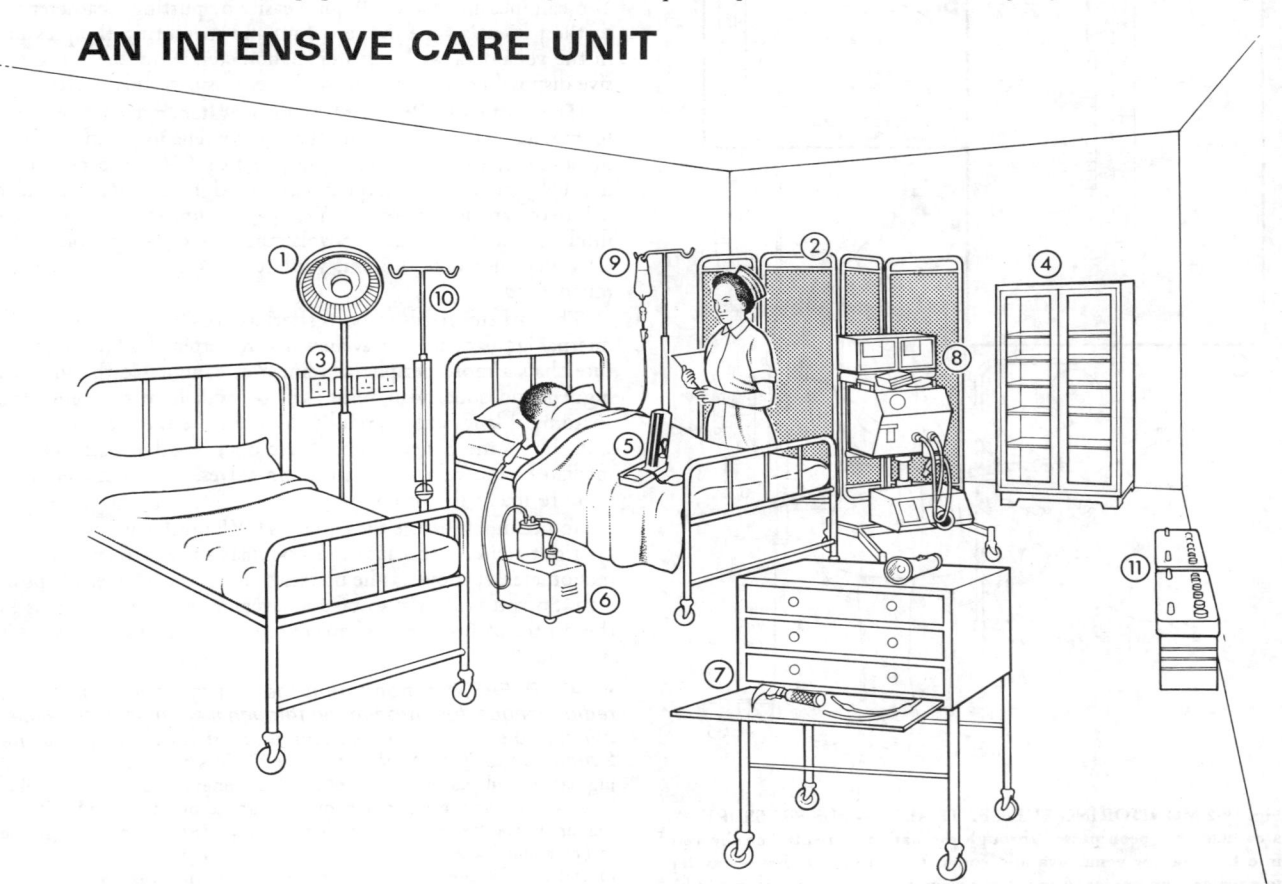

Fig. 19-1 AN INTENSIVE CARE UNIT. The equipment has been disposed around the room for ease of illustration. (1) a good light, (2) washable screens for separating the patients, (3) electric sockets, (4) equipment cupboard, (5) sphygmomanometer, (6) sucker, (7) trolley with equipment for resuscitation, (8) ventilator, (9) drip stand, (10) CVP monitor, (11) emergency batteries for the ventilator. *Kindly contributed by John Farman and Alan Kisia.*

tant it is for a bed or two to be reserved for patients who need special care. Some very minimal hospitals have done this with very good effect.

To begin with you may have so little equipment that your ICU may hardly seem to deserve its name. Nevertheless, it is the human skills that matter—constant care—and you may be able to improve on the equipment later. In a larger hospital the ideal intensive care unit has up to 10 beds, isolation facilities, equipment, stores, and a laboratory, etc.

If your hospital is a small one, your ICU is unlikely to be full all the time so staff it flexibly. The main requirement is that there should be one skilled person with these very sick patients all the time. Assuming there are eight hour shifts, and allowing for leave and sickness, this means that an ICU requires at least four nurses. Ideally there needs to be at least one nurse for every patient during the day and night, but many ICUs accept a ratio of one nurse to two patients. If you don't have enough nurses for this, any special care for the critically ill is valuable. The staff need special skills, so you will probably need to train them on the job. Many of these skills are anaesthetic ones, so it is natural that if there is anyone with special anaesthetic experience, he should play a large part in the ICU.

SETTING UP AN ICU
Choose a large side ward near the theatre, or one or two beds in a main ward. You will need plenty of space round the beds, and a good light. Care for both sexes together, and provide washable curtains between them. Ideally, keep infected patients separate. The beds should have hard boards and means to raise a patient's head and his legs. Provide several electric sockets for each bed. It is a good idea to provide a strong shelf along the wall above the heads of the beds, wide enough to hold an ECG monitor.

EQUIPMENT This includes syringes, drugs, a sphygmomanometer, a sucker, and equipment for intubation, which must *always* be ready beside each bed. Equipment for ventilation and an oxygen unit. All the infusions listed in Section 15.1 and drip stands. A monitor for the CVP. If you have only one ventilator, keep it in the theatre, and fetch it as required. A humidifier. Measuring cylinders for urine. A transportable adjustable light. A battery torch or lantern in case the mains supply fails. These are easily stolen, so put them in a glass fronted cupboard beside the drug cupboard. Two 12-volt car batteries for the ventilator, and a charger.

A chest drain set (S 65.4), a cut-down set (15.2), and a tracheostomy set with cuffed ('Portex') tracheostomy tubes (S 52.2), also plain tubes for infants and children.

19.2 Monitoring the central venous pressure (CVP)

If a patient bleeds and his blood volume falls, he maintains the volume of the blood in his arteries at the expense of that in his veins. So the first sign of a low blood volume is a low central venous pressure (CVP). A rise in his pulse rate and a fall in his arterial blood pressure are later signs of hypovolaemia. Being able to measure the CVP is thus of great value in treating the hypovlaemic shock that may follow a severe injury. Measuring the jugular venous pressure clinically is much less reliable. You can measure the CVP quite easily by putting a catheter into the patient's superior vena cava and measuring the pressure in the vena cava with a water manometer. Now that inexpensive disposable catheters are available, this is readily practicable.

The normal CVP is 0 to 5 cm of water, but it is not easy to measure changes within this range reliably with a water manometer, so aim to raise the patient's CVP to 5 cm. This is usually beneficial, except in cases of right or left ventricular failure or cardiac tamponade. You may be suprised by how much fluid you need to treat hypovolaemic shock, but provided the CVP does not exceed 5 cm, you are unlikely to be giving too much fluid.

The catheter needs to be as short as possible, so the patient's internal jugular and subclavian veins are better sites for venipuncture than a more peripheral vein. You cannot see the internal jugular and subclavian veins, so you will have to follow the anatomical landmarks carefully. You can use the median basilic vein, but some patients don't have one; in other patients, the median basilic vein has obstructing valves, and in any event it is more likely to thrombose.

You cannot measure the patient's CVP until you know where his right atrium is because this establishes the zero level for the manometer. It moves as he breathes and as he changes his position. So you will have to take its average position, which is in the centre of his chest where his mid axillary line crosses his fifth rib.

• CATHETERS, for monitoring the central venous pressure, radio-opaque, for introduction through a cannula, disposable, but capable of being boiled and re-used. (a) 20 cm. (b) 60 cm. 2 mm. Ten only of each size. The 20 cm size are for his internal jugular and subclavian veins and the 60 cm ones for his median basilic. These catheters are for introduction through a cannula. Don't buy those that are introduced through needles, because these can cut through the catheter and leave the cut end of the catheter inside the vein. They must be wide enough, preferably 2 mm, and not less than 1.6 mm.

• MANOMETERS, for central venous pressure, disposable, but capable of being boiled and re-used, with 3-way tap, side arm and delivery tube for connection to catheter. Ten only. You will also need a piece of wood and a spirit level.

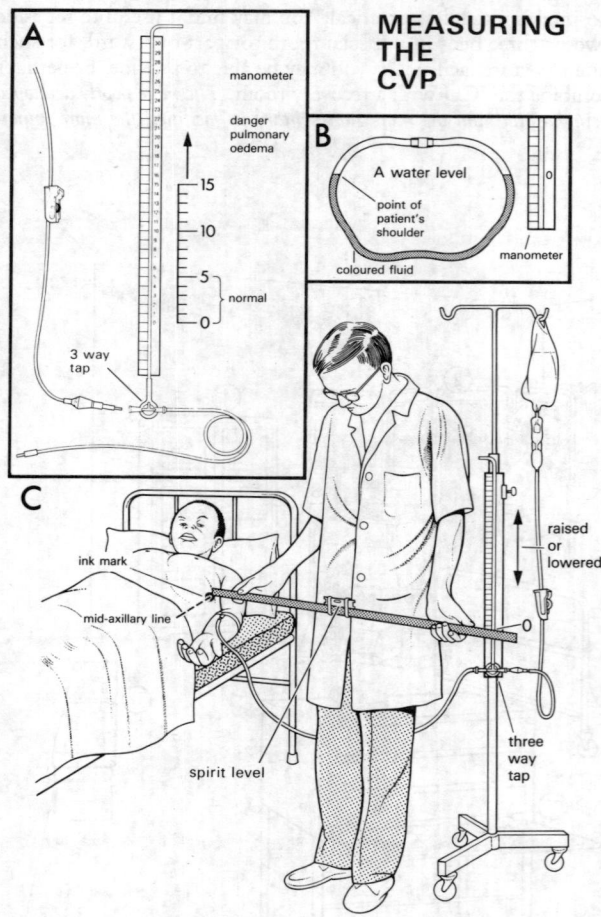

Fig. 19-2 MONITORING THE CENTRAL VENOUS PRESSURE. A, a catheter has been passed through the patient's median basilic vein into his superior vena cava and connected through a three-way tap to a water manometer. A mark has been made with a spirit pen in his mid-axillary line and a bar with a spirit level is being aligned with it. The manometer has been adjusted so that zero on the scale is level with the other end of the bar. B, an alternative water level using a plastic tube, half filled with water with its ends closed.

• *CONNECTORS, Y-shaped, disposable.* These are useful when a central venous catheter is in place. Attach one limb of the Y to the manometer and keep this filled ready for reading. Meanwhile the other limb is used for a slow continuous flush from the drip bottle and for fluid therapy, drug infusion, or intravenous nutrition, but not for blood transfusion or blood sampling, because the blood may clot in the catheter and block it.

CENTRAL VENOUS CATHETER

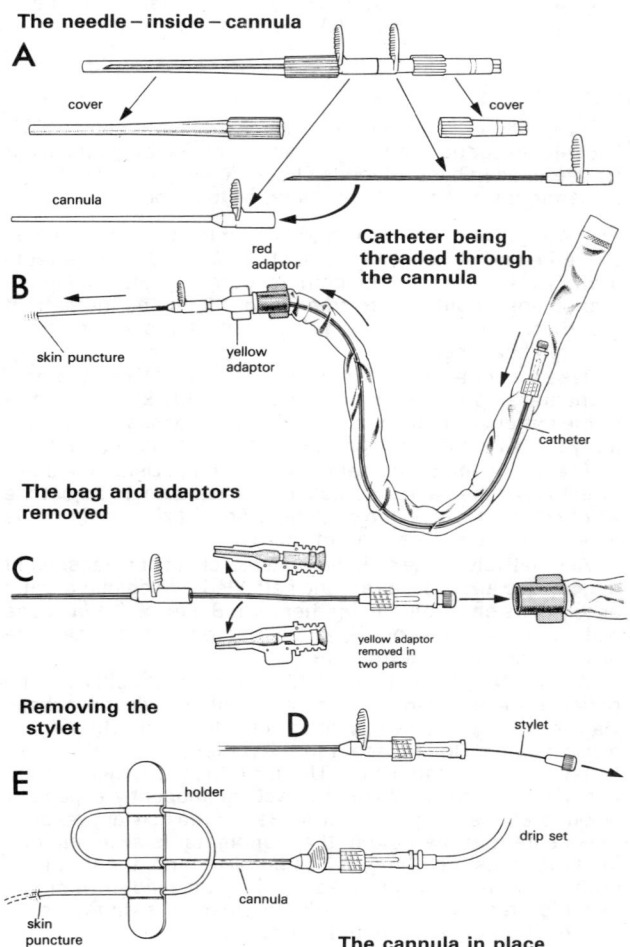

Fig. 19-3 INSERTING A CENTRAL VENOUS CATHETER. A, the cannula with the needle inside it covered by protective guards to keep it sterile. Mount the needle and cannula combination on a syringe to introduce them. B, the cannula has been inserted, and the catheter, in its sterile bag, is being threaded through it. A yellow plastic adaptor, with a rubber grommet in it stops the blood leaking from around the catheter. C, the bag and the adaptors being removed. D, a fine plastic stylet is being withdrawn from the catheter. E, now that the catheter has been threaded through into the vein as far as necessary, the cannula can be withdrawn, and a length of catheter coiled in place in its holder. The drip set has been attatched. This is the 'Cavafix' catheter (BRA), other makes differ. *Kindly contributed by Alan Kisia.*

CATHETERISATION AND THE CVP

You may need to pass a central venous catheter, (1) to maintain a central venous line, (2) to measure the CVP (central venous pressure). For both purposes you have to pass the catheter through a cannula.

CAUTION ! This is a method for the "careful caring operator" who has already done almost everything else in this manual. It is potentially dangerous, so do it for the first time under expert instruction, if you possibly can.

CANNULATION

When you cannulate the great veins of a patient's neck, raise the foot of his bed 20 cm, to distend the veins and reduce the risk of air embolism.

SITES FOR INSERTING THE CATHETER

For all sites, take full aseptic precautions. Use a mask, cap and gloves, and clean the patient's skin carefully. To reduce the risk of infection, don't use "cut downs", and try to keep the site of vein puncture as far as you can from the site of skin puncture. Infiltrate the site of skin puncture with anaesthetic solution using a fine needle.

(1) THE ANTECUBITAL FOSSA This is the safest method to start with. Use a 2mm×60 cm catheter, a 1.6 mm catheter is less satisfactory. Use the patient's right arm. Aim for his basilic not his cephalic vein. Keep his arm extended, and if possible try to enter the vein from above his elbow. If the catheter stops in his axilla, abduct his arm a bit, and try to push the catheter a bit farther. Then "connect the catheter" as described below.

(2) RIGHT OR LEFT SUBCLAVIAN VEIN— INFRACLAVICULAR ROUTE Lay the patient on his back and turn his head to the side opposite to the vein you are planning to cannulate. Sterilise his skin and drape him. Choose a 20 cm catheter. Raise the foot of his bed 20 cm.

Puncture the skin below and just lateral to the mid point of the clavicle. First try to get the general direction using a fine needle and local anaesthetic solution. Point the introducer needle and cannula at 15° to the long axis of his clavicle, and aim it at his sternoclavicular joint. Advance needle and cannula until you enter the vein, as indicated by blood coming from the needle.

Advance the cannula 1 cm further into the vein, while you hold the needle still. Again make sure you aspirate blood, and only now remove the needle.

Pass the catheter through the cannula into his subclavian vein, then through his brachiocephalic vein into his superior vena cava.

If the tip is in his right atrium, it can cause arrythmias, and for this reason, catheter placement should ideally be done under x-ray control. If it is a 2 mm catheter and lies 5 cm inside the his subclavian vein, it will be adequate. Then "connect the catheter' as described below.

(3) SUBCLAVIAN CANNULATION—SUPRACLAVICULAR ROUTE Lay the patient on his back and raise his feet 20 cm. Turn his head away from the side that you are going to cannulate.

Infiltrate anaesthetic solution into the skin over the junction of his clavicle and his sternomastoid, and into the area behind his clavicle. Insert the needle above his clavicle, at the junction of its inner and middle thirds, bisecting the angle between his clavicle and his sternomastoid, as in A, and B, Fig. 19-4. The needle must pass directy behind his clavicle. Aspirate gently as you advance it until blood flows freely. Then "connect the catheter" as described below.

(4) RIGHT INTERNAL JUGULAR VEIN Choose the patient's right internal jugular vein because it is directly in line with his superior vena cava, and you will avoid his thoracic duct. Raise his feet 20 cm (a 30°slope) to make his veins more prominent and air embolism less likely. Sterilise his skin and drape him. Choose a 20 cm catheter.

Tilt his head slightly to the left, as in C, and D, Fig. 19-4. The sternal and clavicular heads of his sternomastoid form a triangle, with its base on his clavicle. His jugular vein runs down the centre of this triangle, immediately lateral to his common carotid artery on a line from his ear to his right nipple. You may be able to feel it as a slight resilience. Insert the cannula at its apex between the two heads of his sternomastoid.

Start by using a 10 ml syringe containing 5 ml of saline attached to a 0.7 mm needle. Use this needle to find the vein, at a point on his ear–nipple line 3–4 cm above his clavicle. Remember the angle of your needle as it lies in the vein.

Then do the same thing with a 1.5 or 2 mm needle–inside– cannula combination attached to a 5 ml syringe filled with saline. When you have entered the patient's internal jugular vein, assure a free flow of blood by repeated aspiration and injection. At the same time bring the cannula to lie flatter against his neck. Then slide the cannula forward into the vein over the needle. You will need practice to learn how to "feel" the vein.

Alternatively, look for filling of the patient's internal jugular vein. It is not usually visible, but you may sometimes see its pulsations separate from those of his carotid. If you see his internal jugular vein, puncture it. If you don't see it, puncture his skin at the apex of the triangle, 3 cm above his clavicle, at about 30° to the coronal plane if his head were in the anatomical position (this is equivalent to about 5 minutes on a clock face). Aim the needle at his suprasternal notch, and advance it under his sternomastoid until you enter the vein. You should find blood at 2 to 3 cm. When you have aspirated blood, push the cannula a few mm further in to make sure it is inside the vein.

When you have entered the vein, advance the cannula ahead of the introducer needle about 1 cm. Then remove the needle and "connect the catheter" as described below.

CAUTION ! (1) The carotid artery lies medially and deep to the vein. (2) A haemothorax, a pneumothorax and arterial injury are rare complications.

CONNECT THE CATHETER (All 4 routes) Connect the drip set, or CVP manometer, and flush it through with intravenous fluid. Anchor the catheter by stitching its hub firmly to the patient's skin. If you don't do this, the catheter is sure to fall out later. Fit the Y-connector (you will need two lines) and join it to the manometer, as below. Then lower the drip container to the floor to confirm that blood runs back into the Y-connection, proving that the tip of the CVP catheter is in the vein. Raise the drip container and immediately flush blood from the tube.

Keep the site of puncture clean and cover it with a dry dressing.

If you need to manipulate the catheter because its tip has become impacted against the atrial wall, clean the site and withdraw the catheter a little way. Don't try to push it further in. The part of the catheter that has remained outside will be contaminated and will promote infection, so don't reintroduce it into the patient.

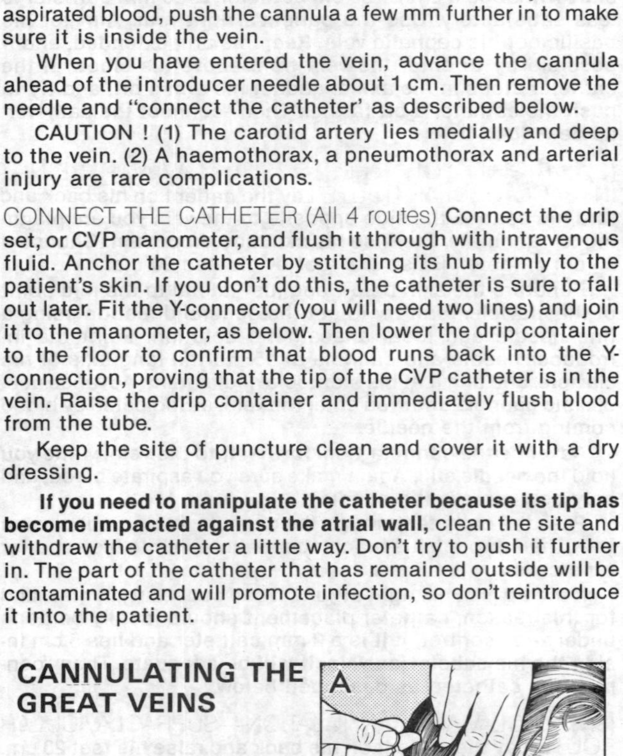

CANNULATING THE GREAT VEINS

Subclavian (supraclavicular route)

Internal jugular

Fig. 19-4 CANNULATING THE GREAT VEINS. A, (frontal view), and B, (lateral view) cannulating a patient's subclavian vein by the supraclavicular route. C, and D, cannulating his internal jugular vein. *After Rutherford, Nelson, Weston and Wilson, with the kind permission of Peter Wilson.*

CAUTION! If the patient's CVP is low, disconnection of the system will not cause visible bleeding. Instead, it will cause air embolism, so keep all connections secure.

X-RAYS Most catheters are radio-opaque. To make sure where the end of the catheter is, take a chest x-ray. If the catheter tip is in the wrong place, you may get a false reading of the CVP and so base a patient's fluid requirements on misinformation.

DIFFICULTIES These are rare if you do the procedure carefully, but they include: (1) Pneumothorax. (2) Puncture of the subclavian artery and a haemothorax. (3) Air embolism. (4) catheter embolus. (5) Arrhythmias. (6) Infection.

MONITORING THE CVP

INDICATIONS (1) Hypovolaemic shock. (2) Monitoring the CVP is useful in septic shock, but it may be misleading and is not as useful as in hypovolaemic shock. A Swan-Ganz catheter is better, but is beyond the scope of this book.

THE MANOMETER Fix the manometer to the central venous catheter, and attach it to a drip stand with adhesive strapping. If you have placed the catheter correctly, the fluid in the manometer should swing freely about 5 mm as the patient breathes. You will also see quicker pulsations synchronous with his heart beat.

Take a wooden bar about a metre long, and fix an ordinary carpenter's spirit level to it. Place an ink mark in the centre of the patient's chest, where his fifth rib crosses his mid-axillary line which is approximately the level of his right atrium.

Place one end of the bar on the ink mark. Using the spirit level to hold the bar horizontal, ask an assistant to adjust the height of the scale on the drip stand, so that zero on the scale is level with the other end of the bar.

Alternatively, make a simple water level out of a transparent plastic tube about 3 metres long half filled with coloured water and with its ends joined together as in B, Fig. 19-2. Place one water level on the tip of the patient's acromnion, and zero the scale on the other water level.

CAUTION ! (1) The tip of the CVP catheter should lie in the patient's superior vena cava, or at its junction with his subclavian vein. If the catheter is incorrectly placed, it will not give true readings. Don't place it in the patient's right atrium, or it may induce arrhythmias. (2) Use the drip for crystalloids only, and not for blood. (3) Check the levelling frequently, especially when he changes his position. (4) Before you take any reading, make sure that the fluid in the manometer is swinging normally with his breathing. If it is not swinging, the tip of the catheter is in the wrong place, or it is blocked. If there are very high readings with very large pressure swings, the tip of the catheter is in his right ventricle.

A normal CVP is 0 to 5 cm of water. For convenience of measurement and monitoring, try to maintain his CVP between 5 and 10 cm of water. If it is over 15 cm, you have overtransfused him, or he has heart failure.

AIM FOR A CVP OF 5 to 10 cm OF WATER

19.3 Equipment for mechanical ventilation (IPPV) and respiratory monitoring

Some contributors have argued that a ventilator would be lethal in many of the hospitals for which we write, in that the discipline necessary to make sure that it is not turned off accidentally, and the necessary nursing and maintenance skills, do not exist. This is correct. Nevertheless there are some hospitals with sufficient continuity and motivation of staff to be able to use a ventilator successfully. This section is for them. Moreover, you need not have expensive apparatus to monitor the blood gases, because you can monitor the carbon dioxide tension quickly and inexpensively with the Campbell-Haldane apparatus, described in the next section. A ventilator, like the East Radcliffe RP4, and the Campbell–Haldane apparatus thus make a good combination.

Although relays of people can ventilate a patient continuously by hand, it is a great help to be able to use a machine for intermittent positive pressure ventilation (IPPV). Use it: (1) Regularly during anaesthesia with relaxants so that you and your staff become familiar with it and know that it is still working. If you keep it in a cupboard and use it for emergencies only, it is sure to fail when you most need it. (2) In the intensive care unit for the indications given in the next section. When you have a patient in intensive care who needs the ventilator, you will have to return to hand ventilation in the theatre.

A patient on a ventilator must either be intubated or have a tracheostomy. You can use a ventilator for short periods during anaesthesia without a spirometer or a humidifier (or condenser), but you will need both of these for the longer periods of ventilation needed for intensive care, although you can do without them for short periods.

You will find that a ventilator which is pressure–limited and time–cycled, like the East Radcliffe RP4 in Fig. 19-4, is the simplest and most reliable. It is also well suited to referral hospitals where maintenance is a problem and where more sophisticated machines are so often out of order. The East Radcliffe RP4 is merely a bellows which driven by a motor that is wired for 220 volts AC and 12 volts DC, so that you can run it from a car battery if the mains should fail. This makes it portable; if necessary, you can run it from the battery of the car that is carrying the patient. The RP4 draws a maximum of 5 amps, so a new fully–charged car battery with a rating of 60 amp hours will power it for about 12 hours before it needs recharging.

The motor of the RP4 ventilator has a gear box that controls the ventilation rate from 12 to 32 cycles a minute in six steps, which you can select. It has a fixed inspiration/expiration (I:E) ratio of 1:2, so that the duration of inspiration is always half that of expiration.

A gauge shows the pressure at the entrance to the patient's airway. You can alter this pressure by placing varying combinations of weights on the lever that operates the bellows, or by varying the distance of these weights from the fulcrum of the lever. They are so arranged that the ventilator cannot deliver a dangerously high pressure to a patient's lungs. Internally, the RP4 has an inlet and a non–return valve, like the Oxford Bellows (10.3). Inspiratory and expiratory tubes lead from the ventilator and join at a Y–piece which fits onto the adaptor cone of a tracheal or tracheostomy tube. A water trap connected to the port of the expiratory tube collects the moisture that accumulates, as it is particularly apt to do if a humidifier is included in the circuit. If necessary, you can fit a PEEP valve to the expired gas port to provide Positive End Expiratory Pressure. If you maintain a positive pressure of 5 to 10 cm of water at the end of expiration, you can improve a patient's oxygenation if he has a pulmonary oedema, the adult respiratory distress syndrome following burns, or shunting from other causes. PEEP increases the resistance to expiration, it holds his alveoli open, and it opens up extra ones.

You can use the ventilator to deliver room air, with added oxygen if necessary, or you can attach the air inlet port to a draw–over vapouriser.

• VENTILATOR, *simple pattern, pressure–limited, class 1, type B, mode of operation continuous, anaesthetic class AP, time–cycled, electric, doubly wound for mains 120 or 220 AC voltage (state which) and 12 volts DC, with patient pressure monitor and handle for manual operation, 20 mm cone fittings on the Y–piece, 30 to 22 mm cone adaptor, and set of spares, as East Radcliffe RP4 pattern or equivalent, one only.* Electric ventilators are the most satisfactory, avoid those powered by oxygen or compressed air. The mains, battery, and hand powered model of the RP4 costs $2,400, the mains and hand powered model costs $1,000.

• SPIROMETER, *Wright's, with 22 mm male cone, (EAS) pattern. One only.* You will need this to measure the patient's tidal and

A SIMPLE VENTILATER

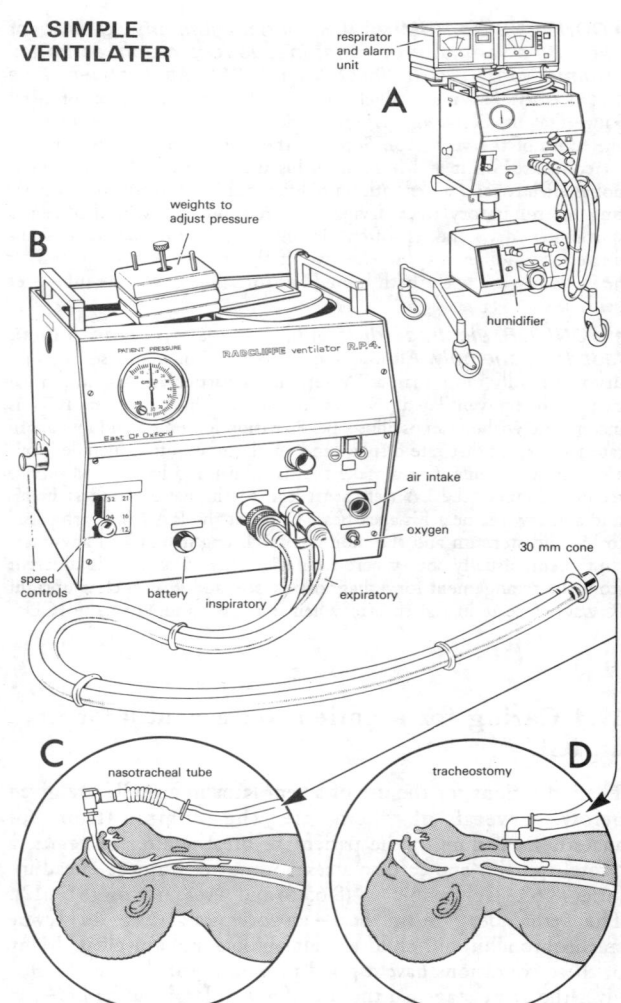

Fig. 19-5 A SIMPLE PRESSURE–LIMITED TIME–CYCLED VENTILATOR. This is the East Radcliffe RP4. It has bellows on which weights are placed to adjust the pressure, which is measured with a gauge, and two gear levers to vary the respiratory rate. Tubes to and from the patient end in a Y–piece, which fits onto a tracheal or tracheostomy tube. There is also an air intake that you can connect to a draw–over vapouriser or an anaesthetic machine, and an expired air outlet to which you can atttach a PEEP valve. A, the complete expensive version of the ventilator on its trolley with a respirometer, an alarm unit, and a humidifier. B, The RP4 itself. C, a patient being ventilated through a nasotracheal tube. D, a patient with a tracheostomy.

minute volume. A spirometer is fragile, and it may be safer if you fix it permanently to the casing of the ventilator and only connect it to the outlet of the ventilator with corrugated hose when you take a reading. Wright's spirometer costs $500. East's supply an electronic respirometer for the RP4 with battery and charger for $660.

• HUMIDIFIER, *electrically heated, water bath type, autoclavable, 110 or 220 AC mains voltage (state which) with double thermostat, (EAS) pattern. One only.* If you ventilate a patient with ordinary room air, his tracheal and bronchial mucosa will rapidly dry out and become infected. Prevent this by using a humidifier to moisten his inspired air. This will cost you about $750. Or, use a much cheaper condenser–humidifier as described below.

If a patient has secretions in his chest, a humidifier will help to supply addditional water to his inspired air; this will liquefy the secretions and make them easier to suck out. Place the humidifier between the patient and the ventilator so that air passes through the humidifier before it reaches his lungs. A humidifier is heated electrically to 37°C, and must have a double thermostat to prevent overheating. If it does overheat, he will inhale pure water vapour without any oxygen and he will die rapidly. Even if it is fitted with two thermostats the temperature of the water bath must be checked half hourly.

• **CONDENSER–HUMIDIFIER**, *thermal humidifying filter, for use with a ventilator or spontaneous respiration, as Portex "Humidi-vent" (POR) 100/580, each $1.2, pack of ten. Five packs only.* This is a small chamber containing a thick piece of metal gauze that fits between a patient's tracheal or tracheostomy tube and the tubes of the ventilator. Some of the water vapour in his expired air condenses on it and humidifies his incoming air. A condenser is not as effective as a water bath humidifier, but it is some help in preventing his respiratory tract drying out. A condenser will also keep a spirometer dry, and is often useful during anaesthesia. A condenser–humidifier is quite effective, if the patient is not infected. If he is, he needs a water bath humidifier (or saline down the tube—see below).

• **MONITOR**, *electrocardiograph, oscilloscope type, robust, fade free, one only.* Although an ECG monitor might seem a luxury it is hardly more than a TV set, and is particularly useful if a patient is being ventilated. Nurses are apt to think that an ICU is incomplete without an oscilloscope. Provision for a high and low alarm rate setting, a heart rate display, and an alarm are often included, but are of limited value. Get a make that is robust and has a good service record. Connect the LA (left arm) lead to the patient's chest in his mid axillary line near his apex beat. Connect the RA (right arm) lead to his mid sternum and the indifferent RL (right leg) lead anywhere convenient, usually somewhere near the other two. This is different from the arrangement for a diagnostic trace, and gives a clear upright R wave. Use it in the theatre when it is not wanted in the ICU.

19.4 Caring for a patient on a ventilator in an ICU

The indications for the use of a ventilator in an ICU are given below. Several of them are the complications of anaesthesia—failure of the patient to breathe after relaxants, a "total spinal", and cardiac arrest. Some are surgical—head injuries (S 63.1), chest injuries (S 65.6) and severe tetanus (S 54.12). The remainder are medical—an occasional case of severe tracheobronchitis in children, and bulbar poliomyelitis. Many of these conditions have a good prognosis—if the patient survives the acute stage, so the use of a ventilator can be life-saving. One of its great advantages is that it removes the extra workload from an exhausted patient. The care of such patients for a few days is the purpose of this section. Use a tracheal tube with a soft cuff with a large residual volume to prevent damage to his trachea.

Ideally, you need a condenser, a spirometer and equipment to measure the blood gases from the beginning of the period of ventilation, but equipment to measure the blood gases is expensive and needs a well-trained technician. Much cheaper and easier to manage is the Campbell–Haldane rebreathing apparatus (19.5), which will measure the PCO_2 reliably and quickly. The pO_2 and the pH are less essential and have the disadvantage of needing a sample of arterial blood.

The first decision you will have to make is whether the patient is in sufficiently severe respiratory failure to need ventilating. You will not be able to measure his blood gases, so you will have to evaluate him clinically.

If he shows several of the following signs, his respiration is probably failing: (1) Jerky, irregular, shallow, laboured, rapid breathing. (2) Restlessness. (3) "Tracheal tug" (11.2). (4) Involvement of his accessory muscles of respiration, including his alae nasae. (5) An open mouth, lip biting and an anxious expression. (6) Cold extremities. (7) Sweating. (8) Drowsiness, leading to unconsciousness. (9) A rising pulse rate and a falling blood pressure. As his respiratory failure gets worse, he becomes increasingly cyanosed. He coughs, sputum accumulates in his chest, and you can hear rhonchi in it. The following special tests, if you have a spirometer and can do them, indicate the need for controlled ventilation: (a) A vital capacity of less than 15 ml/kg body weight. (b) A minute volume of less than 100 ml/kg body weight. A patient who shows these signs will probably die unless you quickly intubate him, or do a tracheostomy, and connect him to a ventilator.

When a patient is properly settled on a ventilator, he should be quiet and allow himself to be completely controlled by it rather than by his own respiratory efforts, which must be in abeyance. To help achieve this, you can paralyse his respiratory muscles peripherally with a long-acting relaxant, such as alcuronium, tubocurarine or pancuronium, any of which you can give intramuscularly to prolong its effect. Or, you can deliberately depress his respiration centrally with opioids, which have the additional advantages of being analgesic and euphoric. If he becomes unsettled as the drug wears off, you are probably underventilating him.

The great danger is that the ventilator may stop unnoticed. This means that it must be watched *constantly,* particularly if it is not fitted with an alarm. So: (1) There should be one nurse for each patient *all* the time, and never less than one nurse for 2 patients. (2) She should *watch for chest expansion* and *listen* to the ventilator. (3) She must be taught how to ventilate by hand immediately if the ventilator fails. (4) The alarms must be checked regularly. (5) If the patient is conscious, he will indicate his need for ventilation.

If a patient's chest expands with every breath, it is being ventilated. If it does not expand, either: (1) the tube is kinked or otherwise obstructed, or (2) the ventilator has become disconnected or stopped working. In either case, his respiration stops, and his heart will stop in less than two minutes unless he is immediately ventilated somehow. There may be some obvious cause such as failure of the ventilator, disconnecting it or switching it off accidentally. Hand ventilation with the handle on the RP4 ventilator or ventilation with a self-inflating bag must start immediately.

The patient will probably have some intrapulmonary shunting and be hypoxic, even if you are ventilating him correctly for his carbon dioxide excretion, so give him oxygen. If you are going to ventilate him for days or weeks, you will have to measure his minute volume regularly. Ideally, you should take arterial blood to measure its carbon dioxide and oxygen tensions, which will confirm that his minute volume is correct and that he is receiving enough oxygen. If possible, do this frequently on the first day, and repeat it daily thereafter. If you cannot sample his blood gases, use the rebreathing method for pCO_2, or use the signs we give below for under and over ventilation.

A patient who wakes up and finds himself on a ventilator is scared. Reassure him, and tell your nurses to do so too. Tell him you are going to help him to breathe for a day or two (or longer), and tell him everything you are going to do to him before you do it.

USING A VENTILATOR

The following description applies to a time-cycled pressure-limited ventilator, of the type described in Section 19.3.

INDICATIONS These include severe respiratory failure due to (1) Head injuries (S 63.1). (2) Severe chest injuries (S 65.6.) (3) Tetanus. Although many patients with tetanus would benefit from IPPV, the extensive nursing care it involves makes it impracticable in most of the hospitals for which we write. Other methods of managing tetanus are described in Section S 54.12. (4) Failure to recover from relaxants (14.4). (5) Cardiac arrest (3.5). (6) A "total spinal" or an epidural that has spread too high (7.2). (7) An occasional case of acute tracheobronchitis in children. (8) Bulbar poliomyelitis, and some cases of polyneuritis. (9) Some cases of poisoning.

EQUIPMENT In addition to the ventilator itself you will want a spirometer and humidifier, if the patient is to be on the ventilator more than a few hours. The ability to monitor blood the blood gases is increasingly useful, the longer ventilation lasts.

CAUTION ! (1) If the ventilaror fails, you must be able to inflate the patient instantly by hand. If it does not have a manual control, have a self-inflating bag instantly available; it is easier to manage than the handle of a ventilator. A bag also gives you a better impression of a patient's airway resistance and his lung compliance. (2) Even if the ventilator does have an automatic alarm, someone must be near by to hear it, and with patient constantly in case the alarm fails.

TESTING Do this before you connect the ventilator to the patient.

(1) Obstruct the patient end of the tubing. Check that the pressure rises when you start the machine and that there is no air leak.

(2) Use corrugated tubing to connect the downstream end of the Oxford Bellows (with its outlet valve immobilised by the magnet) to the ventilator. Like this the bellows acts as a "test lung" and allows you to see if the expiratory valve of the ventilator is working properly. Or, connect a 1.5 or 2 l anaesthetic rebreathing bag to the patient's end of the ventilator, and use this as a "test lung".

NASOTRACHEAL AND TRACHEOSTOMY TUBES For short periods—up to about 48-72 hours—you can use an orotracheal tube, which should be cuffed for adults, and for children over 10 years. For longer periods, use a cuffed nasotracheal tube. The cuffs should be of the low pressure type. Keep the pressures in them as low as posible. Record the volume you use to inflate the cuff and use the same syringe on each occasion. Inflate the cuff until the leak in the patient's trachea is only just obliterated.

If you don't have special low pressure cuffs, which have their own problems and are not so easy to insert, you can use ordinary ones.

CAUTION ! (1) Check that the tube has not gone too far by listening to the air entry over the lungs. (2) Any of the complications of intubation (13.3), or tracheostomy (S 52.2) may occur. (3) Make the tracheostomy with a flap, as in S 2.2.

NASOGASTRIC TUBE Insert this when the patient is intubated, and leave it in.

CONNECTING THE VENTILATOR Make sure that the connections are secure. They must not come apart accidentally.

HUMIDIFICATION This is essential if the patient is to be ventilated for more than a few hours. If he is not infected, a condenser-humidifier is suitable. If he is infected, he will need more water than a condenser-humidifier will provide, so use a water bath humidifier. If you don't have either, instil 1-2 ml of saline into the tube ½ to 1 hourly, to make sure that the patient's respiratory mucosa does not become dehydrated.

SETTING THE VENTILATOR With a time-cycled ventilator, you can change the rate, the pressure, and the volume, although the last two are interconnected.

Add or subtract weights from the bellows to maintain an inflation pressure of 15 to 20 cm of water or less. If the patient's lungs are so severely diseased that they are no longer compliant, you may have to increase this pressure to achieve the desired tidal volume, but a ventilator of this kind is not ideal for "stiff chests" from whatever cause.

Calculate the patient's tidal volume as 6 ml/kg, and aim at mild hyperventilation (a pCO_2 of 30 to 35 mm). So start slighty in excess of the figure you arrive at—say an additional 500 ml in an adult. Start at 12 respirations a minute, and alter the rate on the following clinical indications.

If he shows agitation, tachycardia, ectopic beats or hypertension, you are probably underventilating him. These are all signs of sympathetic activity due to carbon dioxide retention.

If he shows hypotension and pallor, you are probably overventilating him. If he shows tetany, you are grossly overventilating him.

If you can measure his blood gases, aim for a pCO_2 of 30 to 40 mm, and a pO_2 of 90 to 100 mm. Check these values at least daily, and after any change of ventilator variables.

SPIROMETRY Measure the patient's minute volume intermittently. Don't leave Wright's spirometer in the circuit because it easily becomes waterlogged.

RELAXANTS OR SEDATION? If he is very ill or deeply unconscious, he may not need any drugs at all to help him settle on the ventilator. Otherwise he may need a relaxant or a sedative, or a combination of both.

Relaxants. Give him any of the long-acting non-depolarising relaxants described in Chapter 14. Be cautious with these drugs until the nurses are familiar with them.

Sedation. Sedatives are contradicated when you are interested in assessing a patient's level of consciousness, as after a head injury or cardiac arrest. Otherwise, if he is in pain, give him a small dose of pethidine or morphine. When necessary, supplement this with diazepam into a central vein (where it will be painless), or lorazepam (which is longer acting).

Diazepam emulsion is less likely to cause thrombophlebitis. Or, you can give a finely crushed tablet down his nasogastric tube.

When you have relaxed and sedated him correctly, he will lie quietly, with his ventilation fully controlled.

If he is very frightened, uncooperative or restless, give him diazepam.

If he is in pain, give him a pain-relieving drug.

'PEEP' (POSITIVE END-EXPIRATORY PRESSURE)

INDICATIONS (1) Pulmonary oedema. This presents as a stiff chest, a low pO_2, and a characteristic chest x-ray. The detailed diagnosis still largely depends on Swan-Ganz catheter findings. It usually starts after a few days when the patient has been progressing well. (2) ARDS, the adult respiratory distress syndrome, is suggested by the late onset of x-ray changes in the absence of pulmonary oedema or collapse.

METHOD Either connect a PEEP valve to the outlet of the ventilator, or lead a corrugated tube from its outlet port under 10 cm of water.

CAUTION ! (1) Watch with care for a fall in blood pressure (2) Don't use more than 10 cm of water, or the increase in his intrathoracic pressure will depress his cardiac output.

OXYGEN If possible, give the patient a litre of oxygen a minute. This will probably raise the oxygen content of the air he breathes to about 25%. If he has a very abnormal chest, he may need more. If you can measure his pO_2 try to keep it between 90 and 100 mm Hg. High concentrations of oxygen may be dangerous if he has good lungs and you give them for more than 72 hours.

CAUTION ! 100% oxygen is harmful.

SUCTION Suck secretions from the patient's chest at least every 6 hours, or more often if they are copious; use the sterile technique shown in Fig. 13-10. Physiotherapy will also help to clear pulmonary secretions. Turn him so that the infected part of his lung is uppermost, and then pummel his chest during expiration to dislodge the secretions, which you can then suck out. Ask an assistant to use a self-inflating bag to make the patient cough.

FLUIDS AND ELECTROLYTES Prescribe these as in Chapter 15. If the patient needs an indwelling balloon catheter, insert it under the strictest asepsis, and collect his urine into a graduated 250 ml plastic cylinder or bag. Record the volume hourly.

Electrolyte problems are complicated and there are few simple rules. If you can maintain a good fluid intake and an adequate urine output, most of his electrolyte problems will look after themselves. Potassium is the most important electrolyte to check, but remember that metabolic acidosis will raise it, and metabolic alkalosis will lower it. If you can measure his serum sodium reliably each day, it is likely to be a good guide to the water he needs—a high serum sodium probably indicates the need for more water, and a low serum sodium for less.

If your laboratory can measure the sodium and potassium in a patient's serum, it can probably measure them in his urine too. If so, record his sodium and potassium balance in addition to his fluid balance.

FOOD A patient who has had a major operation, a serious accident, burns, tetanus, or septicaemia, rapidly consumes his body tissues, and especially his muscles, to provide the energy he needs for metabolism. If he can absorb food from his gut, you can reduce the breakdown of his tissues by giving him a high energy, high protein diet through a nasogastric tube. These diets are mostly needed in burns, so consult Section S 58.12. Intravenous feeding is likely to be expensive and impractical. The best you may be able to do is to give him 10% dextrose through a central vein.

TURNING Turn the patient to prevent bed sores and help keep his chest clear. Turn him onto one side then onto his back, and then onto the other side every two hours. Record this by writing R, B, and L on the chart.

If the patient is not accepting nasogastric feeds, he will be safest if you nurse him on his sides only, with a slight head–down tilt.

OTHER TREATMENTS He may also need antispasmodics, antibiotics, physiotherapy, and treatment for cardiac failure.

X-RAYS If you have a portable x-ray, use it. Hold the patient's lungs still and fully inflated with the ventilator or bag, while you take an AP x-ray of his chest. If his lungs move during the exposure, the film will be blurred. With a good AP film you will be able to confirm that: (1) His central venous catheter has its tip in his superior vena cava (that is between his sternal notch and his heart shadow). (2) His tracheal tube is correctly placed with its tip in his trachea. (3) You will also get useful information about his lung fields, and you may see air or fluid in his pleural cavity.

RECORDS Record his pulse, and his blood pressure, etc., and also the settings on the respirator, and the volumes and pressures you have measured. If possible use a special chart.

ENDING VENTILATION ON A VENTILATOR

Choosing the right time to discontinue mechanical ventilation needs skill and patience. The signs that a patient is ready for it are: (1) A generally favourable clinical state. (2) Satisfactory tidal volume, minute volume, and respiratory rate during spontaneous breathing. (3) A satisfactory blood gases with minimal oxygen enrichment. (4) A satisfactory chest x-ray.

Try taking him off the ventilator when he is no longer under relaxants or sedatives. You can usually do this in one step, but he may continue to need oxygen by mask. If he shows cyanosis, sweating or tachypnoea, reconnect him to the ventilator. If necessary, try leaving it off for longer periods each day.

CAUTION ! Don't remove his tracheal tube until you are absolutely sure he no longer needs the ventilator.

STERILISING THE VENTILATOR

You will probably be unable to sterilise the ventilator itself, but at least boil or autoclave the tubes.

DIFFICULTIES WITH MECHANICAL VENTILATION

If a patient tries to breathe against the ventilator: (1) You may be underventilating him. (2) The tube may have slipped into a bronchus. (3) The ventilator may not be working properly. (4) Part of his lung may have collapsed. (5) He may be febrile and have an increased oxygen demand. (6) He may need further sedation. (7) He may be well enough to breathe on his own. (8) There may be an obstruction, or his respiratory tract may be full of secretions.

If he "fights on the ventilator", he will become hypoxic, which may have a disastrous effect on his circulation. Struggling will increase his oxygen consumption, and make his condition worse.

If his blood pressure falls seriously, you may be hyperventilating him, and so impeding his venous return and his cardiac output. Another possible cause is a tension pneumothorax. Check that his trachea and apex beat are in their right places. If they are not, he probably has a tension pneumothorax, and needs a chest drain–this is a dire emergency!

If he is cyanosed or distressed, give him oxygen while you try to find out the reasons for distress. If this fails try PEEP.

If the pressure on the gauge rises sharply, suspect that the tubing has kinked, or that it is blocked by mucus or secretions. Change in the compliance of his lungs is another cause, but this usually happens gradually, unless it is due to a tension pnuemothorax.

If he has poor or absent chest movements, the air passage between the ventilator and his airway may be obstructed—see Fig. 13-16. The causes are similar to those of respiratory obstruction during anaesthesia.

IF THE ELECTRICITY FAILS, THINK FIRST OF THE PATIENT ON THE VENTILATOR

19.5 Measuring the pCO_2 with a modified Campbell–Haldane apparatus

The information you need most when a patient is being ventilated continuously is the carbon dioxide tension in his blood. Measuring the carbon dioxide tension in a liquid is difficult, which is why the standard equipment for blood gas analysis costs about $15,000 and needs a technician to work it. By contrast, measuring the carbon dioxide tension of a gas, such as alveolar air, is easy. You can do it with the Campbell–Haldane apparatus, which costs only about $225 and is quick and is accurate to about 1 mm of mercury which is enough for clinical purposes.

In this method the patient breathes from a bag containing oxygen and carbon dioxide and in doing so he brings the carbon dioxide tension in his alveolar air into equilibrium with that in his oxygenated venous blood. You then take a sample of his alveolar air from the bag, and measure the carbon dioxide tension in it by observing the volume change that occurs when you absorb it with potassium hydroxide.

You use the reading on the burette to calculate the pCO_2 of his mixed venous blood. If you want the pCO_2 of his arterial blood, you can get a useful approximation of it by deducting 6 mm Hg. This is the average difference between the arterial and mixed venous pCO_2 of a resting subject. It also takes into account the fact that 'oxygenated' mixed venous blood has a pCO_2 about 2 mm higher than 'true' venous blood.

You will need a bag full of oxygen and CO_2 at the right tension. The easiest way to get this is to use the patient's own alveolar air by asking him to breathe in and out of the bag. He has therefore to breathe into the bag on two occasions: once to fill it with CO_2, and once to equilibrate his alveolar air with it.

• APPARATUS, Campbell–Haldane, modified, for measuring the the alveolar CO_2 with PTFE stopcocks, in case, complete with: (a) a 2 litre nominal capacity rebreathing bag to BS 3353, with mouthpiece, mouthpiece–tap, (b) 50 ml of mercury, (AIM), $225one only. You will also need some 20% potassium hydroxide and some 5% sulphuric acid.

Campbell EJM, Simplification of Haldane's apparatus for measuring CO_2 concentration in respired gases in clinical practice. Brit med J 1960 : 457-458.

MEASURING THE pCO_2

SETTING UP

Filling the Campbell–Haldane apparatus with mercury. Take the plunger out of the syringe: pour about 12 ml of mercury into the barrel: replace the plunger: lower and invert the syringe to allow air to collect at the nozzle end: eject the air through the burette: replace the syringe in the clip on the backboard: adjust the volume of mercury by drawing excess off through the tap A with a fine needle and a small syringe: arrange the position of the plunger so that, with tap C open, the mercury in the burette is just below the zero (10 ml) mark. The volume of the mercury should be such that with the plunger pushed home the mercury level is just below tap A. You can bring it exactly to the level of the bottom of tap A with the screw clip.

THE CAMPBELL–HALDANE APPARATUS

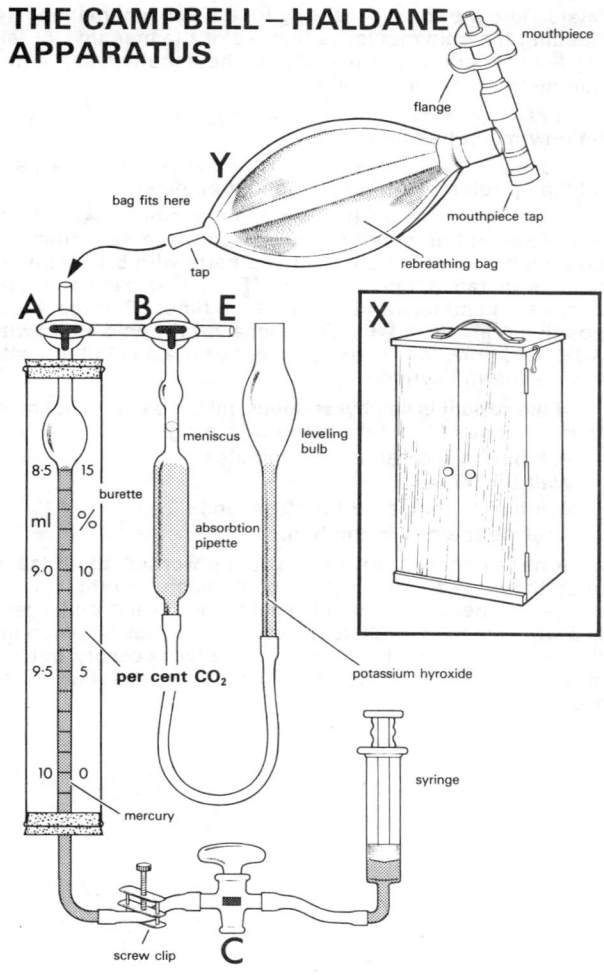

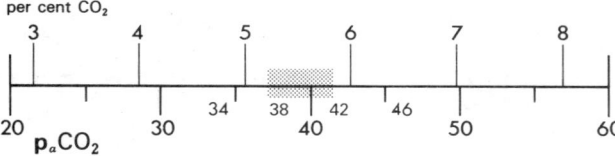

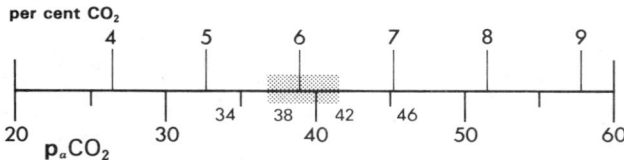

Fig. 19-6 THE CAMPBELL–HALDANE APPARATUS. X, the complete apparatus in its wooden box. Y, the rebreathing bag. Z, the parts of the apparatus. *Kindly contributed by Frank Prior.*

Adding acid. Add 1 ml of 5% sulphuric acid containing some phenolpthalein to the burette. The acid will rest on top of the mercury and keep the burette acid. If the solution goes red (alkaline) change it for some fresh acid, after washing with water.

Do a few blank analyses on room air. There should be no detectable CO_2.

EQUILIBRATIING THE CAMPBELL–HALDANE APPARATUS

Fill the bag with 1.5–2 litres of oxygen. In practice a bag about half full is enough. This is enough for the largest tidal volumes that you are likely to meet, and is satisfactory for an adult with normal ventilation. It should not be much more than about three times his tidal volume, which is about 400–500 ml. If you don't add oxygen, the patient will become anoxic.

You will probably have intubated him or have done a tracheostomy. If so, fit the female cone of his tube onto the male cone of the bag. If he has been paralysed by disease or drugs, ventilate him by squeezing the bag. If he does not have a tracheal tube or a tracheostomy tube, use the mouthpiece and nose clip supplied with the equipment; avoid using a mask.

Ask the patient to rebreathe into the bag for 90 seconds. If the movements of the bag are small, prolong this period to 2 minutes.

If he has difficulty, be firm and encourage him to breathe deeply at an instructed rate.

If he cannot breathe for 1 minute under these conditions, **use two separate periods which are as long as he will tolerate.**

If the movement of the bag at the end of half a minute indicates that his tidal volume is less than half his bag volume, **start again with a smaller volume of gas.**

Wait 2 minutes.

Ask him to rebreathe into the bag for 20 seconds. If he is cooperative and you think his circulatory rate is increased, you can ask him to breathe deeply and stop after 4 breaths in about 10–12 seconds. If he is breathing shallowly, prolong rebreathing for 30–40 seconds.

Analyse the gas in the bag.

CAUTION ! He must be resting, or his mixed venous CO_2 will not reflect his ventilatory status.

ANALYSIS WITH THE CAMPBELL–HALDANE APPARATUS

(1) Turn tap B to position ⊢

(2) Bring the KOH to the meniscus.

(3) Turn tap B to position ⊥

(4) Fill the burette with mercury to the base of tap A.

(5) Close tap C.

(6) Connect the cone or the tubing from the bag to inlet A.

(7) Turn tap A into position ⊥

(8) Blow 20 ml of gas from the bag, so that it issues out through outlet E.

(9) Turn tap A into position ⊣

(10) Draw the gas in the bag into the burette by lowering the mercury until the meniscus is at the zero mark. Do this by using the syringe with tap C open. Use the clamp for fine adjustment. When the mercury meniscus is at the zero mark, close tap C.

(11) Turn tap A to position ⊤ , and tap B into position ⊣

(12) Wait for 10 seconds. If the level of the KOH starts rising, the burette is contaminated with KOH. Wash the burette out with 5% sulphuric acid and start again.

(13) Pass the gas sample to and fro into the absorption chamber about 6 times. Do this by opening tap C and then using the syringe.

CAUTION ! Watch the rising mercury and the rising KOH, and don't let them go too high.

(14) Bring the level of the KOH to its meniscus. Then close tap C. Read the level of the mercury in the burette.

(15) Push the sample over twice more to check that absorption is complete.

(16) Read off the level of the mercury meniscus in the burette. It will give you the %CO_2.

(17) IMPORTANT Leave the apparatus with the KOH level below the meniscus to prevent a deposit of potassium carbonate forming at the meniscus.

Leave tap B in position ⊢

Leave tap A in position ⊣ Other positions are possible, but this will prevent the KOH contaminating the mercury, and leave both sides of the apparatus open to the atmosphere.

CAUTION! If your apparatus has glass taps, and you are not going to use it for 12 hours or more, withdraw the keys from taps A and B, to clean and regrease them. This will prevent them seizing up, if by any chance they have become contaminated with KOH during use. If they stick, and you try to free them forcefully, they may break. If they do stick, tap them lightly with a screwdriver or try to soak them free with water over some days. Plastic taps do not have this difficulty.

RESULT In the following calculation paCO$_2$ is the partial pressure of the patient's arterial CO$_2$. The figure 46 is the water vapour pressure in mm Hg at 37°C. The following calculation assumes that the barometric pressure minus 46 is 700 mm Hg. If you assume that the barometric pressure is constant for each place, it will produce very little error. For convenience Fig. 19-6 includes an approximate conversion scale.

paCO$_2$ = [(700 × % CO$_2$) ÷ 100] − 6

For example, if the %CO$_2$ is 6, then the paCO$_2$ = (7×6) − 6 = 36 mm

NORMAL VALUES are questionable on a ventilator, but you should know these values.
paCO$_2$ = 38–42 mmHg, or 5.06–5.60 kPa

ALTERNATIVELY If you have an anaesthetic machine of the Boyle's type with rotameters, you can make a 5% mixture of CO$_2$ in oxygen, and bypass the first rebreathing. Better, you can get a cylinder of 5% CO$_2$ in oxygen.

DIFFICULTIES WITH THE CAMPBELL–HALDANE APPARATUS

If you have trouble, the common mistakes are: (1) Failure to test for leaks by an occasional blank test with room air. (2) Failure to maintain a trace of acid in the burette. (3) Misreading the volume marking for the per cent marking. (4) Reading the acid meniscus instead of the mercury. (5) Taking the per cent CO$_2$ as the pCO$_2$ without multiplying by (the barometric presssure − 47).

If KOH goes over into the mercury, removing it depends on how much has gone over.

If only a little KOH has gone over, clean the burette, tap, and adjoining tubing with a syringe and catheter.

If more has gone over, turn tap A into position ⊥ . Empty the absorption pipette by pouring off the KOH from the leveling bulb. Fill the absorption pipette with 5% sulphuric acid. Turn tap A into position T , and pass the acid backwards and forwards two or three times. Turn tap A into position T or ⊢ , and pour away the acid. Refill with KOH, and draw the excess acid out of the gas burette with a catheter and syringe.

If the patient is emphysematous, fill the bag with not more than 1½ times his tidal volume with oxygen.
Ask him to rebreathe for 2 minutes.
Wait 3 minutes.
Ask him to rebreathe for 40 seconds.
Analyse the gas in the bag.

If he is uncooperative and you are worried about leaks, slide the large flange of the mouthpiece up to the smaller flange, and put it in his mouth. Peel his lips over it, pull it gently away from his mouth, and sandwich his lips between the flange and your hand. This is not usually necessary, but you may sometimes need to do it, and it may be useful when you are demonstrating.

20 Evaluating the quality of anaesthesia

Death as the result of disease may be inevitable, but death as the result of anaesthesia is a tragedy. The only satisfactory anaesthetic mortality is zero. Mortality, morbidity, and the satisfaction of both the patient and the surgeon are the conventional indicators as to whether anaesthesia is good or bad. Of these, mortality is the crudest and most useful indicator. There are district hospitals (not in Kenya) where the mortality associated with major surgery and anaesthesia is said to be 20% and twice this in children. Much of this mortality is due to the high proportion of gravely ill patients who are operated on late. Fortunately, this represents the extreme, but there are many district hospitals where anaesthetic deaths are unnecessarily common, and occur in at least 1% of major operations.

Prior describes how the anaesthetic mortality at Ludhiana was reduced over a period of years from 0.07% to 0.03% and for major surgery this is probably a suitable target to aim for. Using the EMO methods described here, the Kilimanjaro Christian Medical Centre in Moshi, Tanzania, achieved an anaesthetic mortality for Caesarean section of 0.003%, almost all anaesthetics being given by assistants. Alas, most district hospitals keep no anaesthetic records, so it is not possible to know what their anaesthetic mortality is. The existence of records of almost any kind is in itself an important indicator of good anaesthesia.

One contributor (Julian Bion) reporting the experience of a surgical team on the Thai—Cambodian border, recalls 10 deaths in 600 operations requiring general anaesthesia. Of these patients, 9 died from their injuries and only one from anaesthesia. The one patient who died—needlessly—from aspiration while being given ketamine demonstrates that this can happen. There were, of course, many near misses, and it is these marginal cases that increase anaesthetic mortality in inexperienced hands. These figures represent wartime emergency anaesthesia at its best.

There are two major causes of anaesthetic death, which need to be carved on the back of every anaesthetist's right hand—hypovolaemia and aspiration. After these come failure to intubate, hypoxia and drug overdose. The common factor in all of them is failing to think before acting!

There are many other causes of anaesthetic death, expecially where anaesthetic standards are low. Many are simple and avoidable, and most are the result of very poor practice indeed. A common cause of anaesthetic mortality is not examining patients before anaesthetizing them, so that gross anaemia or diabetes are not diagnosed. Some patients are given too much thiopentone too fast (12.1). Deaths from vomiting and regurgitation (16.5) are much less common if the proper precautions are always taken. Although technical difficulties are less likely with an ether vapouriser like the EMO, than with an anaesthetic machine of the Boyle's type, it is still possible to use a non—rebreathing valve without immobilising the outlet valve of an Oxford Bellows (10.3), and to kill a patient that way. If the oxygen on an anaesthetic machine runs out without anyone noticing, the patient will certainly die. Finally, a patient can die because his tongue has fallen back and obstructed his airway, either in the theatre or afterwards, when not even the simplest precautions have been taken to prevent it. It is one of the purposes of Primary Anaesthesia to prevent anaesthetic deaths from these and many other causes.

Here are some of the more obvious characteristics of anaesthetic care that can be used to evalute its quality. Some are things that should happen (positive targets), and others are things that should not happen (negative targets).

TARGETS FOR GOOD ANAESTHESIA

POSITIVE TARGETS
These are the things that should happen.

INFORMATION Anaesthetic records are kept (4.7). The hospital analyses its records so that it knows the mortality associated with surgery and anaesthesia performed there.

STAFF The person who gives the anaesthetics has been properly trained. Anaesthetic staff in district hospitals are regularly visited and supervised. There is a programme of continuing education to update knowledge and maintain their interest. Anaesthetic mishaps are discussed sympathetically and not vindictively, with the aim of preventing similar mishaps in future. This is best done at a regular mortality and morbidity meetings.

METHODS Patients are *always* examined before they are scheduled for surgery; poor risk cases are identified and anaesthetized appropriately (1.6).

A full range of appropriate anaesthetic methods is employed, including local anaesthesia and ketamine.

No anaesthetic is given unless resuscitation equipment is available.

All patients having a major operation under general anaesthetic are intubated.

Anaesthetized patients are never left alone on the operation table but are always monitored by a competent person.

Patients are treated with courtesy as people, even when anaesthetized; they are handled gently and not subjected to iatrogenic injury.

Proper attention is paid to where and how anaesthetized patients recover.

EQUIPMENT All anaesthetics are given on a table that can be tilted head down, and with suction always available (3-1).

The essential anaesthetic drugs and equipment are present so that there is no unnecessary improvisation. (There are hospitals without oral airways, let alone tracheal tubes).

Equipment is appropriately cleaned and sterilised to prevent nosocomial infections, regularly serviced and maintained in good working order.

Spare oxygen cylinders, suckers, valves, a laryngoscope, bulbs and batteries, are available.

A well labelled supply of resuscitation drugs is always at hand.

NEGATIVE TARGETS FOR EVALUATING ANAESTHESIA

Thiopentone drips are not used by inexperienced people, nor is any operation lasting more than a minute or two ever done under thiopentone alone.

When a bottle of intravenous fluid is empty, the drip is either taken down, or a new one is put up. Empty drip bottles hanging over a patient's bed are a sign that the management of intravenous fluid therapy is very bad indeed. If there is a strip of paper down the side of the bottle marked where the fluid level should be each hour, care is probably very good.

21 Multiple choice questions

21.1 What do you know? One

Here are some multiple choice questions. They are taken from all over the book, and ask only things that it mentions. When you have read it, test your knowledge. Any, all, or none of the answers may be correct. The answers are in Appendix D. Fifteen is a good score, and 20 is a very good score.

1. SITA (31 years) is to have A Caesarean section under subarachnoid anaesthesia with heavy cinchocaine. Which of these things would you do?

A, "Preload" her with a litre of saline. B, Give the table moderate head down tilt. C, Put a wedge under her right buttock after completing the subarachnoid injection? D, Atropinise her. E, Do an augmented saddle block.

2. JOHN (3 years) is to be circumcised, and you have all the drugs and equipment you need. You are a very inexperienced anaesthetist. Which SINGLE method would be the safest?

A, Sacral epidural anaesthesia. B, Halothane in air from a vapouriser. C, Topical anaesthesia of his urethra with lignocaine. D, Intramuscular ketamine. E, Inhalation anaesthesia with ethyl chloride from a vapouriser.

3. Which of these are among the 'Ten golden Rules of Annaesthesia''?

A, There must be someone in the room who can apply cricoid pressure. B, You must have a sucker instantly ready. C, You must be able to control the patient's ventilation. D, You must monitor the patient's pulse and blood pressure continually. E, He must be starved.

4. AYRAM (75 years) needs his left leg amputated above his knee for diabetic gangrene. His diabetes has been controlled by oral hypoglycaemics. You decide to use subarachnoid anaesthesia. Which of the following could you safely you do?

A, Give him an infusion of 0.9% saline and continue his oral hypoglycaemic agent. B, Stop his oral hypoglycaemics, starve him overnight and operate on him in the early part of the morning. C, Give him 1.5 ml of hyperbaric chinchocaine in the left lateral position with his spine horizontal. D, Give him 5 ml of isobaric bupivacaine. E, Give him insulin alone during the operation.

5. You have decided to give a subarachnoid anaesthetic with 0.5% isobaric bupivacaine. Which of the following would you expect to be correct?

A, Giving the table a a head down tilt will increase the level of the block. B, 4 ml will give a higher block than 3 ml. C, Adequate analgesia may take about 15 minutes to develop. D, Analgesia will probably last 4 hours. E, As soon as you have injected the bupivacaine you can turn him into any position you like for the operation.

6. You are an inexperienced anaesthetist. Which of the following patients are suitable for subarachnoid anaesthesia? You have all the equipment and drugs you need, except intravenous fluids.

A, SANJAY (6 years) with a laceration of his foot. B, TITI (7 years) who is to have a supracondylar fracture reduced. C, BUDI (65 years) who needs a herniorrhaphy and is known to be asthmatic. D, KADI (24 years) who also needs a herniorrhaphy but has multiple septic lesions on his back. E, JADI (26 years) with a ruptured spleen that needs removing and is in severe hypovolaemic shock?

7. You have given child PATEL (1 year) an intravenous ketamine drip for a long operation for the correction of scars. Immediately after it he becomes restless and confused. Which of the following would you suspect as being the likely cause of these symptoms?

A, Pain. B, The atropine used for premedication. C, Nausea. D, An overdose of ketamine. E, Hypoglycaemia.

8. VJAY (21 years) is to receive ketamine anaesthesia for the surgical toilet of a wound. Which of the following would you use to reduce the emergence reactions that might follow?

A, Chloral hydrate. B, Diazepam. C, Promethazine. D, Phenobarbitone. E, Pethidine.

9. Which of the following patients would you consider suitable for ketamine anaesthesia?

A, TOPO (29 years), a schizophrenic, who is to have a biopsy taken from his leg. B, SIMON (6 years) an otherwise healthy child who is to have an ulcer on his leg grafted. C, RADHILKA (19 years), a diabetic who is to have her burns dressed. D, EVA (19 years) who is in labour and is to have an internal version for the correction of a malpresentation. E, MARTA (31 years) who needs a Caesarean section and has PIH (pregnancy induced hypertension or pre—eclamptic toxaemia).

10. You have no oxygen and no muscle relaxants. PAUL (33 years) needs a laparotomy which requires good muscle relaxation. Which of these could you safely use?

A, Ether. B, Halothane. C, Thiopentone by infusion. D, Ketamine by infusion (a ketamine drip). E, Trichloroethylene.

11. You have just started to induce MUKERJEE (41 years) by injecting 2.5% thiopentone into a vessel in his antecubital fossa, when he complains of a sudden pain in his arm. What would you do?

A, Immediately take the needle out. B, Stop injecting but leave the needle in the vessel. C, Continue the injection. D, Inject 10 ml of 0.5% procaine through the needle. E, Inject heparin through the needle.

12. For which of the following patients would you add adrenaline to the local anaesthetic that you would use?

A, JOE (24 years) who is to have a digital block for the amputation of the distal phalanx of his right index finger. B, UNG (14 years) who is to be circumcised using a ring block of his penis. C, TERESA (18 years) who is to have an axillary brachial plexus block for the repair of cut tendons. D, JIM (30 years) who is to have an intravenous forearm block for the surgical toilet of a hand injury. E, MAY (40 years) who is to have a retrobulbar block for the repair of a corneal laceration.

13. Which of the following agents form inflammable or explosive mixtures when mixed with oxygen, nitrous oxide or air under the conditions used during anaesthesia?

A, Diethyl ether. B, Trichloroethylene. C, Halothane. D, Ethyl chloride. E, Chloroform.

14. MURMU (30 years) is to have an urgent operation under general anaesthesia. Which of the following features would lead you to suspect that intubation might be difficult?

A, Protruding upper teeth. B, A short neck. C, A large tongue. D, A receeding jaw. E, Kyphoscoliosis of his thoracic and lumbar spine.

15. When is it advisable to give a patient 100% oxygen?

A, Before laryngoscopy. **B**, Before intubating him under thiopentone and suxamethonium. **C**, Before your assistant applies cricoid pressure for a "crash induction and intubation". **D**, If you suspect a patient has cardiopulmonary arrest. **E**, Before you extubate him.

16. You have intubated KINOTTI (26 years) and you want to know if you have been successful. Which of the following tests would help you to decide?

A, Seeing the tube go through his cords with a laryngoscope. **B**, Seeing his chest expand when you inflate his lungs. **C**, Hearing air enter his chest when you inflate his lungs with a bellows or bag. **D**, Watching to see if his abdomen moves on respiration. **E**, Pressing on his chest while you listen for breath sounds through the tracheal tube.

17. In which of these patients would the use of suxamethonium for intubation be dangerous?

A, ASLAM who has appendicitis. **B**, LEOPOLD who is hypertensive. **C**, SANDRA who was severely burnt a few days ago. **D**, LATIM who has pulmonary TB and is being treated with isoniazid. **E**, TARUN who has pyloric obstruction.

18. You have successfully given TERESINA a general anaesthetic, intubated her, and given her a long acting relaxant. Which of the following conditions should be met before removing the tube? You should remove the tube—

A, After giving her neostigmine. **B**, After giving her extra oxygen for 2 or 3 minutes. **C**, After sucking out any secretions in her pharynx and trachea. **D**, After deflating the cuff of her tracheal tube. **E**, After waiting until she starts to inspire.

19. Which of the following are suitable for producing epidural analgesia?

A, 2% pethidine. **B**, 0.5% bupivacaine. **C**, 1.5% lignocaine plus adrenaline 1:200,000. **D**, 2% cinchocaine. **E**, 5% ketamine.

20. You have just given a 43 year old man an epidural anaesthetic. As you position him for surgery he stops breathing. What would you do?

A, Wait until he starts to breathe again spontaneously. **B**, Give him a central respiratory stimulant such as nikethamide. **C**, Intubate him and control his ventilation until he starts to breathe again. **D**, Raise the head of the table. **E**, Measure his blood pressure and give him a rapid intravenous infusion if it is low.

21. You have just given an adult woman a mid–subarachnoid hyperbaric anaesthetic. Ten minutes later she becomes unconscious, stops breathing and is almost pulseless. You have neglected most of the "Ten golden rules" and have no equipment for controlled ventilation. What would you do?

A, Raise the foot of the table. **B**, Raise her legs, while keeping her body supine. **C**, Ventilate her mouth–to–mouth. **D**, Give her an intravenous infusion as fast as you can. **E**, Give her intravenous ephedrine.

22. Which of the these drugs are useful for their central analgesic properties?

A, Pethidine. **B**, Morphine. **C**, Diazepam. **D**, Trichloroethylene. **E**, Ketamine.

23. Which of these stimulate a patient's respiration?

A, Halothane during light anaesthesia. **B**, Intravenous pethidine 1 mg/kg. **C**, Intravenous morphine 0.5 mg/kg. **D**, Trichloroethylene during light anaesthesia. **E**, Ether during light anaesthesia?

24. Which of these would reduce a patient's anxiety before an operation?

A, Aspirin. **B**, Diazepam. **C**, Pethidine. **D**, Naloxone. **E**, Paracetamol.

25. You are anaesthetizing Mrs WANJOHI with ether. After some difficulty, she is asleep, but she is also completely silent and is rapidly becoming cyanosed. Her jaw and trachea show downward twitching movements, her intercostal spaces are sucked in, and her abdomen balloons outwards. Which of these might help her?

A, Giving her more thiopentone. **B**, Giving her more ether. **C**, Raising the angles of her jaw. **D**, Intubating her. **E**, Inserting Guedel's airway.

Answers in Appendix D

21.2 What do you know? Two

1. Which of these are rational combinations of drugs?

A, Suxamethonium and atropine. **B**, Procaine and lignocaine. **C**, Lignocaine and adrenaline. **D**, Pethidine and diazepam. **E**, Neostigmine and atropine.

2. Which of these are rational sequences of drugs?

A, Pethidine followed by thiopentone. **B**, Ether followed by thiopentone. **C**, Trichloroethylene followed by ether. **D**, Diazepam followed by ketamine. **E**, Suxamethonium followed by thiopentone.

3. Why is adrenaline sometimes added to a local anaesthetic solution?

A, To increase the rate at which it is absorbed from the tissues. **B**, To increase the maximum safe dose of some local anaesthetic agents. **C**, To improve the shelf life of a local anaesthetic agent. **D**, To prevent a local anaesthetic from causing hypotension. **E**, To shorten the latent interval before local analgesia starts.

4. Which of these patients would you consider suitable for anaesthesia with ketamine alone?

A, LITETA (23 years) in hypovolaemic shock who needs a surgical toilet for lacerations of her leg. **B**, LUAMPA (7 years) who is to have a tonsillectomy. **C**, LORENZA (51 years) who is to have a large lipoma excised from her back. **D**, LUKULANYA who needs a laparotomy for an acute abdomen. **E**, LUAPULA who needs her arm amputated and in whom you expect intubation may be difficult because he has a receeding jaw.

5. KENYI (39 years) needs his burns dressed under ketamine. Which of these would you do?

A, Starve him. **B**, Be prepared for airway problems. **C**, Give him atropine before anaesthetizing him. **D**, Intubate him as soon as he loses consciousness. **E**, Treat any emergence reactions with intravenous pethidine.

6. Your vote for anaesthetic drugs and equipment has just been cut by 50%. Which would be the cheapest way of anaesthetising a patient who needs a hernia repaired?

A, Subarachnoid anaesthesia. **B**, Nitrous oxide, oxygen and ether from a vapouriser. **C**, Ether, oxygen, suxamethonium and a long acting relaxant. **D**, Intramuscular ketamine. **E**, Halothane from a vapouriser with added oxygen.

7. BARDI had a road accident soon after a large meal. Three hours later he was admitted to hospital and needed some severe lacerations of his trunk sutured. Which ONE of these would be the safest way to anaeshetize him?

A, Open ether. **B**, Continuous thiopentone. **C**, Nitrous oxide, oxygen and halothane from a mask. **D**, Intravenous ketamine. **E**, Infiltration anaesthesia with 1% lignocaine.

8. Which of these is the least painful way of giving parenteral diazepam?

A, Intramuscularly. **B**, As a bolus injection into a freely flowing intravenous drip. **C**, Subcutaneously. **D**, Intradermally. **E**, As a slow bolus injection through a small vein on the dorsum of the hand.

9. Which of these are the correct indications for the use of diazepam in anaesthesia?

A, To treat postoperative pain. **B**, As premedication for ether. **C**, To control the convulsions that may complicate local anaesthesia. **D**, As an intravenous induction agent. **E**, to treat and prevent the emergence reactions that may complicate ketamine anaesthesia.

10. ZOYA (7 years) is to be given ether for a major operation and is to be allowed to breathe spontaneously. What would you do?

A, Induce him with with ethyl chloride. **B**, Premedicate him with atropine. **C**, Starve him. **D**, Premedicate him with morphine. **E**, Intubate him.

11. Which of the following are rational anaesthetic "cocktails"?

A, Pethidine with diazepam. B, Morphine with pethidine. C, Pethidine with promethazine. D, Thiopentone and naloxone. E, Ketamine with phenobarbitone.

12. You have decided to use vapourisers in series. In the alternatives below the vapourisers are represented by their respective agents, starting at the the most upstream one. Which of these are correct?

A, Ether, trichloroethylene. B, Ether, halothane, trichloroethylene. C, Ether, halothane. D, Halothane, thrichoroethylene. E, Ether halothane, trichloroethylene.

13. Which of the following anaesthetics can safely be prolonged for an hour or more without changing the basic method?

A, Intramuscular ketamine. B, A low subarachnoid block with a single injection of heavy chinchocaine through a needle. C, Epidural anaesthesia through a catheter. D, Pethidine and diazepam through an intravenous cannula. E, Intravenous thiopentone through a cannula.

14. You are about to give intubate DIVYA under suxamethonium for a short orthopaedic operation. Which of these would you expect?

A, Her tongue will fasciculate? B, The suxamethonium will make her unconscious. C, She should be given atropine. D, Her ventilation will need to be controlled. E, She may develop postoperative pain.

15. ABDULLAH (30 years) needs to have his ventilation controlled with an EMO vapouriser and an Oxford Bellows. What would you do?

A, Intubate him. B, Paralyse him with suxamethonium and follow this with a long acting relaxant. C, Pause after the upward stroke of the bellows. D, Work the bellows about 15 times a minute. E, Choose an expiratory spill valve of the Heidbrinck type rather than a non—rebreathing valve like the AMBU valve.

16. Which of the following methods, when used alone can produce safe and adequate muscle relaxation for abdominal surgery?

A, Ether anaesthesia. B, Trichloroethylene anaesthesia. C, Nitrous oxide anaesthesia. D, Anaesthesia with a thiopentone infusion. E, An intravenous cocktail of pethidine and diazepam.

17. CHARLES (30 years) has severe bronchitis and needs an urgent appendicectomy. What will be the safest way of anaesthetizing him?

A, Open ether. B, Anaesthesia using a thiopentone infusion. C, Ether and air from a vapouriser. D, Thiopentone, suxamethonium, halothane and tubocurarine. E, Lumbar epidural anaesthesia.

18. MARY (20 years) has a haemoglobin of 6.5 g/dl and needs an emergency laparotomy. You cannot transfuse her or transfer her to another hospital. What method would you use to anaesthetise her?

A, High subarachnoid anaesthesia. B, Intravenous ketamine followed by ether from a vapouriser. C, Intravenous thiopentone followed by ether from a vapouriser. D, An intravenous cocktail of pethidine and diazepam. E, An epidural block.

19. After careful consideration you have decided that you must make intravenous fluids in your district hospital. Which of the folowing precautions are critical?

A, Recently washed bottles must be placed upside down to drain. B, Freshly distilled water must stand for a couple of days before being used to make up solutions. C, Any freshly prepared solution must stand overnight before being autocalved. D, When the bottles are in the autoclave, it should be held at 121°C for at least 40 minutes. E, The autoclave should be opened immediately the holding time at 121°C is completed.

20. CHLOE (2 years) is to have a laparotomy. Which of the following anaesthetic techniques would be best?

A, A high subarachnoid block. B, A ketamine drip and relaxants. C, Trichloroethylene from a Schimmelbusch (open) mask. D, Intravenous pethidine and diazepam. E, Sacral epidural anaesthesia.

21. Which of these things would you expect when you anaesthetize a child of 6 months?

A, He can easily become hypoglycaemic. B, His normal respiration rate will be about 15 per minute? C, His blood volume will be about 85 ml/kg? D, Atropine could seriously increase his temperature if the theatre is very hot. E, If you don't take proper precautions, he can easily become hypothermic.

22. There are many pieces of anaesthetic equipment in your hospital, but no Ayre's T-piece, so you have decided to rig one up. Which of the these features should it have?

A, The limb between the junction of the T and the child, should be longer than the distal limb. B, The volume of gas flowing through it should be less than 4 litres a minute. C, It should have a large dead space. D, It should have a non—return valves. E, It should have a high internal resistance.

23. Which of these are acceptable methods of anaesthetizing a child?

A, Intramuscular ketamine. B, Open ether. C, Ether from an EMO vapouriser using Farman's entrainer and Ayre's T-piece. D, Inhalational induction and intubation using intramuscular suxamethonium. E, The AMBU "Paedivalve" and some means of providing ether vapour and air under a small pressure (plenum).

24. Which of these are the correct reasons why nitrous oxide and oxygen, an adult mask and an expiratory spill valve are unsuitable for children?

A, There will be too lare a dead space between the child's alveoli and the valve. B, The high resistance of an adult spill—valve. C, The high gas flow that these machines will deliver. D, The difficulty of warming the incoming gas. E, The difficulty of making adequate compensation for a young child's high metabolic rate.

25. You have decided to intubate SHANTI (13 months) and to anaesthetize her using an AMBU "Paedivalve". How would you fix it up?

A, By fixing the adaptor of the tracheal tube into the 15 mm female cone of the "Paedivalve". B, By putting a catheter mount between the "Paedivalve" and the tracheal tube. C, By supplying it with gas under a very small positive pressure (plenum). D, By trying to make the dead space between the valve and her alveoli as small as possible. E, By keeping the valve as close to her lips as possible.

Answers in Appendix D.

21.3 What do you know? Three

1. ANITA has bronchial asthma and is in hypovolaemic shock due to the rupture of an ectopic pregnancy. Which of these methods would be most suitable for the emergency laparotomy that she needs?

A, A subarachnoid block. B, An epidural block. C, Thiopentone, suxamethonium, cricoid presure, intubation, ether and alcuronium or gallamine. D, Ketamine, suxamethonium, cricoid pressure, intubation, ether and alcuronium or gallamine. E, Ether induction, intubation, and then maintenance on ether.

2. Which of these can cause hypotension and bradycardia during anaesthesia?

A, Halothane. B, A repeat dose of suxamethonium without atropine. C, Traction on a patient's gut. D, Light anaesthesia. E, Hypovolaemia.

3. Which of these are common causes of anaesthetic disaster?

A, The failure to maintain a clear airway. B, Hypovolaemia. C, Failure to monitor a patient adequately. D, Failure to take a history from a patient and examine him carefully before operating on him. E, Drug overdose.

4. Mr. MAYIM (72) needs his prostate removed. He has a blood urea of 34 mmol/l (200 mg/dl). Which of these would be suitable?

A, A low subarachnoid block. **B,** A low epidural block. **C,** Thiopentone, suxamethonium, ether and gallamine. **D,** A liberal infusion of 0.9% saline. **E,** Gentamicin 5 mg/kg daily for 7 days.

5. SAID (24 years) has jaundice, ascites, a large liver, and a leg which needs amputating after a road accident. Which of these would be suitable for him?

A, Suxamethonium. **B,** Vitamin K. **C,** A transfusion of fresh blood. **D,** Induction with the minimum quantity of diazepam and maintenance with a low dose of ether and tubocurarine. **E,** A thiopentone infusion.

6. JOHN (30 years) is being anaesthetized with ketamine. Which of the following statements are correct?

A, There is no risk of him inhaling his gastric contents. **B,** You can control the depth of anaesthesia more easily if you give the ketamine as an infusion. **C,** You are using one of the safest anaesthetics there is. **D,** He is likely to become hypotensive. **E,** His abdominal muscles will be well relaxed.

7. RAMCHANDRAN was severely hypertensive but his hypertension is being controlled with thiazides and beta blockers, so that his blood pressure is now 120/90. He needs his hernia repaired. What methods would be suitable for him?

A, High subarachnoid anaesthesia. **B,** Anaesthesia using a field block. **C,** Premedication with pethidine. **D,** Local anaesthesia of his larynx after thiopentone and suxamethonium but before intubation. **E,** Stopping his antihypertensive drugs several days before the operation.

8. HERNOKO (37) has a metabolic acidosis as shown by deep panting respiration (hyperventilation), an acid urine, hypotension, generalised muscle weakness and an irregular pulse. He needs an emergency exploratory laparotomy under general anaesthesia. Which of these is he in particular danger from?

A, Failure to breathe after a long acting relaxant. **B,** Death on the operating table. **C,** Convulsions. **D,** Awareness under anaesthesia. **E,** Hypertension.

9. Which of these patients will be in no danger of the acid aspiration syndrome?

A, ROBIA who is having a Caesarean section. **B,** BUROO who is having a laparotomy soon after a traffic accident. **C,** LECK (20 years) with intestinal obstruction whose stomach has just been emptied with a large tube. **D,** Baby MARY who has been starved for the last two hours. **E,** JURG with an acute abdomen who has had a nasogastric tube passed on the ward.

10. Which ONE of these patients, all of whom are to have elective operations, is most in need of cricoid pressure during induction?

A, FIFI who is having a Caesarean section. **B,** KENYI who is having a routine hernia repair. **C,** MULEME who is having a lipoma removed from her calf. **D,** GWEMBE who is having a mastectomy. **E,** OSAMU who is having an operation for piles.

11. JOSIAH was knocked over by a car as he staggered out of a bar, and now needs an urgent laparotomy. Which of the following procedures would be appropriate for him?

A, Rectus block. **B,** High subarachnoid anaesthesia. **C,** The passage of a nasogastric tube, induction with ether with the table tipped head downwards. **D,** Cricoid pressure, thiopentone, suxamethonium and intubation. **E,** Thiopentone, suxamethonium and intubation without cricoid pressure.

12. ZOYENKA (17 years) has been given thiopentone, and paralysed with suxamethonium. You are about to intubate him. Which of these things are true?

A, He cannot now vomit. **B,** He cannot regurgitate. **C,** You should wait to intubate him until his tongue has stopped fasciculating. **D,** His muscle paralysis will need reversing with neostigmine. **E,** He needs a few breaths of pure oxygen.

13. You have just induced MANUEL with ether. There is a gurgling noise from under the mask, and a loud wheezing. He is difficult to inflate. What would you do?

A, Quickly wash out his stomach. **B,** Quickly tip the table head down. **C,** Suck out his pharynx. **D,** Intubate him and suck out his trachea through the tube. **E,** Postpone the operation if this is possible and observe him carefully.

14. Which of the following measures help to prevent vomiting or regurgitation during the induction of anaesthesia?

A, Starving a patient preoperatively. **B,** Emptying his stomach with a large tube before you induce him. **C,** Intubating him with cricoid pressure. **D,** Identifying patients who are at particular risk. **E,** Operating under local anaesthesia where you can.

15. An otherwise normal adult is losing blood slowly. Which of these statements is true about him?

A, The first sign of hypovolaemia is a fall in his blood pressure. **B,** Constricted peripheral veins and delayed capillary refilling usually occur before a serious drop in blood pressure. **C,** He may show no signs until he has lost 500 ml of blood or more. **D,** If you induce him with thiopentone, he may suddenly become seriously hypotensive. **E,** His haemoglobin level is a reliable early guide to the volume of blood that he has lost.

16. Which complications are mothers who are being anaesthetized for Caesarean section particularly liable to?

A, Laryngospasm. **B,** The acid aspiration syndrome. **C,** A catastrophic rise in blood pressure as the baby is delivered. **D,** A rise in blood sugar as the baby is delivered. **E,** The supine hypotensive syndrome.

17. You have all the fluids you need. Which of these are appropriate indications for giving a patient an intravenous drip of 0.9% saline?

A, To maintain "an open vein" during a major operation. **B,** To "preload" a mother who is having a Caesarean section under subarachnoid anaesthesia. **C,** To provide a patient with his water needs in the immediate postoperative period. **D,** As the only fluid with which to rehydrate a patient who is dehydrated as the result of intestinal obstruction. **E,** As the first fluid to give a severely shocked patient while you wait for blood.

18. You have all the fluids you need. Which of these are acceptable indications for giving a patient 0.18% saline in 4.3% dextrose?

A, To supply a balanced combination of water and electrolytes in the immediate postoperative period. **B,** To maintain an "open vein" during a surgical operation. **C,** To hydrate a mother having a Caesarean section. **D,** To maintain the hydration of a patient who cannot take fluids by mouth. **E,** To maintain the entire energy needs of a patient who cannot take food by mouth.

19. SOPHIE had a normal blood pressure preoperatively. She is now having a Caesarean section. When you measure her blood presure you are alarmed to find that it is only 65 mm systolic. What might be the reasons for this?

A, The supine hypotensive syndrome. **B,** Too large a dose of lignocaine for infiltration anaesthesia or intercostal blocks. **C,** Blood loss. **D,** Hypoxia. **E,** Reaction to a blood transfusion.

20. BARDI (34 years) is a 60 kg man who has had a successful laparotomy for intestinal obstruction. The weather is hot and you are giving him 3 litres of fluid a day. How much urine would you expect him to pass if he is in normal fluid balance?

A, 0.3 ml/kg/hour. **B,** 1 ml/kg/hour. **C,** 3 ml/kg/hour. **D,** 500 ml/day. **E,** 1500 ml/day.

21. Which of these will quickly raise a patient's blood pressure?

A, The rapid infusion of 0.9% saline. **B,** The rapid infusion of a plasma substitute. **C,** Methoxamine intravenously. **D,** Digoxin intramuscularly. **E,** Raising his legs well above the level of his trunk.

22. You have paralysed YASSER with suxamethonium and have then given him alcuronium after the signs of paralysis by the suxamethonium have worn off. After the operation he will not start to breathe. What might be the cause?

A, He might still be deeply anaesthetised. **B,** You might have forgotten to reverse the residual paralysis produced by the alcuronium. **C,** He might still be paralysed from the effects of the suxamethonium, if he happens to be one of the few patients who lacks the enzyme that destroys it. **D,** He might be hypothermic. **E,** He might be acidotic.

23. You have intubated LUKE under suxamethonium and thiopentone, and then given him alcuronium. You are about to remove the tube at the end of the operation when you notice that his intercostal movement is poor, he has tracheal tug and is fighting for breath. What might be the cause of all this?

A, You have tried to reverse the action of the alcuronium too early. B, You have not given him and adequate dose of neostigmine. C, The neostigmine you have given him might not yet have had time to act. D, He might have been given gentamicin before the operation. E, He might be severely alkalotic.

24. You have been warned that intermittent suxamethonium is a dangerous method of producing sustained abdominal relaxation. Yet you have given XANTHE (21 years) a total of 500 mg of suxamethonium for this purpose. You should not be suprised therefor, when, at the end of the operation, she fails to breathe. What are you going to do now?

A, Give her a double dose of neostigmine? B, Give her more atropine? C, Keep relays of nurses ventilating her until she eventually recovers. D, Give her naloxone. E, Give her hydrocortisone.

25. Which of the following drugs cross the placenta in sufficient quantity to affect a baby significantly in the doses used in anaesthesia?

A, Ketamine. B, Pethidine. C, Diazepam. D, Gallamine. E, Thiopentone.

Answers in Appendix D.

21.4 What do you know? Four

1. You have learnt to intubate adults and now wish to intubate children. Which of the following statements are correct?

A, A child's respiratory tract is narrowest at his cricoid ring. B, He needs a plain non–cuffed tracheal tube. C, He may need to be intubated with a pillow under his neck. D, If he he is less than a month old, you could intubate him while he is awake. E, If he is an infant and you do not have a special infant's laryngoscope, you can use the tip of the blade of an adult instrument.

2. Under what conditions is it it dangerous to anaesthetize the vocal cords of a patient who is to have an anaesthetic?

A, If he is to have an intraocular operation. B, If he is likely to vomit or regurgitate. C, If an operation is to be done on his nose, mouth or pharynx. D, If he is a child. E, If he is very old.

3. You are ventilating a patient's lungs with a bag and a mask, when this suddenly becomes difficult and requires high pressures. What might be the cause of this?

A, His airway might be blocked anywhere. B, He might have bronchospasm. C, His larynx might be in spasm. D, If you have been giving him a general anaesthetic, he may be waking up. E, The effect of the relaxant may be wearing off.

4. You are ventilating a patient with bellows and a face mask when it suddenly feels as if his lungs have lost their normal compliance so that he becomes abnormally easy to ventilate. What might be the cause of this?

A, There may be a leak between the mask and his face. B, The corrugated breathing tube may be disconnected from the anaesthetic circuit. C, His level of anaesthesia may have become too light. D, He may be dead. E, He may have developed a pneumothorax.

5. When does a patient need extra potassium?

A, After prolonged vomiting. B, After prolonged nasogastric suction. C, When he is oliguric. D, When he has diarrhoea. E, When he has a small gut fistula.

6. Which of these are indications for intubating a patient?

A, Coma with airway obstruction. B, Prolonged respiratory failure. C, A patient whom you have to induce yourself and then hand to a minimally trained assistant while you operate. D, A patient who has to be operated on in some unusual position. E, Subarachnoid anaesthesia which has spread too high.

7. What are the acceptable ways of finding out if you have placed a tracheal tube correctly in a patient's trachea?

A, Listening for the air entry over both his lungs. B, Seeing the tube lying between his vocal cords. C, Hearing air coming out of it when you press his chest. D, Passing a catheter down it. E, Listening for air going in and out of it as he breathes.

8. What is the major danger of intubation?

A, Infecting a patient's lower respirstory tract. B, Injuring his cords. C, Attempting it and failing. D, Attempting it and not recognising that you have failed. E, Death from the inhalation of vomit.

9. Which of the following provide suitable conditions for tracheal intubation?

A, Ether in the stage of surgical anaesthesia. B, Intravenous ketamine. C, Trichloroethylene anaesthesia. D, Deep unconsciousness following a head injury. E, Thiopentone followed by suxamethonium.

10. Which of the following is true about a non–rebreathing valve such as the Ambu E valve?

A, You can switch quickly and easily from spontaneous to controlled ventilation at any time without changing the circuit. B, You can use it with a flow of nitrous oxide and oxygen. C, You don't have to remove it from a patient's face when you control his respiration manually with it. D, You can use the same valve for all sizes of patient. E, It has less compressible dead space than an expiratory spill valve of the Heidbrinck type.

11. You want to anaesthetize a patient with ether. Which of these would make induction the smoothest and fastest?

A, Ether and air from a vapouriser. B, Open ether. C, Thiopentone followed by ether from a vapouriser. D, Thiopentone, followed by suxamethonium, tracheal intubation and ether from a vapouriser. E, Thiopentone followed by halothane, and then ether from a vapouriser.

12. During the course of an anaesthetic a patient's pupils become widely dilated and do not react to light. What could be the reason for this?

A, The level of anaesthesia might be too light. B, Anaesthesia might be too deep. C, He might be dead. D, He might have been given intravenous morphine. E, He might have been given intravenous neostigmine.

13. Patient JAMES is being anaesthetized with ether. The movement of his chest lags behind that of his diaphragnm. Each time he breathes his trachea is pulled downwards. Which of the following are true about this stage of anaesthesia?

A, He has reached the optimum level of anaesthesia for surgery. B, You could intubate him quite easily without using a muscle relaxant. C, It is similar to moderate halothane anaesthesia. D, You can safely give more ether. E, He would show similar signs if he was breathing spontaneously when only partly under the influence of relaxants.

14. Which of the following, when used as the sole anaesthetic agent, either leaves the respiration unchanged, or stimulates it enough during light surgical anaesthesia to make added added oxygen unnecessary in a fit patient?

A, Trichlorethylene. B, Ether. C, Halothane. D, Ketamine. E, Chloroform.

15. Which of the following are true about the EMO vapouriser?

A, It has a high internal resistance. B, It is temperature compensated. C, It is flow compensated. D, It has a small mechanical dead space. E, You can use it to vapourise any volatile agent.

16. Which of these agents have no effect on the protective power of a patient's laryngeal reflexes?

A, Ketamine. B, Pethidine. C, Thiopentone. D, Diazepam. E, Ether.

17. In which of the following conditions is it useful to measure the central venous pressure?

A, Hypovolaemic shock. B, Septic shock. C, Severe placental abruption. D, Surgical dehydration. E, Diabetic acidosis.

18. You have decided to do a Caesarean section under ketamine.

Which of the following are true?

A, Provided you give a low dose of ketamine, you need not worry about its effect on the baby. **B**, You can wait to give diazepam or promethazine until after he is delivered. **C**, You will get good muscular relaxation. **D**, You will not need to worry about the supine hypotensive syndrome. **E**, You need not put up an intravenous drip.

19. Which of the following disadvantages of ketamine are prevented or reduced by atropine?

A, Its slow recovery period. **B**, Increased salivation. **C**, Emergence reactions. **D**, The risk of respiratory arrest. **E**, Increased muscle tone.

20. Which of the following statements are true about the use of intravenous morphine?

A, It should be given in a standard dose to all patients. **B**, It is useful when given with thiopentone as a cocktail. **C**, It provides excellent analgesia. **D**, It is a a powerful respiratory depressant. **E**, It is an excellent anaesthetic for evacuating incomplete abortions.

21. Which of the following statements are true about local anaesthesia?

A, It is more reliable than general anaesthesia. **B**, It is often indicated in patients with lung, liver or kidney disease. **C**, It can safely be given by injecting through infected tissue? **D**, It needs the patient's co-operation? **E**, It is particularly useful in children?

22. Turn to Fig. 2-4. For what drugs is the dose for a 50 kg patient 10 mg?

A, Thiopentone. **B**, Morphine. **C**, Intramuscular methoxamine. **D**, Intravenous ephedrine. **E**, Intravenous ketamine for induction.

23. Turn to Fig. 5-1. For what drugs is the maximum dose for a 50 kg patient 15 ml?

A, 1% plain lignocaine. **B**, 2% lignocaine with adrenaline added to it. **C**, 0.25% bupivacaine. **D**, 0.5% bupivacaine. **E**, 2% plain lignocaine.

24. COSMO is having fits while he is anaesthetized. Which of these measures would help to control them?

A, Making sure he is adequately oxygenated. **B**, Giving him diazepam intravenously. **C**, Giving him intravenous thiopentone. **D**, Giving him morphine intravenously. **E**, Maintaining him on ether anaesthesia until they stop.

25. Which of the following are true about epidural anaesthesia?

A, It requires a smaller dose of anaesthetic drug than a subarachnoid one. **B**, It can be given through the sacral hiatus. **C**, It is more reliable than a subarachnoid one. **D**, It requires that the drug be given in a hyperbaric solution. **E**, It can be given through a catheter.

Answers in Appendix D.

21.5 What do you know? Five

1. Which of the following drugs react to form cloudy precipitates when they are mixed together in the same syringe and so should be given in separate syringes?

A, Diazepam and pethidine. **B**, Thiopentone and atropine. **C**, Ketamine and diazepam. **D**, Promethazine and pethidine. **E**, Suxamethonium and atropine.

2. Pethidine is a useful drug for treating postoperative pain, but it does have some side effects. Which ones?

A, Hypotension. **B**, Nausea and vomiting. **C**, Raised CSF pressure. **D**, Hypertension and tachycardia if a patient is also having a monoamine oxidase inhibitor. **E**, Constipation.

3. Which of the following are signs that you have given a patient too much intravenous fluid?

A, Warm hands and feet. **B**, A low urine output. **C**, Sacral oedema. **D**, Prominent neck veins. **E**, Crepitations at his lung bases.

4. Which of the following statements are true about intravenous local anaesthesia?

A, Prilocaine is the best drug to use. **B**, It is suitable for operations on the shoulder. **C**, The cuff you have used should be deflated as soon as the operation is over. **D**, If necessary you can prolong the operation for as long as you like. **E**, It is contraindicated if a patient with a full stomach needs an emergency operation.

5. AKU (17 years) has been admitted with an open eye injury and multiple lacerations. Which of these drugs would be safe?

A, Morphine. **B**, Suxamethonium. **C**, Atropine. **D**, Gallamine. **E**, Ether.

6. KWAME (19 years) is semiconscious and restless with a head injury, for which he needs a craniotomy. Which of these might further raise his intracranial presure?

A, Pethidine for controlling his restlessness. **B**, Controlled hyperventialtion to lower his pCO$_2$ to about 30 mm. **C**, Thiopentone induction. **D**, Coughing when you intubate him. **E**, Straining during light anaesthesia.

7. You have only the minimum list of drugs and no specialist anaesthetist. Which of the following patients would you refer for skilled anaesthesia if you could?

A, CHRISTIAN who has a history of abnormal bleeding and who needs circumcision. **B**, KWANTA (38 years) with a short history of frequent angina who is to undergo oesophagoscopy and gastroscopy because of dysphagia. **C**, KWANSA (38 years) who is being treated for myasthenia gravis and who needs a laparotomy for the removal of an intra-abdominal mass. **D**, KIMI (19 years) with untreated mild hypertension who needs a sequestrectomy for his tibia. **E**, AMA (20 years) with moderate anaemia who needs her leg amputated.

8. Which of the following are true about ketamine emergence reactions?

A, They are particularly common in children between the ages of 2 and 7. **B**, You can reduce their incidence by premedicating patients with diazepam. **C**, They are more likely to occur if patients are disturbed as they recover from anaesthesia. **D**, You can reduce their incidence if you give the maximumum safe intravenous dose slowly as a bolus injection. **E**, They seldom cause serious problems.

9. Which of these drugs would you include in your cardiopulmonary resuscitation trolley?

A, Atropine. **B**, Adrenaline. **C**, Calcium chloride. **D**, Lignocaine. **E**, Sodium bicarbonate.

10. SEWA (34 years) needs an urgent operation for rupture of her uterus and the death of her baby. She is severely shocked. Which of the following are correct?

A, She may develop disseminated intravascular coagulation. **B**, She needs intramuscular pethidine immediately to settle her while the theatre is being made ready. **C**, She is a suitable patient for an epidural block. **D**, A blood sample should be taken for grouping and cross matching before she is given dextran or some other plasma expander. **E**, An indwelling catheter will be helpful.

11. Which of the following statements are true about the quantities of drugs contained in particular volumes of solutions?

A, 2.5% thiopentone solution contains 25 mg/ml. **B**, 2% lignocaine contains 200 mg/ml. **C**, 0.5% bupivacaine with adrenaline 1:200 000 contains 5 mg/ml of bupivacaine. **D**, 8.4% sodium bicarbonate contains 1 mmol/ml. **E**, A litre of 5% dextrose contains 50 g of dextrose.

12. Which of the following patients would be likely to be difficult to intubate through their mouths?

A, KEIL with trismus due to tetanus. **B**, OLUWA with burns contractures of his neck. **C**, FRANCIS with ankylosis of his temporomandibular joints. **D**, WAMBUI with dentures. **E**, CHUKWE with arthritis of his neck.

13. Which of the following are true about anaesthetizing an infant?

A, He can readily develop bradycardia. **B**, He has a large surface area relative to his weight. **C,** He should preferably be intubated with a plain tracheal tube. **D,** He cannot be intubated under suxamethonium. **E,** Anaesthesia can be monitored reliably with a precordial stethoscope.

14. Which of these have clinically useful antagonists?

A, Ketamine. **B,** Ether. **C,** Alcuronium. **D,** Halothane. **E,** Pethidine.

15. An adult is to have a laparotomy for which he needs good muscle relaxation. After premedicating him with pethidine and intubating him under thiopentone and suxamethonium, you are going to give him ether and air from a vapouriser. Which of the things you have done will reduce his need for alcuronium, or any other long acting relaxant?

A, Intubation. **B,** Pethidine. **C,** Controlled ventilation. **D,** Atropine. **E,** Ether.

16. Which of the following anaesthetic methods would be sure not to cause postoperative vomiting or nausea?

A, An epidural block. **B,** A subarachnoid block. **C,** Ketamine anaesthesia. **D,** Trichloroethylene anaesthesia. **E,** Ether anaesthesia.

17. When would you use extra oxygen with an ether vapouriser?

A, When a patient is anaemic. **B,** At altitudes of over 1000 metres. **C,** When a patient has a history of angina or dyspnoea. **D,** When he is critically ill. **E,** When his blood looks poorly oxygenated during surgery.

18. What are the indications for premedicating a patient with promethazine?

A, To prevent the emergence reactions of ketamine. **B,** To treat postoperative vomiting. **C,** To prevent hypothermia. **D,** To prevent hypotension. **E,** To reduce anxiety.

19. You have done bilateral intercostal nerve blocks on a patient who is to have a Caesarean section. What would you expect?

A, It will provide some muscle relaxation. **B,** It will provide adequate analgesia. **C,** There will be no need to inject oxytocin after the delivery of the baby. **D,** Bilateral pneumothoraces as a possible complication. **E,** There is no need to worry about the supine hypotensive syndrome.

20. Which of the following methods are suitable for operating on a patient who has injured the second and fourth fingers of his hand?

A, Digital nerve blocks. **B,** An axillary block. **C,** An intravenous forearm block. **D,** Combined median and radial nerve blocks. **E,** Ketamine anaesthesia.

21. You have just anaesthetised OGECHI (17 years) with ether and have given her a full relaxing dose of tubocurarine. Just before her abdomen is opened you are told that the planned laparotomy that she was to have must now be postponed beause the blood that had been cross matched for he has been given to someone else. What would you do?

A, Immediately reverse her paralysis with a normal dose of atropine and neostigmine. **B,** Immediately reverse her paralysis with a double dose of atropine and nesotigmine. **C,** Give her a neostigmine drip, and continue to control her ventilation. **D,** Turn off the ether, control her ventilation and reverse her paralysis as soon as she shows any spontaneous muscular activity. **E,** Continue with light ether or sedation and controlled ventilation for 30 or 40 minutes until she shows obvious signs of breathing spontaneously.

22. You are taking a history from ACHIENG (68 years) and examining him before you operate. He tells you that he has frequent attacks of fainting and dizziness. What might be the cause?

A, Anaemia. **B,** Aortic stenosis. **C,** Hypoglycaemia. **D,** Heart block. **E,** Bronchial asthma.

23. AGNES (21 years) complains of nausea and vomiting. She has just had a Caesarean section during which she was given ether in air from a vapouriser. Which of the drugs she has had could be responsible for her nausea and vomiting?

A, Pethidine. **B,** Atropine. **C,** Alcuronium. **D,** Ergometrine. **E,** Ether.

24. LULU (39 years) is to have a haemorrhoidectomy. Which of the following anaesthetic methods would be suitable for her?

A, Deep ether anaesthesia from a vapouriser. **B,** Light ether anaesthesia with a muscle relaxant. **C,** Sacral epidural anaesthesia. **D,** Low subarachnoid anaesthesia. **E,** A bilateral sciatic nerve block.

25. You are an inexperienced anaesthetist. Which of the following methods are suitable for young children?

A, Ketamine. **B,** Subarachnoid anaesthesia. **C,** Epidural anaesthesia. **D,** Open ether. **E,** Intravenous pethidine and diazepam as an anaesthetic "cocktail".

Answers in Appendix D.

Appendices

Appendix A Making your own intravenous fluids

Bottles of sterile intravenous fluids are one of the most essential commodities in medicine. They are heavy and are almost entirely water. If they have to be transported over long distances, it is a great economy, and a great security, to prepare them regionally, or to be able to make them in your own hospital. One hospital calculated that whereas 500 ml of saline cost $1.5 to buy, it only cost 1c to make. *Making intravenous fluids with anything less than the ideal equipment is potentially dangerous, but not to have any intravenous fluids is even more so.*

You can make these fluids satisfactorily on a small scale, but only *if vigilance and discipline are constant*. All may go well for 10 years until, suddenly, there are several deaths from infected fluids. There are two dangers—

(1) Bacteria in the bottles causing septicaemia. Prevent this by following the sterilizing regimes meticulously.

(2) Dead bacteria or their products or foreign matter in the bottles causing pyrogenic reactions. These reaction are less often fatal, but avoid them if you can. Be aware that bacteria can grow in distilled water, and make all solutions in *freshly distilled* water, in which bacteria have not had time to grow.

Ideally, intravenous solutions should be made in a sophisticated plant with careful bacteriological, biological and chemical control. But you can, if necessary, do without many of these ideal facilities before your solutions kill more patients than they save. Life—saving intravenous fluids can be made under very simple conditions. For example, Nangina Hospital, a mission hospital in the Busia district of Kenya, has been making intravenous fluid for several years over a wood fire, and has never had any serious reactions. So it can be done—but only with perpetual vigilance!

As this story shows, you will have to balance the risks of not having any fluids, or not having enough fluids, with those of fluids that have not been prepared under ideal conditions.

A STORY "Our trouble at the moment is fluids. We are supposed to get them from the teaching hospital, but that is 250 km away. Each trip costs us about $100 in petrol and servicing alone, and they will only give us 16 boxes at a time. Sometimes they don't have any, so we have to buy a few Swiss—made plastic bottles from our local pharmacy for $2 each—imagine it, water imported from Switzerland! All the voluntary agency hospitals here make them, but the goverment won't let us make our own. It is more than my job's worth to try".
LESSON The government is probably right. Supervision is probably good enough in the voluntary agency hospitals to justify the risk.

You will probably be unable to test your fluids bacteriologically, so we only describe methods of testing the autoclave. Much more important is: (1) cleanliness, (2) the use of only freshly distilled water, (3) the sterilization of all fluids immediately they have been prepared, as soon as the chemicals are dissolved, and (4) the careful supervision of the sterilizing process. If there are few bacteria in your bottles when they go into the autoclave, the safety margin of your sterilization process is increased, and the risk of contamination with pyrogens is reduced.

Here are the instructions for making fluids for a large hospital or a small region. This method is more elaborate than smaller district hospitals will be able to manage, so you may have to omit some of the less critical details details, such as the use of a sintered glass filter. Firstly, the equipment:

• *AUTOCLAVE, downward displacement model, with pressure gauge and thermometer in the discharge line, one only.* Although this is the best kind of autoclave for intravenous fluids, you can use an ordinary theatre autoclave. An autoclave with a quick cooling system will let you process more batches. Buy a type in which the cooling water is sterilized during the sterilization cycle.

• *STILL, electric, state voltage, capable of being operated by gas or a kerosene pressure stove, capacity 5 litres an hour, able to make a distillate of BP standard, as (MAN) or (BOC) with spare parts including 4 spare heating elements, 4 spare water connections and 4 spare splash heads, one only.* Stills vary in capacity. Estimate your demands and order a still of a size that will allow you to fill them by distilling on 3 days a week. If you need more water, you can run 2 or 3 stills at the same time. If you need a licence to operate a still, get one.

• *FILTER, sintered glass, grade 3, pore size 15–40μm, three only.* Before a solution is put in a bottle it should be filtered to remove all particulate matter. You can use: (1) A sintered glass filter, which is the best because you can clean and reuse it many times. Grade 4 pore size 5–15μm filters retain more particles, but the flow rate is low and you need a vacuum. The difficulty with sintered glass filters is that they clog up with particles and need cleaning with concentrated sulphuric acid, and potassium or sodium nitrate. (2) An ordinary funnel and filter paper. (3) A filter candle of the Berkfeld type.

• *Alternatively, FILTER PAPER, Whatman 540, box of 100 sheets, one box only.* Many hospitals find fine filter paper and an ordinary funnel is quite adequate.

• *VACUUM PUMP, water operated, or electric, one only.* This is not essential. A water pump will be practical only if you have a good head of water. Put a wash bottle between the pump and the filter.

• *BOTTLES, glass, for intravenous fluids, 500 ml, 37 mm neck, as (SHU) "Capsulot" No 2-114 or equivalent, 500 only.* You will want bottles, stoppers and caps that fit one another.

• *SCREW CAPS, aluminium, with "Capsulot" screw threads and centre hole, to fit bottle with 37 mm neck, as (SHU) 'Capsulot' No. 375 or equivalent, three thousand only.*

• *RUBBER STOPPER, to fit transfusion bottle with 37 mm neck, as (SHU) "Capsulot" No.37-83, six thousand only.*

• *OVERSEALS, alminium, 5000 only.* Ideally, once a rubber cap has been pierced with the needle of a giving set it should be discarded, but if you use a disc of aluminium on top of the stopper, you can use it again.

• *MISCELLANEOUS MINOR EQUIPMENT* You will also need 5 and 10 litre plastic containers, a 5 or 10 litre aspirator jar, a hot plate, funnels, and tubing.

• *USEFUL ADDITIONAL EQUIPMENT A bottle scrubber, a sprinkler.*

• *CHEMICALS (1) Sodium chloride BP, 10 kg only. (2) Dextrose anhydrous BP (or dextrose monohydrate for intravenous use BP), 20 kg only. (3) Sodium citrate $2H_2O$ BP 2 kg. (4) Citric acid monolydrate BP (or, anhydrous citric acid BP) 1 kg (5) Potassium chloride BP, 5 kg. (6) Sodium acetate BP 5 kg. (7) Calcium chloride $2H_2O$ BP, 500 g. (8) Sodium bicarbonate BP or AR 1 kg. (9) Disodium edetate AR 50 g.* These are the chemicals you will need in the appropriate proportions. Ten kg of sodium chloride will make about a thousand litres of saline. The grade of chemicals you specify should be pure enough, but not unnecessarily pure, which will make them expensive. For example, there is no need to buy AR (Analytical Reagent) grade dextrose. BP (British Pharmacopoeia) grade is good enough. Ringer's lactate (Hartman's solution) is easier to make with sodium acetate (a dry powder) instead of sodium lactate, which is a sticky syrup.

A SIMPLE INTRAVENOUS FLUID PLANT

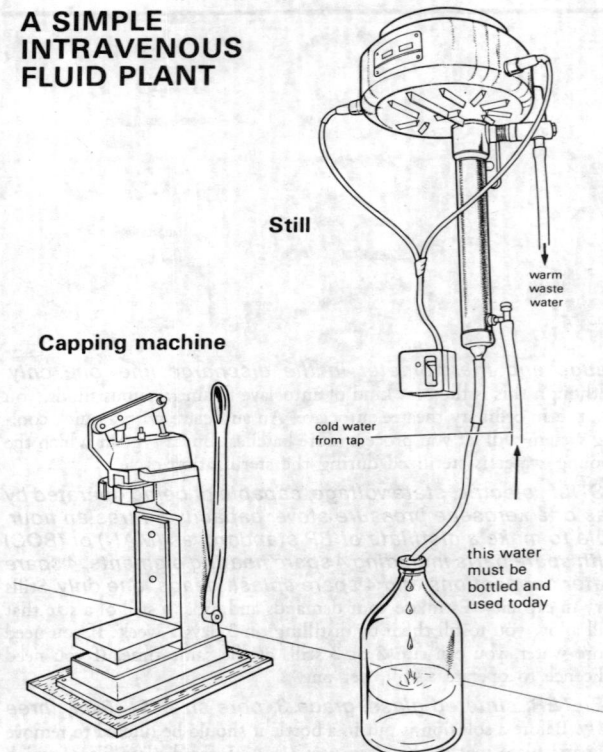

Fig. A-1 SIMPLE EQUIPMENT FOR INTRAVENOUS FLUIDS *You should ideally have much better equipment than this, but you can make life–saving fluids with only simple equipment.*

PREPARING INTRAVENOUS FLUIDS

ACCOMMODATION
If possible, set aside two rooms, painted with washable paint, and equipped with a supply of tap water and tables (preferably terazzo) with a smooth washable surface. The first room is for cleaning bottles, and the second a sterile laboratory. Provide it with a simple boot barrier made from a plank across the door.

STERILE TECHNIQUE Change your shoes before you enter the sterile room, wash your hands, and disinfect them with 70% spirit. Wear a cap, a mouth mask and gloves. Always use a non-touch technique and don't touch anything that comes into direct contact with the intravenous fluid, the raw materials or the distilled water. Always consider your hands as bacteriologically dirty. Clean the laboratory thoroughly after work.

RINSING Rinse your equipment three times with fresh distilled water before using it. When you have finished work, wash it, rinse it with distilled water, and dry it. Open all screw caps and stopcocks so that water can drain and air can circulate and dry them. Put small items into a hot air oven. Slowly raise the temperature to avoid damage to sintered glass filters. Put bigger equipment into a position in which it can drain off easily.

BOTTLES Avoid bottles that have dried before you can wash them. Soak them first in water containing a detergent, remove the label and wash the outside first. Only then can you remove the stopper without the risk of fibres from the lable entering the bottle.

Wash the bottles with tap water containing a weak household detergent. Clean their insides with a brush. Rinse them with tap water, if possible using a sprinkler, and afterwards with freshly distilled water.

If possible, presterilise your bottles at 160°C for 2 hours. Cover them loosely with an aluminium overseal to protect them from dust. Close the cool sterile bottles with clean sterile stoppers. You can store sterile bottles for a long time.

If a dry bottle has not been presterilised, rinse it with distilled water before filling.

CAUTION! (1) Don't use excessive quantities of detergent. (2) Let all equipment, especially bottles, drain upside down on a wire rack. If necessary make one from wire netting.

NEW RUBBER STOPPERS Wash these with a warm weak (less than 1%) detergent, rinse them with tap water, and boil them in several changes of distilled water. Then sterilise them in a drum. If they are not completely dry afterwards, put them in a hot air oven, at a temperature not exceeding 105°C until they are dry.

USED STOPPERS If possible, use a new stopper each time. If you cannot always use new stoppers, soak used ones in a 1:30 solution of Savlon Hospital concentrate, rinse them with tap water and treat them like new stoppers.

Put an aluminium disc overseal directly on top of the used stopper.

CAUTION! Don't use stoppers with visible, open holes. If you want to test a stopper, put a warm bottle of intravenous fluid into a cool concentrated solution of methylene blue. Discard the stoppers of any bottles which show a bluish colour—the methylene blue solution will have been sucked through the hole.

SCREW CAPS AND OVERSEALS Screw caps have the advantage that you can reuse them, but they have the disadvantage that you never know if a bottle has been opened or not. So use overseals if you can. Wash them in a hot detergent solution, rinse them in tap water and freshly distilled water, to remove any particles that could be introduced into the intravenous fluid through the spike of the giving set. Dry and store them in a closed container.

DISTILLED WATER Reject the first portion of the distillate, and rinse the storage container with the second portion before you fill it full. Connect the still and the storage container with a plastic tube. To keep out the dust, lead this tube into the container through a stopper with a hole in it.

CAUTION ! *Use freshly distilled water only,* if possible made that day; if this is not possible don't keep it more than one day. You can if necessary keep plain distilled water overnight. *Never keep prepared solutions overnight!*

In an emergency, you can use rain water, preferably that caught off an aluminium roof. Discard the first catchings after a dry spell and use it fresh.

FILTERING Filter your solution through a sintered glass filter, or filter paper. If you use paper, refilter the first portion so as to remove the fibres that have got into the filtrate from the outside of the paper.

After use, clean a sintered glass filter with fresh distilled water, and dry it in a hot air oven, slowly increasing the temperature.

When a glass becomes dirty, clean it with hot (about 80°) concentrated sulphuric acid, containing 1 2% of potassium or sodium nitrate.

CAUTION (1) In order to avoid breakage of the glass, add acid at a lower temperature, stepwise to acid at a higher temperature. (2) Use acid with great care and have the doors and windows open.

After treating a filter in acid, wash it many times in distilled water, and dry it. You can reuse the acid many times, but add more potassium nitrate. Or, you can clean the filter with potassium permangnate and hydrogen peroxide. Make a 10% solution of potassium permanganate, and let it dry on the filter. Add some 20-volume hydrogen peroxide, wash with water, then distilled water, and dry it.

COMPOSITION With all the fluids below, dissolve the powder in freshly distilled water, add more water to make the required volume, mix thoroughly, filter, distribute the solution into bottles, seal and sterilize them without delay.

0.9% saline Sodium chloride 90 g, distilled water to 10 litres.

5% dextrose Anhydrous dextrose 500 g (or dextrose monohydrate for parenteral use BP 550 g), water to 10 l. Put the dextrose into water, heat it on a hot plate and shake it from time to time. Dextrose solutions are sometimes slightly brown (caramelized). This is harmless.

0.18% sodium chloride in 4% dextrose ("Dextrose saline") Sodium chloride 18 g, dextrose anhydrous 400 g (or dextrose monohydrate for parenteral use BP 440 g), distilled water to 10 litres. Dissolve the dextrose in hot distilled water.

Modified Ringer's lactate (Hartman's) solution Sodium chloride 60 g, potassium chloride 4 g, calcium chloride $2H_2O$ 2.7 g, sodium acetate ($3H_2O$) 40 g, distilled water to 10 litres.

Acid citrate solution for blood storage (ACD) BP Formula A. Sodium citrate $2H_2O$ BP 22 g, citric acid monogydrate 8 g (or anhydrous citric acid 7.3 g), dextrose anhydrous 22.4 g (or dextrose monohydrate for parenteral use BP 24.5g), distilled water to 10 l. 120 ml of this will prevent clotting in 800 ml of blood.

Sodium bicarbonate 1 mmol/ml (8.4%) Sodium bicarbonate) 84 g, disodium edetate 100 mg, distilled water to one litre. Disolve the powders without heating. Don't heat the sodium bicarbonate solution, to encourage it to dissolve, or you may drive off some CO_2 and convert part of it to sodium carbonate solution. Theoretically, you should pass carbon dioxide through this solution, to bring its pH to between 7.5 and 8, but in practice there is no need to—the patient will supply it! Also, small harmless particles may form, due to interaction with the glass of the bottle.

Potassium chloride 1 mmol/ml (7.45%) Potassium chloride 74.5 g, distilled water to one litre.

Sodium chloride 1 mmol/ml (5.85%) Sodium chloride 58.5 g, distilled water to one litre.

CAUTION ! (1) Distribute these 1 mmol/ml solutions into 50 or 100 ml bottles. Don't distribute them in 500 ml bottles, because someone is sure to give a patient a whole bottle by mistake. You can also use 50 ml vials, 20 mm stoppers and overseals, but you will need an additional tool for your sealing machine. (2) Make sure you autoclave the bottles immediately after you have prepared them.

USE OF CONCENTRATED SOLUTIONS You can make 0.9% saline, and Ringer's lactate 10 times more concentrated, filter it, distribute it into bottles with a measuring cylinder and then add the required volume of distilled water.

INTRAVENOUS FLUIDS

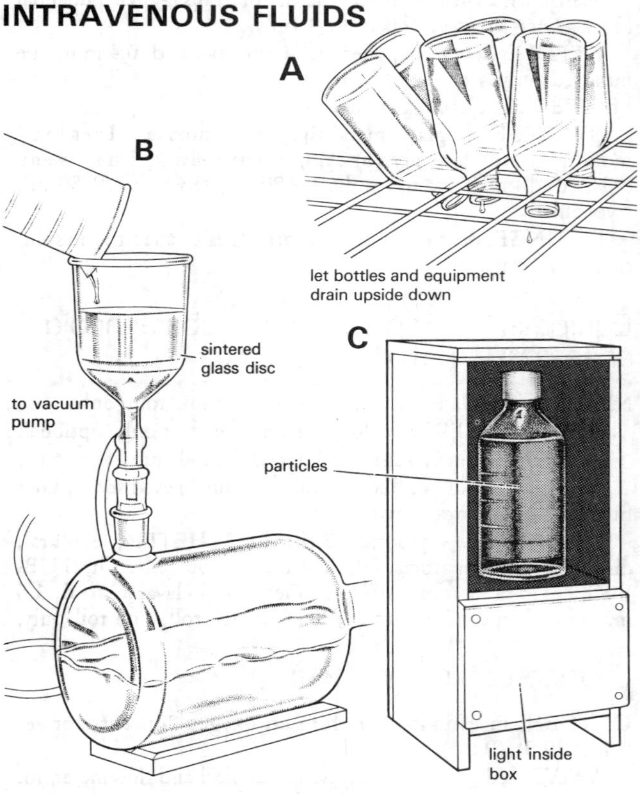

Fig. A-2 MAKING INTRAVENOUS FLUIDS. A, allowing washed bottles to drain. **B,** filtering through a Seitz filter. **C,** inspecting bottles for particles. *Kindly contributed by Ruediger Killian.*

If you do this with dextrose saline, the concentrated solution should only be five times more concentrated than the final one.

AUTOCLAVING INTRAVENOUS FLUIDS
Immediately before autoclaving, close the bottles airtight. Make sure there is the correct amount of water in your autoclave, so as not to form superheated steam or damage the heating elements.

DISCHARGING AIR Be sure that the vent is open to discharge all the air during the initial heating up period. Let steam issue from the vent for 3 to 5 minutes before you close it. At this stage the thermometer should read 100°C and the pressure gauge zero.

HEATING UP Let the pressure rise to 1 kg/cm^2 (15 pounds per square inch), and the thermometer in the discharge channel to 121°C. You can then be sure that there is no air or superheated steam in the chamber. For efficient sterilization the steam should be saturated and wet.

HEAT PENETRATION TIME This is the time needed for the solution in the bottles to reach 121°C. It varies from one autoclave to another and also depends on the size of the load. If possible, ask the manufacturer for the exact data.

Here is a rough guide—50 ml bottles 6 mins, 100 ml bottle 10 mins, 500 ml bottles 15 mins, 1000 ml bottles 18 to 20 mins.

MINIMUM HOLDING TIME This is 15 minutes and starts when the heat penetration time ends. It is the time during which sterilization takes place, and is the same for all sizes of bottle.

So the total time for which you have to keep the load at 1 kg/cm^2 is:—

For 50 ml bottles, 6+15 = 21 minutes.
For 100 ml bottles, 10+15 = 25 minutes.
For 500 ml bottles, 15+15 = 30 minutes.
For 1000 ml bottles, 20+15 = 35 minutes.
CAUTION ! Be on the safe side and add 5 minutes.

COOLING Switch off the heat and let the autoclave cool down. Don't open it until the pressure is zero.

CAUTION ! (1) Don't let it cool so much that the pressure goes below zero. (2) Don't apply the post–sterilization vacuum that you would use with dressings. If you do either of these things, the bottles may burst.

If you can measure only the chamber temperature, wait to open the autoclave until it reads 50°C. If you can measure the temperature inside the bottles with a thermocouple, you can open the autoclave when it reads 75°C.

LOOKING FOR PARTICLES Build a simple black box with a light a the bottom. Illuminate each bottle and look carefully for particles. If you examine the bottles before autoclaving, you can refilter those with particles. This will reduce the number you reject. But, always check all bottles after sterilization and reject any with particles.

Instruct anyone who uses a bottle of solution to inspect it carefully for cloudiness before he gives it to a patient. Bacteria may have grown meanwhile, particularly in solutions containing glucose.

STERILITY TESTING There are three possibilities, none of which is completely adequate and practical (see above). But you may wish to use them. (a) Add some soil to the central bottle and test that. (b) Use Oxoid (OXO) test papers impregnated with the spores of Bacilus stearothermophilus, a particularly heat resistant organism, and culture them with Oxoid tryptone soya broth. This shows that sterilization really is reliable. (c) Use autoclave test paper. This is useful for distinguishing treated and untreated packages but are not reliable for testing the safely of the autoclaving process.

**THE DISTILLED WATER MUST BE FRESH
AUTOCLAVE THE SOLUTIONS THAT DAY**

Appendix B Drugs and equipment

Here is all the equipment required for the methods that have been described in earlier pages, except for preparing intravenous fluids, which is in Appendix A. If possible, a medical service should choose one particular vapouriser and standardize on that choice. In many cases the supplier mentioned is not the original maker, and better and cheaper equipment may be available elsewhere. The codes used in the descriptions refer to the following suppliers. Hopefully, all items will become increasingly available locally. We have deliberately given the makers of only a few items of less easily obtained equipment. When quantities have been specified, they are those appropriate to fitting out a district hospital. Not all of this equipment is essential (an oxygen concentrator for example). All equipment is further described and discussed elsewhere in the text.

Addresses of suppliers

(AIM) Aimer Products, Rochester Place, Campden Town, London NW1. (Haldane apparatus)

(AMB) AMBU International, 32 Marielundvej, DK-2730, Copenhagen, Denmark.

(BOD) Ludwig Bodemer KG, 7702 Gottmadingen (KR Konstanz) Postfach 30, West Germany. (Stills)

(BOC) British Oxygen Ltd., Hammersmith House, London W6, England.

(DRA) Drägerwerke AG, Postfach 1339, Moisinger Alee 53/55, D2400 Lubeck, West Germany.

(EAS) H G East and Co Ltd, Sandy Lane West, Littlemore, Oxford OX4 5JT England. (Ventilator, spirometer, humidifier)

(JAM) Jambotkar Enterprises, Anand Niwas, 164/C, Dr. Ambedkar Road, Dadar, Bombay 400 014, India.

(MAN) Mannesty Machines Ltd., Liverpool 24, England. (Stills)

(MAR) Gerbrüder Martin, Bahnhofstrasse 124, Postfach 60, D-7200 Tuttlingen, West Germany.

(LOO) Hack Loos, Export Department, 3100 AB, Scheidam, The Netherlands.

(MED) BOC Medishield, Priestley House, Priestley Way, London NW2 7AG, England.

(MIE) Medical and Industrial Equipment Ltd., 26-40 Broadwick Street, London W1A 2AD, England.

(PEN) Penlon Ltd., Abingdon, Oxfordshire OX14 3PH, England.

(POR) Portex Ltd., Hythe, Kent CT21 6YL, England.

(RIM) Rimer Birlec Ltd., Melingriffith Works, Whitchurch, Cardiff CF4 7XT, England. (Oxygen concentrator)

(SHU) Schubert and Co. Ltd., 24 Vallens Backvej, DK-2600 Klostrup, Copenhagen, Denmark.

Anaesthetic drugs (2.5)

Anaesthetic agents Ether in cans or bottles of 500 ml. Halothane in 500 ml bottles. Trichloroethylene in 500 ml bottles. Ketamine in vials containing 10, 50 and 100 mg/ml. Morphine in 15 mg ampoules. Thiopentone sodium in 0.5 g ampoules with water for injection to make 20 ml of 2.5% solution, or in 1 g ampoules to make 40 ml of 2.5% solution.

Drugs for inducing and reversing muscular relaxation Suxamethonium bromide powder ("Brevedil M") in 40 mg ampoules. Alcuronium ("Alloferin") 2 ml ampoules containing 5 mg per ml. Neostigmine 2.5 mg in 1 ml.

Drugs for premedication Atropine in tablets of 0.5 mg, and ampoules of 0.6 mg in 1 ml. Diazepam as 2 mg or 5 mg tablets, and in ampoules of 10 mg in 2 ml. Promethazine as 25 mg tablets and 50 mg ampoules. Pethidine as 50 mg tablets, and ampoules of 25 mg in 1 ml. Naloxone 400 micrograms/ml in ampoules of 1 ml, and 20 micrograms/ml in ampoules of 2 ml. Alternatively, nalorphine.

Vasopressors Methoxamine hydrochloride in ampoules of 20 mg in 1 ml. Ephedrine as tablets of 30 mg, and ampoules of 30 mg in 1 ml.

Local anaesthetics Bupivacaine in ampoules of 0.25% and 0.5% solution, without adrenaline or preservative. Lignocaine ampoules of 2% and 4% solution *without* adrenaline. Lignocaine with adrenaline in dental cartridges, 1.8 or 2.2 ml. Lignocaine in pressurised aerosol cans delivering 10 mg at each puff. Cinchocaine heavy spinal solution with dextrose 6% in ampoules of 3 ml. Adrenaline in ampoules of 1 mg in 1 ml.

Miscellaneous anaesthetic equipment (4.2)

AIRWAYS, Guedel, transparent plastic, (a) size 000, two only, (b) size 00, two only, (c) size 0, two only, (d) size 1, four only, (e) size 2, eight only, (f) size 3, eight only, (g) size 4, four only.

AIRWAY, nasal, two only.

GAG, mouth, Fergusson, with Ackland jaws, adult size, one only.

WEDGE, anaesthetic, boxwood or plastic, one only.

TUBES, stomach, plastic, 76 cm Sizes 10 Ch, 20 Ch, 24 Ch, and 30 Ch, six only of each size.

SUCKER, operating theatre, electric, state voltage, with two 1000 ml plastic bottles and tubing, two only.

SUCKER, foot-operated with two wide-mouthed 100 ml plastic bottles, and metal tubes, two only.

SUCKER TUBE, metal, Yankauer, wide bore, fixed nozzle, three only.

Equipment for local and regional anaesthesia (5.1)

NEEDLE, hypodermic. (a) 0.45 × 16 mm, one hundred needles only. (b) 0.65 × 30 mm, one hundred needles only. (c) 1.45 × 60 mm, as one hundred needles only. (d) 0.8 × 100 mm fifty needles only.

NEEDLE, with bulbous guard, for transvaginal pudendal block, Luer fittings, 140 mm, 4 only.

NEEDLE, dental, hypodermic, double pointed, 0.4 mm, one hundred only.

NEEDLE, diaphragm, five only.

SYRINGE, all glass, metal tip, central nozzle, "Luer lok" mount, (a) 1 ml, ten only. (b) 2 ml, twenty only. (c) 5 ml, twenty only. (d) 10 ml, twenty only. (e) 20 ml, ten only. (f) 50 ml, two only.

SYRINGE, dental, for 2.2 ml cartridges of anaesthetic solution, two only.

Equipment for epidural and subarachnoid anaesthesia (7.1)

NEEDLE, spinal, Pitkin, Luer, 0.6 × 83 mm, four only.

INTRODUCER, Sise, for spinal needle, four only, optional.

NEEDLE, spinal, Pannett, Luer, 0.9 × 100 mm, four only.

NEEDLE, epidural, Tuohy, Huber mount, keyed stylet, Luer fitting, 1.6 × 76 mm, two only.

CATHETER, epidural. Either, CATHETER, epidural, disposable but reautoclavable if necessary, 50 only. Or, TUBING, epidural, 1 mm outside diameter, autoclavable, to fit 1.6 mm ext. diameter, Tuohy needle, 5 metre roll, one roll only.

Oxygen equipment (9.3)

OXYGEN, in cylinders, or from an oxygen concentrator see below (9.3) (RIM).

VALVE, reducing, with screw handwheel and flowmeter, for oxygen cylinder, one only of each.

OXYGEN CONCENTRATOR, water-cooled, closed system with oxygen boost, and alarms for low pressure, low vacuum, or low oxygen concentration, one only. Extra equipment, not for routine supply.

OXYGEN ANALYSER, one only. Extra equipment, not for routine supply.

Valves and bags etc. (10.1)

VALVE, simple expiratory spill valve, Heidbrinck type, with angled connector and 20 mm 1SO cone fittings, one only.

VALVE, adult, non–rebreathing, anaesthesia type, for controlled or spontaneous respiration, AMBU E, with 22 mm male inlet cone, 22/15 mm patient cone, and 22 mm male outlet cone, complete with 4 spare leaflets, as (AMB) 21-00, two only.

MASK, face, sizes 1 to 5, two only of each size.

HARNESS for face mask, two only.

TUBE, corrugated, anaesthetic, 12 mm, length of one metre, two lengths only.

Adult equipment for a drawover vapouriser (10.3)

VAPOURISER, ether, draw–over type, flow and temperature automatically compensated, in case complete, one outfit only. The outfits supplied with each vapouriser vary. Here is that for the EMO. You will need the equivalent equipment with other vapourisers.

EMO PORTABLE OUTFIT, with 15/22 mm connections, as (PEN) 51022, one only. This consists of (a) an EMO ether inhaler, (b) 2 male breathing tube connectors, (c) two female breathing tube connectors, (d) two 30 mm breathing tubes, (e) one head harness, (f) one connector mount, (g) 9 cm of plain connecting tube, (h) one Oxford inflating bellows, (i) one 105 cm breathing tube, (j) one Heidbrinck expiratory valve, (k) one angle connector, and (l) one facemask size 3, all in a carrying case.

OXYGEN ATTACHMENT KIT, for EMO, (PEN) 51200, one only.

VAPOURISER, Oxford Miniature, "OMV Fifty", right to left flow, with halothane scale as standard, also trichloroethylene and chloroform scales, one only. If possible, supply two.

VAPOURISER, uncalibrated, for halothane only, Bryce–Smith, one only. Optional.

INHALER, trichloroethylene, hand held, as (MED) "Cyprane" pattern, one only.

BAG, AMBU, self–inflating, adult size, with 22 mm female inlet cone, and 22/15 mm patient cone, ISO specification, in plastic pouch, with nipple for oxygen inlet at one side, as (AMB) type "R" 96-03-00, one only.

Equipment for intubating the trachea (8.2)

LARYNGOSCOPE, large handle, American hook–on fitting, to take D type cells (also called U2 or R 20) and 3 volt bulbs with No. 8 ANC threads, two only.

BLADE, laryngoscope, Macintosh, large, and extra large, hook–on fitting, to take standard bulb, one only of each size.

BLADE, laryngoscope, Seward or Robertshaw type, child, hook–on fitting, to take the standard bulb, one only.

BULB, spare, for laryngoscope, 3 volt, No. 8 ANC thread, three only.

TUBE, orotracheal, with cuff, Magill, red rubber, and following, (a) 7 mm, five only. (b) 8 mm, ten only. (c) 9 mm, ten only. (d) 10 mm, five only.

TUBE, orotracheal, plain with out cuffs, rubber, Oxford non–kink, (a) 3 mm, three only. (b) 3.5 mm, three only. (c) 4 mm, three only. (d) 4.5 mm, three only. (e) 5 mm, three only. (f) 5.5 mm, three only. (g) 6 mm, five only.

TUBE, nasotracheal, cuffed, rubber, 6 mm, 7 mm, 8 mm, and 9 mm, six only of each size.

TUBE, nasotracheal, uncuffed, rubber, 2.5 mm, 3.0 mm, 3.5 mm, 4.0 mm, 4.5 mm, 5 mm, 5.5 mm, two only of each size.

ADAPTOR, tracheal, plastic, 3 mm to 10 mm, with male cone fitting, one only of each size, set two sets only.

CONNECTOR, tracheal, angled, 15 mm female cone combined with 22 mm male cone at one end and 15 mm male at the other, one only.

CATHETER MOUNT, connecting tube, 9 cm, with 15 cm female cone and 22 mm female cone, plain, anti–static, as (PEN) 50067, one only.

INTRODUCER, for adult tracheal tubes, malleable copper, two only.

INTRODUCER, for infant and child tracheal tubes, one only.

FORCEPS, anaesthetic, Magill, adult size, one only.

FORCEPS, anaesthetic, Magill, child size, one only.

CATHETERS, tracheal, suction, plastic, 8 Ch, 12 Ch, 16 Ch, 20 Ch, fifty only of each size.

BRUSHES, for cleaning tracheal tubes, small, medium and large, three only of each size.

SPRAY, Macintosh or Forrester, oral, with malleable rubber covered tube, one only.

Equipment for intravenous infusion (15.1)

SOLUTION, intravenous, 500 ml bottles. (a) 0.9% saline. (b) 0.18% saline in 4.3% dextrose. (c) Ringer's Lactate (Hartman's solution). (d) 5% dextrose. One hundred bottles of each only.

POTASSIUM CHLORIDE, SODIUM CHLORIDE, SODIUM BICARBONATE, 50 ml bottles, 1 mmol/ml, sterile, for local preparation, 10 bottles of each solution.

MANNITOL, 10%, 500 ml, 10 bottles only.

GIVING SET, intravenous, plastic, to deliver 15 drops per ml, with soft rubber segment for injections, one hundred sets only.

NEEDLE, hypodermic, short bevel, 3×40 mm, one hundred needles only.

NEEDLE, Mitchell, intravenous. 0.9 mm, three only.

CANNULA, "needle inside cannula" venous, teflon, autoclavable, Luer fitting, (a) 0.5 m. (b) 1 mm (c) 1.5 mm. Ten only of each size.

NEEDLE, intravenous, 0.9 mm, type to be specified.

Paediatric equipment for general anaesthesia 18.3

VALVE, paediatric, non–rebreathing, anaesthesia type, for controlled or spontaneous respiration, as AMBU "Paedivalve" with 15 mm male inlet cone, 22/15 mm patient cone, and 15 mm outlet cone, complete with 4 spare leaflets, and 15 mm male to 22 mm female plastic adaptor, as (AMB) 101-00, two only.

AYRE'S T-PIECE CHILD CIRCUIT KIT, for EMO vapouriser, complete, as (PEN) 51543, one kit only. This consists of: (a) 15 mm to 15-22 mm elbow connector, (b) 15 mm Ayre's T-piece, (c) 15 mm male tube mount, (d) 15 mm female tube mount, one of which is used as a bag mount, (e) 500 ml reservoir bag with tail, (f) 1 metre of 6 mm gas feed hose, (g) 22-6 mm gas feed adaptor, (h) 21 cm of 10 mm reservoir hose.

FACE MASK, child, Rendell–Baker, as (PEN) 50345 and following, size 0, 1, and 2, three only of each size.

ENTRAINER, Farman's paediatric, for use with EMO children's circuit, as (PEN) 50332, one only.

Equipment for intensive care 19.2

All the equipment in this section is optional.

CATHETER, for monitoring the central venous pressure, radio–opaque, for introduction through a cannula, (a) 20 cm. (b) 60 cm. 2 mm. Ten only of each size.

MANOMETER, for central venous pressure, disposable, but capable of being boiled and re–used, with 3–way tap, side arm, and delivery tube for connection to catheter. Ten only. You will also need a piece of wood and a spirit level.

CONNECTOR, Y–shaped, disposable.

VENTILATOR, simple pattern, pressure–limited, class 1, type B, mode of operation continuous, anaesthetic class AP, time–cycled, electric, doubly wound for mains 120 or 220 AC voltage (state which) and 12 volts DC, and handle for manual operation, 20 mm cone fittings on the Y-piece, 30 to 22 mm cone adaptor, and set of spares, as East Radcliffe RP4 pattern or equivalent, one only.

SPIROMETER, Wright's, with 22 mm male cone, (EAS) pattern. One only.

HUMIDIFIER, electrically heated, water–bath type, autoclavable, 110 or 220 AC mains voltage (state which) with double thermostat, (EAS) pattern. One only.

CONDENSER–HUMIDIFIER, thermal humidifying filter, for use with a ventilator or spontaneous respiration, as Portex "Humidi–vent" (POR) 100/580, pack of ten. Five packs only.

MONITOR, electrocardiograph, oscilloscope type, robust, fade–free, one only.

MODIFIED CAMPBELL–HALDANE APPARATUS, for measuring alveolar CO_2, in case, complete with: (a) a 2 litre nominal capacity rebreathing bag to BS 3353 with mouthpiece, mouthpiece–tap, and 15 mm female cone for connection to a tracheal or tracheostomy tube, (b) 50 ml of mercury, (AIM), $225, one only. Extra equipment, not for routine supply. You will also need some 20% potassium hydroxide and some 5% sulphuric acid.

Appendix C References

Material has been assembled from very many sources, here are a few of them.

Ajao OG, Ladipo OA. The use of local anaesthetics for emergency abdominal operations. Tropical Doctor 1978; 8: 73-75.

Bewes PC. Surgery. African Medical Research and Education Foundation, Box 30125, Nairobi, Kenya, 1984.

Boulton TB. Recent Advances in Anaesthesia: Anaesthesia and resuscitation in difficult enviroments, 1975.

Cory CE, Bewes PC. Proceedings of the Sixth KCMC Postgraduate Seminar, Anaesthesia. Mimeo, 1975.

Corti L, Corti P. Epidural Anaesthesia in an upcountry hospital. Tropical Doctor, 1978;8:119-122.

Farman JV. Anaesthesia and the EMO system. English Universities Press, 1973.

Galbraith JEK. Basic Eye Surgery. Churchill Livingstone, 1979.

Kamm G, Bewes PCB. Ketamine. Tropical Doctor 1978.

Kamm Georg, Graf–Banermann T. Machame Anaesthesia Notebook for Medical auxiliaries. Springer Verlag: Berlin, 1982.

Lweno H, Proceedings of the Association of Surgeons of East Africa. 1980:22-25.

Prior FN, and others, Household Hints in Anaesthesia. Bharati Press: Vellore, South India, 1970.

Prior FN. Manual of Anaesthesia for the Small Hospital. Giani Printing Press: Chaura Bazar, Ludhiana, 1976.

Vaughan AB. Anaesthetics, The Oxford Handbooks for Medical Auxiliaries. Oxford University Press: 1969.

Appendix D, answers to the multiple choice questions in Chapter 21

What do you know? One 1, ACDE. **2,** D only. **3,** All of them. **4.** B and C. **5,** All except A. **6,** C only. **7,** E only. **8,** B and C. **9,** B and C. **10,** A only. **11,** B, D, and E. **12,** C only. **13,** A and D. **14,** All except E. **15,** All of them. **16,** A, B, and C. **17,** C, only. **18,** All of them. **19,** B, and C. **20,** C, and E. **21,** All except A. **22,** All except C. **23,** E only. **24,** B and C. **25.** C, D, and E.

What do you know? Two 1, All except B. **2,** A, C, and D. **3,** B only. **4,** A, C, and E. **5,** A, B, and C. **6,** A only. **7,** E only. **8,** B only. **9,** All except A. **10,** B, C, and E. **11,** A and C. **12,** All of them. **13,** A and C. **14,** All except B. **15,** All except E. **16,** A only. **17,** E only. **18,** B only. **19,** A and D. **20,** B only. **21,** All except B. **22,** None of them. **23,** All of them. **24,** A, and B. **25,** All except B.

What do you know? Three 1, D only. **2,** A, B, and C. **3,** All of them. **4,** A, and B. **5,** B, C, and D. **6,** B, and C. **7,** B, C, and D. **8,** A and B. **9,** None of them. **10,** A only. **11,** A, C and D. **12,** A, C, and E. **13,** All except A. **14,** All of them. **15,** B, C and D. **16,** B and E. **17,** A, B, and E. **18,** All except E. **19,** All of them. **20,** B and E. **21,** All except D. **22,** All except C. **23,** All except E. **24,** C only. **25,** All of them.

What do you know? Four 1, All of them. **2,** B and C. **3,** All of them. **4,** A and B. **5,** All except C. **6,** All of them. **7,** A, B, and E. **8,** D only. **9,** A, D, and E. **10,** A, and C. **11,** D only. **12,** B, and C, only. **13,** B, and E. **14,** B and D. **15,** B and C. **16,** None of them. **17,** All of them. **18,** A and B. **19,** B only. **20,** C and D. **21,** B and D. **22,** B, C, and D. **23,** A and B. **24,** A, B and C. **25,** B and E.

What do you know? Five 1, A and C. **2,** All of them. **3,** C, D, and E. **4,** A only. **5,** All except B. **6,** A, D and E. **7,** A,B and C. **8,** B, C and E. **9,** All of them. **10,** A, D and E. **11,** All except B. **12,** B, C, and E. **13,** All except D. **14,** C and E. **15,** E only. **16,** None of them. **17,** All of them. **18,** A, B and E. **19,** A, B, and D. **20,** All except D. **21,** E only. **22,** all except E. **23,** A, D and E. **24,** All except E. **25,** A, and D.

Index

With this index we have included an explanation of the words that may be unfamiliar to some of our non–doctor readers. References with a dash in them, as for example 10-10, refer to figures. Those section numbers that have a D after them, as for example, 16.6D, refer to the "Difficulties" at the end of a particular section.

abdominal operations
   epidural anaesthesia for, 7.2
   local anaesthesia for, 6.7, 6.8
abscesses, 5.8
acid aspiration sydrome, a disease caused by the acid in a patient's stomach getting into his lungs, 16.3
acid citrate solution, a solution which stops blood clotting, Appendix A
active vomiting, 16.2
adaptor, a plastic fitting that joins a tracheal tube to a tracheal connector, 13.2
addresses of suppliers, Appendix B
adrenaline, a drug that causes blood vessels to constrict and slows the absorption of local anaesthestic drugs, 3.31, 5.3
   dangers in intravenous forearm blocks, 5.3, 6.19
AFYA ether vapouriser, 10.7, 10-10, 10-11, 10-12
air as carrier gas, 1.1, 9.1
airway, a path from the outside air to a patient's lungs, 3.1, 3.2, 4-1, 4.2, 4.6, 4-2, 13.2
   anatomy in children, 18.1
   Guedel, 4.2, 4-1, 4-4
alcoholic, 4.1
alcuronium, a drug that makes the muscles relax, 2.7, 14.3, 17.4
   dose of, 2-4
alveolar nerve block, 6.3
AMBU, a firm that makes anaesthetic equipment
   'Paedivalve", a special non-return valve for children, 18.3
   E valve, a non-return valve for adults, 13-1, 10-2, 10-7
amputations of arm, local anaesthesia for, 6.17
anaemia, not enough haemoglobin in the blood, 4.1, 17.1
analgesia, not being able to feel pain in part of the body (local analgesia), or the whole body (general analgesia)
   with ether, 11.2
   intravenous 8.6, 8.9
   trichloroethylene, 11-6, 11-7
antecubital fossa cannulation, 19.2
anaesthesia, anaesthetics, 2.6, 2.7
   assistants, Preface, 2.1
   Caesarean section, 6-11
   in children, Chapter 18
   for the conjunctiva, 5-4
   dangers of, 1.1
   deep, 4.3
   dose of, Figure 2-4
   for the ear drum, 5-4
   with the patient in an unusual position 16.12
   fitness for, 4.1
   history, 4.1
   infiltration, 5.4
   intravenous 4.4
   local, see local anaesthesia, Chapter 5
   machines, 1.1, 9.2, 9-2
   monitoring, 20.1
   objectives in planning, 1.1
   on the floor, 16.12
   ordering 2.5
   principles, 5.4
   quality of, Preface, 20.1
   standards of, 1.1
   surface, 5-4
   urethra, 5-4
   with a full stomach, 16.5
   with neck in flexion, 16.12
   with patient on his side, 16.11, 16.12
anaesthetists, anaesthesiologists, 1.1
ankle block, 6.24, 6.19, 6-28
antepartum haemorrhage, 16.6D
anoxia, lacking oxygen, 3.4
anus, 6.16, 6-16
apnoea, postoperative, 4.6
arm, 6.18
arrest, respiratory, the patient stops breathing, 3.4
aspiration, stomach, the contents of the stomach get into the lungs, 3.3
assessment, preoperative, checking the the patient before operating on him, 3.1
assistants, anaesthetic, 2.1
asthma, 3.31, 4.1, 7.2, 2.6, 17.8, 18-3
atomic war, Preface
atropine, the drug used to prevent the side effects of some autoclave, a steel vessel in which things can be sterilized at high temperatures and pressures, Appendix A
awareness during anaesthesia, 4.3
awake intubation, 13.6
axillary block, a block high up on the patient's arm, 6.18, 6-18
Ayre's T-piece, the piece of anaesthetic equipment for children, 10-7, 18-2, 18.3

bags, anaesthetic, 10.3
barbotage, mixing a anaesthetic solution with the patient's cerebrospinal fluid (CSF) before injecting it, 7.5
bellows, 10.6
bicarbonate, intravenous, 3.5
biopsy, a piece of tissue taken for analysis, anaesthetic for 6.15
bladder, emptying before operation, 4.1
bleeding, see haemorrhage, 4.3
blind nasal intubation, 13.4
block in a tracheal tube, 13-16
block, anaesthetic, injecting an anaesthetic solution close to a nerve to prevent it working and so prevent the patient feeling pain, Chapter 6
   abdomen, 6.7
   anus, 6.16
   ankle, 6-27, 6.24
   axillary, 6.18
   brachial plexus, 6.17
   eye, 6.5
   fingers, 6.21
   hernia, 6.12
   has failed, 6.22
   inferior alveolar nerve, 6-3, 6.3
   for inguinal operations, 6.11
   intravenous forearm, 6.19
   intercostal, 6.9
   lingual nerve, 6-3, 6.3
   mouth and teeth, 6.3
   paracervical, 6.14
   for penis, 6.15
   pterygopalatine, 6.4
   pudendal, 6.13
   of rectus muscle 6.8
   scalp, 6.6
   sciatic nerve, 6.23
   "Three–in–one", 6.22
   teeth 6.3
   wrist, 6.20
blood,
   gases, 19.3
   loss, 15.6
   pressure, 4.3, 4.5, 5.9
   replacement, 15.6
   transfusion, 15.1
   volume in children, 18.1
bolus intravenous ketamine, a bolus intravenous injection is one given over a minute or two with a syringe, an intravenous injection can also be given in a drip, 8.2
bouginage, a way of dilating the urethra with an instrument   local anaesthesia for, 5.8
Boyle's machine, a kind of anaesthetic machine, 1.1, 9.2, 9-2
brachial plexus, the nerves of the arm as they run through the neck, 6-17
brachial plexus block, 6.17
brain damage, 3.5
breast, local anaesthesia for, 6.10
breath–holding, voluntary refusal to breath, 3.4, 11.3D
breathing, spontaneous, 4.3
breathing has stopped, 3.4, 5.9
breech delivery, local anaesthesia for, 6.13
bronchospasm, contraction of the bronchi making breathing difficult as in asthma, 16.3, 17.8, 3.3
bronchitis, 3.3, 4.1
brushes, for tracheal tubes, 13.2
Bryce–Smith Induction Unit, 10.11, 10-16, 10.7
BSIU, see Bryce–Smith Induction Unit
bupivacaine, a drug for local anaesthesia, 1.1, 1.1, 5.3
   dose of, 5-1
   hyperbaric subarachnoid anaesthesia, 7.6
   isobaric anaesthesia, 7.5

Caesarean section
   epidural anaesthesia for, 7.2

ketamine, 8.1
local anaesthesia for, 6.9
lumbar epidural anaesthesia for, 7.2
Caldwell Luc's operation, an operation on the maxillary sinus, 6.4
Campbell–Haldane apparatus, a way of measuring the carbon dioxide in the blood, 19.3, 19.5, 19-6
cannula and needle, a kind of tube, 15.2
cannulation of central vein, 19.2
capital costs of anaesthesia, 2.3
carbon dioxide retention, failure to breath out carbon dioxide, 4.3
cardiac (concerning the heart)—
  arrest, stopping, 3.5, 4.6, 8.5
  arrhythmias, abnormal heart beat, 14.2
  asthma, 3.3
  failure, 7.2, 16.6D
  output, the cardiac output is amount of blood pumped by the heart, 4.3
cardiopulmonary arrest, the heart and breathing stop, 3.-2, 3.5
care
  preoperative (before the operation), anaesthetic, 4.1
  postoperative (after the operation), 4.5
carotid pulse, pulse of a large artery in the neck, 3.5
catastrophies, see disasters, 4.5
catheter mount, a short piece of corrugated tubing that joins a tracheal tube to an anaesthetic machine, 13.2
catheter, a thin rubber or plastic tube
  epidural, 7.2
  for monitoring CVP, 19.2
  tracheal, 13.2
catheter–inside–needle, 15.2
catheterisation, passing a tube into a patient
  anaesthesia for, 5.8
  of bladder, 4.1
  of central vein, 19.2
caudal epidural anaesthesia, anaesthesia by injecting a drug through the hole at the bottom of a patient's sacrum, 7.3, 7-5
central venous—
  catheter, 19-3
  pressure, the pressure of blood as it enters a patient's heart, 19.2, 19-2
charts for fluid therapy, 15-4. 15.6
chemicals for intravenous fluids, Appendix A
chest operations, local anaesthesia for, 6.7
children, Chapter 18
  intubation of, 13.6
  ketamine for, 8.5
"chimney" for ether, 11-4
chlorpromazine, a drug for premedication, 2-4, 2.8, 8.8
chlorpropramide, 17.7
cholinesterase, a substance in the blood that destroys acetyl choline, 4.1, 14.1
cinchocaine, a drug for subarachnoid anaesthesia, 2.5, 7.6
circulatory failure, 15.3
circulation, 3.5, 4.3
circumcision, removal of the foreskin, anaesthesia for, 6.15, 7.3
citrate accumulation, citrate is used to prevent blood clotting; when many bottles of bottles of blood have been given, there may be too much citrate in the body, 4.4
clenched teeth, vomiting behind, 16.2
closed circuit, an anesthetic machine in which the nitrous oxide is goes round and round and is used more than once, 9.2
"cocktails", a mixture of anaesthetic drugs, 8.8
  for Caesarean section, 6.9
colostomy closure, a colostomy is an opening between the gut and the surface of the abdomen, local anaesthesia for, 6.8
common cold, 4.1, 17.8

compliance, the compliance of a patient's lungs is their feel through a bag or bellows when you control a patient's ventilation, 13.7
complications, difficulties or unexpected happenings
  of local anaesthesia, 5.9
  postoperative, 4.6
conjunctiva, the wet mucous membrane of the eye, 5-4
condenser–humidifier, a device for giving the water vapour that a patient breathes out back to him when he breathes in, 19.3
connector, tracheal, a plastic fitting that joins the adaptor of a tracheal tube to a catheter mount, 13.2
controlled ventilation, "breathing" a patient when he cannot breathe himself, 13.1, 13-3, 14.1, 14.4
cost of anaesthesia, 2.3
convulsions, fit, 4.1
  after local anaesthesia, 5.9
  during epidural block, 7.2D
cough,
  extubation, 16.5
  postoperative, 4.6
"crash induction", a rapid method of induction, 16.5
credits, Preface
cricoid, one of the cartilages of the larynx, 16.4, 16.5, 3.1
  membrane, local anaesthesia through, 13.5
  pressure,
CVP, central venous pressure, 19.2
cyanosis, postoperative, 4.6
cystoscopy, looking through an instrument into the bladder, caudal epidural anaesthesia for, 7.3
'Cyprane" vapouriser, a vapouriser for trichloroethylene, 10.12, 11-6

Darrow's solution, a type of intravenous fluid, 15.6
"D & C", scraping out the uterus, anaesthetic for 6.14
dead space, the space between a patient's alveoli and the outer air; if this is too large, oxygen and carbon dioxide cannot leave and enter his blood as they should, 10.1, 10.2
death,
  anaesthetic, 7.1, 4.2, 20.1
  from anoxia, 13.3
  "on the table", death during an anaesthetic, 4.2
  postoperative, 4.5
  under subarachnoid anaesthesia, 7.1
deep peroneal nerve block, 6.24
dehydration, lack of water in the body, 4.1, 15.3
delirium, a violent mental disturbance caused by illness, 11.2
depolarising relaxant, a drug that paralyses the body for a short time, 14.1, 14.2
depth of anaesthesia, monitoring, 11.2
dermatomes, the parts of the body supplied by each spinal nerve, 6-8
. deterioration, (getting worse, becoming more ill) postoperative, 4.6
dextran, a temporary substitute for blood, 17.1
dextrose (glucose, a sugar) solutions, 15.1
"Dextrostix", a text for dextrose (glucose), 17.7
diabetes, a disease in which there is too much sugar in the blood, anaesthesia for, 16.6D, 17.7
diazepam, a drug used for premedication or inducing anaesthesia, 2-4, 2.5, 2.8
  induction with ether, 11.3
  with pethidine, 8.8
digital, concerning the finger, digital nerve block, 6-23, 6-24
digoxin, a heart drug, 4.4
dilatation and curettage, ("D & C") enlarging the external os of the uterus and scraping it out, anaesthesia for, 6.14

disasters, anaesthetic, 3.1, 4.5, 12.2
diseases, undiagnosed, 4.1
disorientation, not knowing where you are in time or place, 5.9
dissociative anaesthesia, the kind of anaesthesia produced by ketamine, 8.1
district hospitals, Preface
diuresis, passing urine, 15.3
draw–over vapouriser, an anaesthetic machine in which air passes over the surface of an anaesthetic agent such as ether, so that it evaporates and mixes with the air, 10.4
"drips", intravenous infusions, 15.2, 15.3
dropping bottle, for ether, 11-4
drug doses for anaesthesia, 2-4
drug(s) for local and regional anaesthesia, 5.3
  list, Appendix B
  medication, 4.1
Dräeger vapouriser, 10.7
d-tubocurarine, a long acting relaxant, 14.3
ear drum, anaesthesia for, 5-4, 5.8

East Radcliffe RP4 ventilator, a machine for breathing, 19.3
ECG, electrocardiogram, or an electrical picture of the heart's action, 4.4
economics of anaesthesia, 2.3
electrolyte disturbance, abnormalities of the salts and water in the body, 15.3
emergence reactions, violent behaviour in a patient recovering form an anaesthetic: with ketamine, 8.1
EMO, the Epstein Macintosh Oxford vapouriser, a machine for giving a patient ether, 10.6
  in children, 18.3
  circuits for, 10-7
  controls for, 10-9
  mechanism of, 10-6
endotracheal, inside the trachea, see tracheal tube, intubation etc.
ephedrine, a drug for treating low blood pressure, 13.4, 2.10, 2-4
epidural anaesthesia (blocks), a method of anaesthtizing a patient by injecting a drug into his spinal canal, but outside his dura, 4.3, 4.6, Chapter 7
  in children 18.2
episiotomies, special cuts made in the perineum to make childbirth easier, anaesthesia for episiotomies, 6.13
Epstein Macintosh Oxford, see EMO,
equipment,
  essential, 16-2
  for epidural and subarachnoid anaesthesia, 7-1
  for ketamine drip, 8-3
  for recovery, 4.5
  for subarachnoid and epidural anaesthesia, 7.1
  list, Appendix B
  standardisation, 2.3
  suppliers, Appendix B
ether, a liquid anaesthetic agent, 1.1, 11.1 11.2, 11.3, 11.4, 11.5
  for children, 18.2
  with improvised vapourisers, 10.13
  with the EMO, 10.6
"Ether-Pac"vapouriser, 10.8
"Etherair" vapouriser, 10.9
ethyl chloride, a dangerous liquid anaesthetic agent, 11.9
examination, before anaesthesia, 4.1
excising a small lesion, 5-3, 5.4
expiratory spill–valve, a valve that allows a patient to breathe out, 10-2, 10.11
  controlled ventilation with, 13.1
explosions with ether, 11.5
extradural anaesthesia, see epidural anaesthesia Chapter 7
extubation, removing a tracheal tube, 16.5
eye, anaesthesia for eye operations, 16.9
  local anaesthesia for, 6.5

face masks, 10.3
  Rendell–Baker, 18.3
facial surgery, anaesthesia for, 16.10
facial nerve block, 6.5
failure,
  cardiac, 4.4, 7.2, 17.4
  left venticular, 3.3
Farman's entrainer, an anaesthetic device for children, 18.3, 10-7
Fergusson's gag, an instrument for opening the mouth in an emergency, 16-1
femoral hernia, local anaesthesia for, 6.12
field block for the breast, 6.10
finger, local anaesthesia for, 6.21, 6-24
fires with ether, 11.5
fitness for anaesthesia, 4.1
fits, see convulsions, 5.9
flame photometer, an instrument for measuring the concentration of sodium and potassium in the blood, 15.3
flow of fluid through a needle, 16-6
flowmeters, 9.2
fluid(s), Chapter 15
  balance, postoperative, 4.5, 15.5
  during operation, 15.4
  intravenous, preparation of, Appendix A
  record of, 4.5
  rectal, 15.6
  replacement, 15.3
  renal failure, 15.7
"Fluo-Pac" vapouriser, 10.8
foot, local anaesthesia for, 6.19, 6.24, 6.27, 6-28
forceps, anaesthetic, Magill, 13.2
  extraction, delivering a baby with forceps, local anaesthesia for, 6.13
forehead, local anaesthesia for, 6.6
foreign body in trachea, 13.7
fracture, anaesthesia for, 5.6
femur, a leg bone, anaesthesia for fractures of, 6.22
frusemide, a drug to make the kidney excrete urine, 14.4
full stomach, anaesthesia for, 16.1

gag, Fergusson, 4.2
gallamine, a long–acting relaxant, 2-4, 2.5, 17.4, 17.8, 14.3
gastric (stomach) fluid replacement, 15.5
general anaesthesia, Chapter 9, 10 and 11 etc.
giving set, some plastic tube and needles for giving a patient blood or fluid, 15.2
glottis, the narrowest part of the lungs oedema of, 13.2
glycogen store in children, glycogen is an energy store in the liver, 18.1
"golden rules of anaesthesia", 3.1
gums, local infiltration of, 6-2

haemoglobin, the red substance in the blood that carries oxygen, 14.1, 17.1
haemorrhage, bleeding, 4.2
haemorrhoidectomy, removing piles, 7.3
halothane, a liquid anaesthetic agent, 2.3, 11.6, 11.8, 1-1
  with an improvised vapouriser, 10.13
  with an OMV, 11.6
hand injuries, local anaesthesia for, 6.19
harness, for face mask, 10.3
head injuries, anaesthesia for, 16.8
health centres, Preface, 2.2
heart, see cardiac,
  beat, 4.32
  stopped, 3.5
Heidbrinck valve, a type of expiratory valve on an anaesthetic machine, 10.11, 13.1
hepatic (liver) failure, anaesthesia for, 17.5
hernia, an abnormal swelling caused by contents of the abdominal cavity protruding through its wall, anaesthesia for 6.11. 6.12, 6-12
how to use this book, 1.1

Huber point, a special curved point, on an epidural needle, 7.2
humidifier, a device for making the air a patient breathes damp, 19.3, 19.4
hydrocoele, a collection of fluid round the testis, local anaesthesia for, 6.11
hyperbaric subarachnoid anaesthesia, a method of anaesthetizing a patient by injecting a heavy solution of an anaesthetic into the fluid round his spinal cord, 7.6
hyperpyrexia, high fever, 2.7
hypertension, high blood pressure,
  after local anaesthesia, 5.9
  postoperative, 4.6
hypoglycaemia, too little sugar in the blood, 8.5
hypotension, low blood pressure, 4.4, 4.6
  in lumbar epidural anaesthesia, 7.2
postoperative, 4.6
  with subarachnoid and epidural anaesthesia, 7.1
hypovolaemia, too small blood volume, 4.4, 4.5, 14.4, 15.7
  preventing recovery from relaxants, 14.4
  signs of, 4.5
hypoxia, too little oxygen in the blood, 4.3, 4.4,

iatrogenic injury, injury caused by health workers, 20.1
ICU, see intensive care unit, a small room in which a few patients are given extra special care, 4.5, 19.1
induction, the first part of anaesthesia, putting a patient to sleep,
  for general anaesthesia, 9.1
  methods for induction with ether, 11.3
"infiltrate–and–cut" anaesthesia, 5.5
infiltration anaesthesia, making part of the body anaesthetic by injecting an anaesthetic drug directly into it, 5.4, 5.4
  for opening abscesses, 5.7
inflammable vapours during anaesthesia, 11.5
infraorbital block, 6.5
infusions, intravenous, to infuse a patient is to inject fluids directly into his blood vessels 15.1
inguinal hernia, local anaesthesia for, 6.12
inguinal (groin) operations, local anaesthesia for, 6.11
inhalation, to inhale is to breathe in, an inhalational anaesthetic is given to a patient in the air he breathes, 10.11
inlet valve, 10.11
intensive care unit or ICU, 4.5, 19.1
intercostal block, a block for the nerves between the ribs, 6.7, 6-9
intermittent positive pressure ventilation (IPPV), a method of making a patient breathe when he cannot breathe for himself, 3.4, 13.1, 13-1, 14.1, 14.4
"intermittent suxamethonium", a rather unsatisfactory way of producing relaxation by giving a patient more than one dose of suxamethonium, 14.2
internal jugular (one of the veins in the neck) cannulation, 19.2
intravenous,
  analgesia, 8.6
  cannula, a tube for putting fluids into veins, 15-2
  fluids 4.1, Appendix A
  infusions, putting fluids into the veins of a patient, 15.1, 15.2
  line, a needle or tube in a patient's veins, 15.2
  morphine, 8.7
  regional anaesthesia, a way of making part of the body anaesthetic, 6.9, 6-19, 6-20
introducer, an instrument for making intubation easier, 13.2
intubation, passing a tube down into a patient's trachea, so that he can be anaesthetised more safely, 4.2, 13.2, 20.1

difficulties with, 13.3D
nasal, 13.4
of babies, 13.6
with an open mask, 11-4
with suxamethonium and nitrous oxide, 9.2
IPPV, see intermittent positive pressure ventilation, 3.4
ISO (International Standards Organisation), an organisation that encourages manufacturers to make equipment of the same size so that equipment from different makers fits together, 2.4
isobaric subarachnoid anaesthesia, anaesthesia by injecting a drug into the fluid round a patient's spinal cord, 7.5

jaundice, anaesthesia for, 4.1
'jungle juice'', a local anaesthetic mixture, 5.4

kanamycin, an antibiotic, 4.1
ketamine, an anaesthetic drug, Preface, 1-1, 2.3, Chapter 8
  bolus intravenous, 8.2
  compared with ethyl chloride, 11.9
  dose of, 2-4
  drip, 8.3, 8.4, 8.9
  induction for ether, 11.3
  in children, 18.2
  in obstetrics, 16.6
  with local anaesthesia for abdominal operations, 6.7
  compared with ethyl chloride, 11.9
  with diazepam, 8.6
  with relaxants, 8.4
Kussmaul's breathing, a kind of deep sighing respiration, 17.2
lungs will not inflate, 13.7
laryngeal spasm,
  during ether anaesthesia 11.3D
  oedema, fluid collecting on a patient's vocal cords, making them swell and stopping air passing through into his lungs; anaesthesia for, 13.5
  reflexes, 8.1
  spasm, 9.3, 4.6, 11.3D
    with ketamine, 8.1
    with thiopentone, 12.1

laryngoscope, an instrument for looking at the larynx, 13.2, 13-4, 13-7, 13-12
laryngoscopy, looking at the lungs, 13.3
larynx, the part of the respiratory tract in which the sounds of speech are made,
  anaesthesia for, 13.5
  view of, 13-8
latent interval of local anaesthetics, the time between injecting the drug and the patient's ceasing to feel pain, 5.3
lateral cutaneous nerve of thigh, block for, 6.22
left lateral tilt, tilting a pregnant mother so that her uterus no longer presses on the large blood vessels at the back of her abdomen, 16.6
leg,
  epidural anaesthesia for, 7.2
  local anaesthesia for, 6.22
lignocaine, a local anaesthetic drug, 1.1, 5.3
  for intubation, 13.5
  causing hypotension, 4.4
  dose of, 5-1
  for hyperbaric subarachnoid anaesthesia, 7.6
  spray, 3.3
  for surface anaesthesia, 5.3
lingual (tongue) nerve block, 6.3
local anaesthesia, a method of making part of the body anaesthetic by injecting it with an anaesthetic drug, Chapter 5
  agents for, 2.5
  complications of, 5.9
  cost of, 2.3

hypotension in 4.4
for intubation, 13.5
maximum doses of, 5-1
overdose of, 5.3
local infiltration, 5-2
long-acting relaxant, a drug that paralyses a patient for about an hour, 13.2, 14.1, 14.3, 14.4
'Luer-lok' syringes, a special fitting for syringes and needles that prevent them from coming apart, 5.4
lumbar epidural anaesthesia, 7.2

magnet for Oxford bellows, 10.1, 10.6, 10-18
malignant hyperpyrexia, a serious complication of anaesthesia in which the patient develops very high temperature and usually dies, 4.1
manometer for CVP, 19.2
markers for local anaesthesia, 5.4
mask, open, for ether, 11-4, 10.6
maximum (largest) dose,
of local anaesthetics, 5-1
of other anaesthetic drugs, 2-4
meatotomy, 6.15
median nerve block, 6.20
medullary paralysis, paralysis of the lowest part of a patient's brain; a patient with this paralysis is in great danger of death, 11.2
Mendelson's syndrome, 16.3
mepivacaine hydrochloride, a local anaesthetic drug, 7.6
metabolic acidosis, too much acid in the body, 3.5, 17.2
metabolic alkalosis, too much alkali in the body, 4.6
metabolic rate, a measure of how fast the tissues of the body are working and how much heat they are making, metabolic rate in children, 18.1
methoxamine, a drug to raise the blood pressure, 2.10, 2.4, 2-4
monitor, electrocardiograph, 19.3
monitoring, to monitor somebody is to watch him very carefully, 3.1
the CVP 19.2, 19-2
the depth of anaesthesia, 14.3, 1.3
a paralysed patient, 14-3
morphine, a powerful drug to prevent pain, 2.9, 2-4, 4.6
drips, 8.9
intravenous, 8.7
motor end-plates, 14.1
mouth, local anaesthesia for, 6.3
mouth-to-mouth ventilation, a method of making a patient breathe by breathing into his mouth, 3-3
muscle relaxants, 14.1

nalorphine, a drug to abolish the action of morphine, 2.5, 6.9
naloxone, another drug to abolish the action of morphine, 5.9, 6.9
nasal polypi, growths in the nose, anaesthesia for, 6.4
nasal mucosa, anaesthesia for, 5.8
nasal intubation, passing a tube from the nose down to the trachea, 13.4
nasogastric tube, a tube from the nose down into the stomach, 16.4
needle,
dental, 5.1
hypodermic, 5.1, 15.2
diaphragm, 15.2
spinal, 7.1
winged, 15.2
needle-inside-cannula, 15.2
neomycin, an antibiotic, 4.1
neonate, a newborn child, anaesthesia for, 18.1
neostigmine, a drug that stops the action of a long-acting relaxants, 2-4, 2.5, 2.7, 14.1, 14.3

neuromuscular junction, the place where the very smallest nerves join a muscle to make it work, 14.1
nitrous oxide, 1.1, 9.2
non-depolarising relaxant, a long-acting muscle-paralysing drug, 14.1
non-rebreathing valve, a valve that allows the patient to breathe out and also prevents him breathing back into the anaesthetic machine, 10-2, 10.2, 10.6, 10.11, 13.1, 13.2, 13-5, 13.7, 18.3
normal delivery, anaesthesia for, 6.13, 6.14, 7.2, 16.16

obstetrics, anaesthesia for, 7.3, 16.6
obstruction respiratory, see airway
oedema, laryngeal, 13.5
OMV, Oxford Miniature Vapouriser, 10-7, 10.10, 10-15, 11-6
open ether, a way of giving ether without using a vapouriser, 11-4
open vein, a tube or needle in a patient's vein so that you can give him an intravenous injection quickly, 3.1, 3.2, 15.2
opioids, drugs like opium or morphine, 4.6
organophosphate, a chemical used for killing insects, poisoning with, 14.2D
outpatients, anaesthesia for, 16.11
over-transfusion, 15.7
overdose of local anaesthetics, 5.3
Oxford bellows, 10.6, 10-7, 10-12, 18.3
Miniature Vaporiser, see OMV, 10.10
tubes, 13.6
bellows, 10.6
oxygen, a gas in the air that is essential for life, 4.3, 9.3, 10.6
concentrator, 9.3, 9-4
cost of, 9.3
economical use of, 1.1, 9.3

"Paedivalve", an anaesthetic non-rebreathing valve for children, 10-2, 10-7, 10-11
paediatric bellows, 18.3
pain,
postoperative, 4.6
after chest wounds, local anaesthesia for, 6.7
pancuronium, a long-acting relaxant, 2-4, 14.3, 17.4
paracervical block, a block beside the cervix of the uterus, 6.14, 6-14
paradoxical breathing, an abnormal form of breathing in which the patient mainly breathes with his diagphram, and his chest contracts during during inspiration instead of expanding, 4.2, 11.2
paramedication, 2.6, 5.1, 5.2
paraphimosis, inability of the foreskin to go back normally over the penis, 6.15
passive regurgitation, fluid from stomach flowing into the lungs, 16.3
pCO$_2$, a measure of carbon dioxide in the blood, 19.3, 19.4, 19.5
pelvic operations, 7.2
penis, 6.15
Penlon bellows, 10.6, 13-1
PEEP, positive end expiratory pressure, a way of keeping a patient's alveoli open when he is being artificially ventilated, 19.4
perineal operations, anaesthesia for, 7.3
perphenazine, 4.6
pethidine, a very useful analgesic drug, 2-4, 2.6, 2.9, 4.6, 8.6, 8.8, 9.2
phenobarbitone, a long acting sedative drug, 4.1
phenytoin, a drug to prevent convulsions 4.1
phosgene, a poisonous gas, 9.2
PIH, pregnancy induced hypertension or pre-eclampsia, 16.6D
piles, swollen veins besides the anus, 6.16
plenum system, a method of anaesthetizing a patient in which the anaesthetic gases are

supplied to him under a small positive pressure, 18.3, 10-2
pneumothorax, air in the pleural cavity, 4.6, 6.7, 13.7, 6.17
position,
during intubation, 13-15
recovery, 4-5, 4.6
positive end-expiratory pressure (PEEP), 19.4
postoperative care, 4.5
potassium, an important element in the body, 15.1, 15.3, 15.5
pO$_2$, a measure of the pressure of oxygen, 19.4
pre-eclampsia, see PIH
preoxygenation, filling a patient's lungs with oxygen before doing something, 9.3, 13.3, 13.4, 13.6, 16.5
"preloading", giving a patient some saline before an anaesthetic that will cause his blood vessels to expand and lower his blood pressure; preloading prevents this fall, 7.1, 7.2
premedication, giving a patient analgesic or sedative drug to calm him before he is anaesthetized, 2.6, 5.2, 6.9, 9.1, 11.3, 14.2
for caesarean section, 6.9
for general anaesthesia, 9.1
for ether, 11.3
for local anaesthesia, 5.1
for suxamethonium, 14.2
prilocaine, a drug for subarachnoid anaesthesia, 6.19, 7.6
procaine, a local anaesthetic drug, 5.3, 5-1
promethazine, a drug for premedication, 2-4, 2.8, 8.8
protective reflexes, reflexes that keep food and fluid out of a patient's airway, 8.1
pterygopalatine the middle part of the face, block for, 6.4, 6-5
pudendal block, a block which is used during labour, 6.13
pulse, 4.3, 4.4, 14.1

radial nerve block, 6.20
records for anaesthesia, 4.5, 4.7, 4-7, 4-8, 20.1
recovery, 4.5, 4-6, 9.1
position, a safe position in which a patient lies as he recovers from an ananesthetic
rectal fluids, 15.6
rectus block, 6.8, 6-10
references, Appendix C
regurgitation, foods and fluids from the stomach flowing into the lungs, 16.3
rehydration, putting the water back into a patient's body after he has lost it, 15.3
reintubation, 4.6
relaxants, drugs that paralyse a patient's muscles, 1-1, 8.4, 11-6, Chapter 14
in children, 18.2
renal (kidney) failure, 4.1, 7.2, 15.7, 17.6
Rendell-Baker child's mask, 10-7
respiratory infections, 3.4, 4.1, 4.6, 17.8, 19.3
restlessness, postoperative, 4.6
resuscitation, bringing a patient who is nearly dead back to life, usually giving by him back the blood and fluids he has lost, 3.5, 3.6
retrobulbar block, a block of the nerves behind the eye, 6.5
ring block for the penis, 6.15, 6-15
Ringer's lactate, an intravenous fluid, 15.1, 16.7, Appendix A
rules, the "ten golden rules of anaesthesia", 3.1
Ryle's tube, a small stomach tube, 16.4

sacral epidural anaesthesia, a method of anaesthetising the lowest spinal nerves, 7.3
saddle block, a method of anaesthetising the saddle part of the body, or the part on which a patient sits, 6.9, 7.7, 7-8
salbutamol, a drug for asthma, 3.3
saline, a solution of salt in water, 15.1, Appendix A

saphenous nerve block, a nerve on the inner side of the leg, 6.24
scalp, anaesthetic for, 6.6
Schimmelbusch mask, this used for giving ether, 11.4
sciatic nerve block, the sciatic nerve is the largest nerve of the leg, 6.23, 6-26
'Scoline'', short–acting relaxant, 2.5, 14.1
sedation, making a patient calm and sleepy, 2.6
self–inflating bags, 10.3
semi–open system, 10.7
septic shock, a kind of shock produced by some very severe infections, 4.4
shock, hypovolaemic, a disease caused by a severe loss of blood or fluid in which a patient becomes cold and sweaty and his blood pressure falls, 16.7
short–acting relaxant, a drug that paralyses a patient for a short time, 14.1
shoulder dislocation, shoulder out of place, 6.17
sickle cell anaemia, 17.1
single–handed operator, methods for, 7.1
Sise introducer, a special needle used during subarachnoid anaesthesia, 7.1
skin graft, 6.22
    traction, 6.22
soda lime, a chemical fo absorbing carbon dioxide, 9.2
sodium bicarbonate, an alkaline intravenous solution, 15.1
sodium chloride, ordinary salt, 15.1, Appendix A
"solid chest", a chest that will not inflate, 3.3
spasm, laryngeal, 3.2
special care, 19.1
spirometer, an instrument for measuring how a patient breathes, 19.3, 19.4
sphenopalatine block, see pterygopalatine block, 6.4
spinal anaesthesia, the old term for subarachnoid anaesthesia, 4.3, 7.1, 7.4, 7.6
spontaneous respiration, breathing without any help, 10.6, 18.3
spray, Macintosh, a spray used for anaesthetizing the larynx, 13.2
sputum, 17.8
staff, anaesthetic, 2.1
stages of ether anaesthesia, 11-2, 11.2
standardizing equipment, 2.4
starvation, 3.1, 4.1, 8.6, 16.4
sterility, something is sterile when there are no living micro organisms on it, 7.1
sternal compression, a way of making a patient's blood circulate when his heart has stopped, 3.5, 3.6
steroids, a group of drugs used to treat some sorts of arthritis and other diseases, 4.4
stethoscope, oesophageal, 4.3
stomach, anaesthesia with a full stomach 1-1, 4.1, 16.4
streptomycin, an antibiotic, 4.1
stridor, breathing noisily, 3.2
subarachnoid anaesthesia, a method of anaesthetizing a patient by putting a drug into the fluid round his spinal cord, also called spinal anaesthesia, 4.3, 7.1, 7.4, 4.6 7.5, 7.6
subclavian cannulation, 19.2

sucker, 3.1, 4.2, 4-2
suction, 4.2, 13.3
superficial peroneal nerve, block for, 6.24
supervision, 20.1
supine hypotensive syndrome, the fall in a mother's blood pressure that occurs when her pregnant uterus presses on the large vessels at the back of her abdomen, 4.4, 16-5, 16.6
suppliers, addresses of, Appendix B
supraclavicular subclavian cannulation, 19.2
    brachial plexus block, 6.17
supraorbital block, 6.5
sural nerve, this is a nerve in the foot, block of, 6.24
surface anaesthesia, a method of anaesthetising a patient's mucous membranes by putting the drug directly onto them 5-4, 5.8
suxamethonium, a short–acting relaxant, 2-4, 2.5, 14.1, 14.2
    intramuscular, in babies, 18.2
symphysiotomy, a method of helping childbirth by cutting the bones at the front of the mother's pelvis, 6.13
syringes, 5-1
system, anaesthetic
    for AFYA vapouriser, 10-11
    for halothane, 11-5

table, tipping, 3.1
tachycardia, a fast pulse, 4.4
targets for anaesthesia, 20.1
teeth, anaesthesia for, 6-1, 6.3
"ten golden rules, of anaesthesia", 3.1, 3-1, 16-2
thiopentone, an important induction agent, 2-4, 3.4, 6.9D, 9.2, 8.6, 8.8, 12.1, 12-1, 12-2, 16.5, 17.8, 20.1
"three–in–one block", a block for three nerves in the groin, 6.22, 6-25
thyroidectomy, removing the thyroid, 4.6
tibial nerve, block for, 6.24
tidal volume, the amount of air a patient breathes in and out each time he breathes, 13.2
"tie–and–cry anaesthesia", 18-1, 18.2
toe block, 6.21, 6-24
"total spinal", subarachnoid or epidural anaesthesia that has been so high that it involves the whole of patient's spinal cord, 7.1, 7.6
"tracheal tug", an abnormal form of breathing in which a patient's trachea moves down each time he breathes, 4.2, 11.2, 11.3, 19.4
tracheal tube, a tube that is put into a patient's trachea to make sure he can breathe, 13.2, 13-6, 13.7
training, 2.1
tranquilisers, drugs that make a patient calm and sleepy, 2.8
transport of patient, 4.5
transvaginal pudendal block, 6.1, 6-13
trichloroethylene, a liquid anaesthetic agent, 1.1, 2.3, 9.2, 10.13, 11-6, 17.4
'triple airway manoevre'', a method of restoring a patient's airway, 3.4
tubal ligation, 6.8
tube, tracheal, 13.2
    corrugated, 10.3
tuberculosis, TB, 4.1, 7.8

tuberosity block, 6.3
Tuohy needle, a needle used during epidural anaesthesia, 7.1, 7.2
twitches, 5.9, 7.2D

ulnar nerve block, 6.2
umbilical hernia, 6.8
uncalibrated vapouriser, 10.11
unusual positions, anaesthesia for, 16.12
unconsciousness, 5.9
"unlimited method of local anaesthesia", 5.5
urethra, a tube that carries urine from the bladder to the outside world,
    anaesthesia for, 5-4, 5.8
urine output, 4.3
urine testing, 4.1
urological (bladder and kidney) operations, 7.3
urticaria, an itchy red rash, 5.9

vacuum extraction, delivering a baby by pulling on a vacuum cup attached to his head, 6.13
valve,
    non–rebreathing, 10.1, 10-1, 10-2
    simple expiratory, 10-1
vapouriser, an anaesthetic machine that turns a liquid such as ether into a vapour or gas, 10.4
    combinations of, 10.6
    "Cyprane", 10.12
    draw–over, 10.4
    EMO, 10.6
    ether, 1.1, 10-10
    "Ether–pac", 10.8
    "Fluo-Pac", 10.8
    for children, 18.2
    for ether, 10.4. 11.3
    Oxford Miniature, 10.10
        simple pattern, 10-5, 10.5
    improvised, 10.13, 10-17
    trichloroethylene, 10.12
    uncalibrated, for halothane only, 10.11
vasomotor tone, normal contractions of a patient's blood vessels, 18.1
vasectomy, an operation for tying the tube that carries a man's sperm from his testis to his penis, 6.11
vasopressors, drugs that raise the blood pressure, 2.5, 2.10
ventilation, breathing, 4.4
    controlled, 3.1, 3.4, 3.5, 13.1
    mouth–to–mouth, 3.4
vomiting
    after local anaesthesia, 5.9
    active, 16.2
    inhalation of, 16.3
    during intubation, 13.3
    ether anaesthesia, 11.3D
    postoperative, 4.6
ventilator, 19.3, 19.4, 19-5

wedge, anaesthetic, 4-1, 4.2
wheeze, wheezing, 3.2, 3.3, 4.6, 13.7
wrist block, 6-21, 6.20, 6-22

xylocaine, see lignocaine

Yankauer sucker, the common kind of surgical sucker, 4.2